The Little Black Book of Psychiatry

Levine

The Little Black Book of Psychiatry

David P. Moore, MD

Associate Clinical Professor
Department of Psychiatry
University of Louisville School of Medicine
Louisville, Kentucky

General Series Editor

Daniel K. Onion, MD, MPH, FACP
Professor of Community and Family Medicine
Dartmouth Medical School
Director of Maine-Dartmouth Family Practice Residency Program
Augusta, Maine

Other titles in the Little Black Book series:

The Little Black Book of Primary Care, Third Edition,
by Daniel K. Onion

The Little Black Book of Geriatrics, by Karen Gershman and
Dennis M. McCullough

Blackwell
Science

© 2000 by Blackwell Science, Inc.

Editorial Offices:

Commerce Place, 350 Main Street, Malden, Massachusetts 02148, USA

Osney Mead, Oxford OX2 0EL, England

25 John Street, London WC1N 2BL, England

23 Ainslie Place, Edinburgh EH3 6AJ, Scotland

54 University Street, Carlton, Victoria 3053, Australia

Other Editorial Offices:

Blackwell Wissenschafts-Verlag GmbH, Kurfürstendamm 57, 10707 Berlin, Germany

Blackwell Science KK, MG Kodenmacho Building, 7-10 Kodenmacho Nihombashi, Chuo-ku, Tokyo 104, Japan

Distributors:

USA

Blackwell Science, Inc.
Commerce Place
350 Main Street
Malden, Massachusetts 02148
(Telephone orders: 800-215-1000 or 781-388-8250; fax orders: 781-388-8270)

Canada

Login Brothers Book Company
324 Saulteaux Crescent
Winnipeg, Manitoba, R3J 3T2
(Telephone orders: 204-224-4068)

Australia

Blackwell Science Pty, Ltd.
54 University Street
Carlton, Victoria 3053
(Telephone orders: 03-9347-0300; fax orders: 03-9349-3016)

Outside North America and Australia

Blackwell Science, Ltd.
c/o Marston Book Services, Ltd.
P.O. Box 269
Abingdon
Oxon OX14 4YN
England
(Telephone orders: 44-01235-465500; fax orders: 44-01235-465555)

Acquisitions: Christopher Davis
Production: Kevin Sullivan
Manufacturing: Lisa Flanagan
Cover design by Leslie Haimes
Typeset by Achorn Graphics
Printed and bound by Edwards Brothers

Printed in the United States of America
01 02 03 5 4 3 2

The Blackwell Science logo is a trade mark of Blackwell Science Ltd., registered at the United Kingdom Trade Marks Registry

Library of Congress Cataloging-in-Publication Data

Moore, David P.
The little black book of psychiatry / by David Moore.
    p. cm.
    Includes bibliographical references.
    ISBN 0-86542-562-0
    1. Psychiatry Handbooks, manuals, etc. 2. Diagnosis, Differential Handbooks, manuals, etc. I. Title.
    [DNLM: 1. Mental Disorders—diagnosis Handbooks. 2. Diagnosis, Differential Handbooks. 3. Mental Disorders—therapy Handbooks. WM 34 M821L 2000]
RC456.M6735 2000
616.89—dc21
DNLM/DLC
for Library of Congress   99-24497
                                 CIP

This book is dedicated to my family, especially my wife, Nancy, who have supported (and tolerated) me during my literary endeavors. It is also dedicated to my teachers, in particular James W. Jefferson, MD, who has inspired many a physician.

Contents

Preface   xii
Medical Abbreviations   xiii
Journal Abbreviations   xvi

1. *Diagnostic Evaluation*   1
    1.1   The Diagnostic Interview and Evaluation   1
    1.2   Format for Reporting the Psychiatric Evaluation   11
    1.3   Common Psychiatric Symptoms and Signs   17

2. *Early Onset Disorders*   25
    2.1   Mental Retardation   25
    2.2   Reading Disorder (Developmental Dyslexia)   28
    2.3   Mathematics Disorder (Developmental Dyscalculia)   29
    2.4   Disorder of Written Expression (Developmental Dysgraphia)   30
    2.5   Developmental Coordination Disorder (Developmental Clumsiness, Clumsy Child Syndrome)   30
    2.6   Expressive Language Disorder (Developmental Expressive Aphasia)   31
    2.7   Mixed Receptive-Expressive Language Disorder (Developmental Sensory Aphasia)   32
    2.8   Phonologic Disorder (Developmental Articulation Disorder, Developmental Dysarticulation)   33
    2.9   Stuttering   35
    2.10 Autism (Autistic Disorder)   36
    2.11 Rett's Syndrome (Rett's Disorder)   38
    2.12 Attention-Deficit/Hyperactivity Disorder   40
    2.13 Conduct Disorder   43
    2.14 Pica   45
    2.15 Rumination Disorder   46
    2.16 Tourette's Disorder (Gilles de la Tourette's Syndrome)   47
    2.17 Encopresis (Functional Encopresis)   49
    2.18 Enuresis (Not Due to a General Medical Condition, Functional Enuresis)   51
    2.19 Separation Anxiety Disorder   53

2.20 Selective Mutism (Elective Mutism) 55
2.21 Reactive Attachment Disorder of Infancy or Early
       Childhood 56

3. *Delirium, Dementia, and Related Disorders* 57
    3.1   Delirium 57
    3.2   Dementia 61
    3.3   Alzheimer's Disease 66
    3.4   Multi-Infarct Dementia 67
    3.5   Lacunar Dementia 68
    3.6   Binswanger's Disease (Subcortical Arteriosclerotic
          Encephalopathy) 69
    3.7   AIDS Dementia 70
    3.8   Dementia Due to Head Trauma 71
    3.9   Parkinson's Disease 72
    3.10 Diffuse Lewy Body Disease (Lewy Body Dementia,
          Senile Dementia of the Lewy Body Type, Cortical
          Lewy Body Disease) 74
    3.11 Huntington's Disease (Huntington's Chorea) 75
    3.12 Pick's Disease 76
    3.13 Creutzfeldt-Jakob Disease 77
    3.14 Alcoholic Dementia (Alcohol-Induced Persisting
          Dementia) 78
    3.15 Inhalant-Induced Dementia 79
    3.16 Amnestic Disorders 80
    3.17 Korsakoff's Syndrome (When Occurring Secondary to
          Wernicke's Encephalopathy in Alcoholics, Known as
          Alcohol-Induced Persisting Amnestic Disorder) 83
    3.18 Transient Global Amnesia 85
    3.19 Catatonia 86
    3.20 Personality Change (Due to a General Medical
          Condition) 89
    3.21 Frontal Lobe Syndrome 91
    3.22 Klüver-Bucy Syndrome 92
    3.23 Interictal Personality Syndrome (Geschwind Syndrome) 94

4. *Substance-Related Disorders* 95
    4.1   Alcoholism (Alcohol Dependence) 95
    4.2   Blackouts 98
    4.3   Alcohol Withdrawal Syndrome 99

4.4 Delirium Tremens (Alcohol Withdrawal Delirium) 101
4.5 Alcohol Withdrawal Seizures ("Rum Fits") 103
4.6 Wernicke's Encephalopathy 104
4.7 Stimulant (Amphetamine, Methamphetamine, Dextroamphetamine)- and Cocaine-Related Disorders 105
4.8 Caffeine-Related Disorders 106
4.9 Cannabis-Related Disorders 108
4.10 Hallucinogen-Related Disorders 109
4.11 Inhalant-Related Disorders 111
4.12 Nicotine-Related Disorders 112
4.13 Opioid-Related Disorders 114
4.14 Phencyclidine-Related Disorders 117
4.15 Sedative-, Hypnotic-, or Anxiolytic-Related Disorders 118

5. *Schizophrenia and Other Psychoses* 122
    5.1 Schizophrenia 122
    5.2 Schizophreniform Disorder 130
    5.3 Schizoaffective Disorder 131
    5.4 Delusional Disorder 133
    5.5 Brief Psychotic Disorder 136
    5.6 Postpartum Psychosis ("Puerperal Psychosis") 137
    5.7 Shared Psychotic Disorder (Folie à Deux) 138
    5.8 Alcoholic Paranoia (Alcohol-Induced Psychotic Disorder with Delusions) 139
    5.9 Alcohol Hallucinosis (Alcohol-Induced Psychotic Disorder with Hallucinations) 141
    5.10 Secondary Psychosis (Psychotic Disorders Secondary to General Medical Conditions, and Substance-Induced Psychotic Disorders) 142

6. *Mood Disorders* 145
    6.1 Major Depression (Unipolar Depression) 145
    6.2 Dysthymia 154
    6.3 Postpartum Depression (Major Depression with Postpartum Onset) 155
    6.4 Postpartum Blues 156
    6.5 Premenstrual Syndrome (Premenstrual Dysphoric Disorder, Late-Luteal-Phase Disorder) 157

6.6   Bipolar Disorder (Manic-Depressive Illness, Circular Type)   158

6.7   Cyclothymia (Cyclothymic Disorder)   164

6.8   Secondary Depression (Mood Disorder Due to a General Medical Condition with Depressive Features)   165

6.9   Secondary Mania (Mood Disorder Secondary to a General Medical Condition with Manic Features)   168

7. Anxiety Disorders   170

7.1   Panic Disorder   170

7.2   Agoraphobia (Including Agoraphobia Without History of Panic Attacks and Panic Disorder with Agoraphobia)   173

7.3   Specific Phobia (Simple Phobia)   174

7.4   Social Phobia   175

7.5   Obsessive-Compulsive Disorder   177

7.6   Posttraumatic Stress Disorder   179

7.7   Generalized Anxiety Disorder   181

7.8   Secondary Anxiety (Anxiety Disorder Due to a General Medical Condition)   182

8. Somatoform and Related Disorders   185

8.1   Somatization Disorder (Briquet's Syndrome)   185

8.2   Conversion Disorder   187

8.3   Pain Disorder   189

8.4   Hypochondriasis   192

8.5   Body Dysmorphic Disorder (Dysmorphophobia)   194

8.6   Malingering and Factitious Illness   195

9. Dissociative Disorders   197

9.1   Dissociative Amnesia   197

9.2   Dissociative Fugue   198

9.3   Dissociative Identity Disorder (Multiple Personality Disorder)   199

9.4   Depersonalization Disorder   200

10. Sexual and Related Disorders   202

10.1   Hypoactive Sexual Desire Disorder   202

10.2   Sexual Aversion Disorder   203

10.3   Female Sexual Arousal Disorder   204

10.4   Male Erectile Disorder   205

10.5   Female Orgasmic Disorder   207
10.6   Male Orgasmic Disorder   208
10.7   Premature Ejaculation   210
10.8   Dyspareunia (Not Due to a General Medical
        Condition)   211
10.9   Vaginismus   212
10.10   Paraphilias   212
10.11   Gender Identity Disorder (Transsexualism)   215

11. *Eating Disorders*   *217*
    11.1   Anorexia Nervosa   217
    11.2   Bulimia Nervosa   219

12. *Sleep Disorders*   *222*
    12.1   Primary Insomnia (Psychophysiologic Insomnia and
            Idiopathic Insomnia)   222
    12.2   Primary Hypersomnia (Idiopathic Hypersomnia)   224
    12.3   Kleine-Levin Syndrome (Recurrent Form of Primary
            Hypersomnia)   226
    12.4   Narcolepsy   227
    12.5   Sleep Apnea (Breathing-Related Sleep Disorder)   230
    12.6   Pickwickian Syndrome (Central Alveolar Hypoventilation
            Syndrome)   232
    12.7   Circadian Rhythm Sleep Disorder   232
    12.8   Restless Legs Syndrome (Ekbom Syndrome)   234
    12.9   Nocturnal Myoclonus (Periodic Limb Movement Disorder
            of Sleep)   235
    12.10   Nightmare Disorder (Incubus)   236
    12.11   Sleep Terror Disorder (Pavor Nocturnus)   237
    12.12   Sleepwalking Disorder (Somnambulism)   238
    12.13   REM-Sleep Behavior Disorder   240
    12.14   Sleep Paralysis (Isolated Sleep Paralysis)   240

13. *Impulse-Control Disorders Not Classified Elsewhere*   *242*
    13.1   Intermittent Explosive Disorder   242
    13.2   Kleptomania   243
    13.3   Pyromania   244
    13.4   Pathologic Gambling   245
    13.5   Trichotillomania   246

14. *Personality Disorders   248*
    14.1   Paranoid Personality Disorder   248
    14.2   Schizoid Personality Disorder   249
    14.3   Schizotypal Personality Disorder   250
    14.4   Antisocial Personality Disorder   251
    14.5   Borderline Personality Disorder   253
    14.6   Histrionic Personality Disorder   255
    14.7   Narcissistic Personality Disorder   256
    14.8   Avoidant Personality Disorder   257
    14.9   Dependent Personality Disorder   258
    14.10 Obsessive-Compulsive Personality Disorder (Compulsive
           Personality Disorder, Anankastic Personality Disorder)   259
    14.11 Passive-Aggressive Personality Disorder   260

15. *Other Conditions   262*
    15.1   Parkinsonism (Including Neuroleptic-Induced
           Parkinsonism)   262
    15.2   Dystonia (Including Acute Neuroleptic-Induced
           Dystonia)   265
    15.3   Oculogyric Crisis   267
    15.4   Akathisia (Including Acute Neuroleptic-Induced
           Akathisia)   268
    15.5   Tremor (Including Medication-Induced Postural
           Tremor)   270
    15.6   Neuroleptic Malignant Syndrome   272
    15.7   Tardive Dyskinesia   274
    15.8   Serotonin Syndrome   276
    15.9   Postconcussion Syndrome   278
    15.10 Adjustment Disorders   279
    15.11 Bereavement   281
    15.12 Suicidal Behavior   282
    15.13 Violent Behavior   286

16. *Psychopharmacology and Electroconvulsive Treatment   292*
    16.1   Psychopharmacology   292
    16.2   Electroconvulsive Therapy   310

Index   322

Preface

This manual is intended as a ready guide to the diagnosis and treatment of psychiatric disorders. Each disorder is covered, with sections on epidemiology, symptomatology, laboratory data, course, complications, etiology, differential diagnosis, and treatment. It is the manual I wish I had a quarter-century ago when I began to see psychiatric patients, and I offer it to the students and residents of today so that they can have a head start in the field. In using this manual, students and residents not only will be able to help their patients, but also will acquire an approach to psychiatric practice that they can build on in the years to come.

I would like to thank and acknowledge my editor, Chris Davis, who was kind enough to introduce me to this project, and who has supported me throughout.

David P. Moore

Medical Abbreviations

AA	Alcoholics Anonymous	DDAVP	desmopressin
ABGs	arterial blood gases	ddx	differential diagnosis
ACE	angiotensin-converting enzyme	dL	deciliter
		DMA	dimethoxyamphetamine
ACTH	adrenocorticotropic hormone	DMT	dimethyltryptamine
		DST	dexamethasone suppression test
AIDS	acquired immunodeficiency syndrome	DTR	deep tendon reflex
AIMs	abnormal involuntary movements	DTs	delirium tremens
		DUI	driving under the influence
ANA	antinuclear antibody	dx	diagnosis
ApoE	apolipoprotein E	DZ	dizygotic
ASO	anti–streptolysin-O antibody	ECT	electroconvulsive therapy
		EEG	electroencephalogram
B_{12}	vitamin B_{12}	EKG	electrocardiogram
BAL	blood alcohol level	ER	emergency room
bid	twice daily	ERP	endoscopic retrograde pancreatography
BP	blood pressure		
BUN	blood urea nitrogen	esp	especially
		ESP	extrasensory perception
Ca	calcium	ESR	erythrocyte sedimentation rate
CA	Cocaine Anonymous		
CBC	complete blood cell count	fhx	family history
CC	chief complaint	FTA	fluorescent treponemal antibody test
CCK	cholecystokinin		
Chem	chemistry	f/u	follow-up
CHF	congestive heart failure		
CNS	central nervous system	GABA	gamma-aminobutyric acid
COPD	chronic obstructive pulmonary disease	GERD	gastroesophageal reflux disease
CPK	creatine phosphokinase	gm	gram
cps	cycles per second		
CRF	corticotropin-releasing factor	h	hour
		HIV	human immunodeficiency virus
CSF	cerebrospinal fluid		
CT	computed tomography	h/o	history of
		HPI	history of the present illness
d	day		
DAI	diffuse axonal injury	hs	bedtime

HVA	homovanillic acid	NA	Narcotics Anonymous
hx	history	nbM	nucleus basalis of Meynert
		NC	noncontributory
ICU	intensive care unit	ng	nanogram
im	intramuscular	NH_3	ammonia
IU	international units	NMDA	N-methyl-D-aspartate
iv	intravenous	NPH	normal-pressure hydro-cephalus
K	potassium	NPO	nothing by mouth
kg	kilogram	NREM	non-REM (rapid eye movement)
L	liter	NSAID	nonsteroidal anti-inflam-matory drug
lb	pound		
LFT	liver function test		
LP	lumbar puncture	OTC	over-the-counter
LSD	lysergic diethylamide		
		PE	physical examination
MAO	monoamine oxidase	PET	positron emission tomog-raphy
MAOI	monoamine oxidase inhibitor		
mcg	microgram	PMH	past medical history
MCV	mean corpuscular volume	po	orally
MDA	methylenedioxyamphet-amine	prn	as needed
		pt	patient
MDMA	3,4-methylenedioxy-methamphetamine	PTSD	posttraumatic stress disorder
mEq	milliequivalent	PVC	premature ventricular contraction
mg	milligram		
Mg	magnesium	q	each
MHPG	methoxyhydroxyphenyl-glycol	qd	daily
		qh	each hour
min	minute	qid	4 times daily
mL	milliliter		
mm Hg	millimeters of mercury	RBC	red blood cell
mo	month	REM	rapid eye movement
MPTP	1-methyl-4-phenyl-1,2,3,6-tetrahydropyridine	RF	rheumatoid factor
		ROS	review of systems
MR	mental retardation	Rx	treatment
MRI	magnetic resonance imaging		
		sc	subcutaneous
MS	multiple sclerosis	SE	side effect
MSA	multisystem atrophy	sec	second
MSE	mental status examination	SGGT	serum gamma-glutamyl-transferase
MZ	monozygotic		
		SGPT	serum glutamic-pyruvic transaminase
Na	sodium		

SIADH	syndrome of inappropriate antidiuretic hormone secretion	TFT	thyroid function test
		TGA	transient global amnesia
s/p	status post	TIA	transient ischemic attack
SPECT	single-photon emission computed tomography	tid	3 times daily
		TSH	thyroid-stimulating hormone
SSRI	selective serotonin reup-take inhibitor	U/A	urinalysis
STP	2,5-dimethoxy-4-methylamphetamine	VDRL	Venereal Disease Research Laboratory
sx	symptom(s)	vs	versus
T7	free thyroxine index	WBC	white blood cell
TB	tuberculosis	wk	week
TCA	tricyclic antidepressant	wnl	within normal limits
TENS	transcutaneous electrical nerve stimulation	yr	year

Journal Abbreviations

Acta Neurol Scand	Acta Neurologica Scandinavica
Acta Pediatr	Acta Pediatrica
Acta Psychiatr Scand	Acta Psychiatrica Scandinavica
Alcoholism: Clin Exp Res	Alcoholism: Clinical and Experimental Research
Am J Med	American Journal of Medicine
Am J Psychiatry	American Journal of Psychiatry
Ann Int Med	Annals of Internal Medicine
Ann Neurol	Annals of Neurology
Arch Dis Child	Archives of Diseases of Childhood
Arch Gen Psychiatry	Archives of General Psychiatry
Arch Int Med	Archives of Internal Medicine
Arch Neurol	Archives of Neurology
Arch Neurol Psychiatry	Archives of Neurology and Psychiatry
Arch Sex Behav	Archives of Sexual Behavior
Biol Psychiatry	Biological Psychiatry
BMJ	British Medical Journal
Br J Psychiatry	British Journal of Psychiatry
Br J Soc Clin Psychol	British Journal of Social and Clinical Psychology
Brain	Brain
Can J Psychiatry	Canadian Journal of Psychiatry
Comp Psychiatry	Comprehensive Psychiatry
Cortex	Cortex
Drugs	Drugs
Epilepsia	Epilepsia
Hosp Community Psychiatry	Hospital and Community Psychiatry
Irish Med J	Irish Medical Journal

J Affect Disord	Journal of Affective Disorders
JAMA	Journal of the American Medical Association
J Am Acad Child Adolesc Psychiatry	Journal of the American Academy of Child and Adolescent Psychiatry
J Am Acad Child Psychiatry	Journal of the American Academy of Child Psychiatry
J Child Neurol	Journal of Child Neurology
J Clin Psychiatry	Journal of Clinical Psychiatry
J Clin Psychopharm	Journal of Clinical Psychopharmacology
J Consult Clin Psychol	Journal of Consulting and Clinical Psychology
J Fam Pract	Journal of Family Practice
J For Sci	Journal of Forensic Science
J Gen Int Med	Journal of General Internal Medicine
J Learning Disabilities	Journal of Learning Disabilities
J Nerv Ment Dis	Journal of Nervous and Mental Disease
J Neurol Neurosurg Psychiatry	Journal of Neurology, Neurosurgery and Psychiatry
J Pediatr	Journal of Pediatrics
J Pers Disord	Journal of Personality Disorders
J Psychiatr Educ	Journal of Psychiatric Education
J R Soc Med	Journal of the Royal Society of Medicine
J Sex Marital Ther	Journal of Sex and Marital Therapy
J Speech Hear Disord	Journal of Speech and Hearing Disorders
J Stud Alcohol	Journal of Studies of Alcohol
Lancet	Lancet
Mayo Clin Proc	Mayo Clinic Proceedings
Med Aspects Hum Sex	Medical Aspects of Human Sexuality
Med J Aust	Medical Journal of Australia
Mov Disord	Movement Disorders

NEJM	New England Journal of Medicine
Neurology	Neurology
Pain	Pain
Pediatr Ann	Pediatric Annals
Pediatr Clin North Am	Pediatric Clinics of North America
Pediatr Rev	Pediatric Review
Pediatrics	Pediatrics
Postgrad Med	Postgraduate Medicine
Psychiatr Clin	Psychiatric Clinics
Psychiatr Med	Psychiatric Medicine
Psychol Med	Psychological Medicine
Psychopharmacol Bull	Psychopharmacology Bulletin
Psychopharmacology	Psychopharmacology
Psychosomatic Med	Psychosomatic Medicine
Psychosomatics	Psychosomatics
Q J Exp Psychol	Quarterly Journal of Experimental Psychology
Q J Med	Quarterly Journal of Medicine
Science	Science
Sleep	Sleep
S Med J	Southern Medical Journal

Notice

The indications and dosages of all drugs in this book have been recommended in the medical literature and conform to the practices of the general medical community. The medications described do not necessarily have specific approval by the U.S. Food and Drug Administration for use in the diseases and dosages for which they are recommended. The package insert for each drug should be considered for use and dosage as approved by the FDA. Because standards for usage change, it is advisable to keep abreast of revised recommendations, particularly those concerning new drugs.

1. Diagnostic Evaluation

1.1 THE DIAGNOSTIC INTERVIEW AND EVALUATION

Am J Psychiatry 1970;126:997. Arch Gen Psychiatry 1973;28:215. Comp Psychiatry 1981;22:500. J Nerv Ment Dis 1980;168:167.

THE INTERVIEW SETTING

The setting should be conducive to the pts' telling of their stories.

Privacy is generally desirable, as many pts are less than forthcoming when others can listen in.

A private interview room or office is preferable; if not available, then ensure as much privacy as possible by pulling the curtains around the bed or retiring to a less traveled part of the ward or ER.

Family and friends should generally *not* be allowed to sit in as their presence may inhibit the pt; tell them you'll speak with them later.

Interruptions, as they disturb the free flow of the conversation, should be avoided, and phone calls and pages should be avoided, if possible.

Seat yourself at an angle to the pt, so that the pt can comfortably look at you or away from you; keep a comfortable distance (1–2 arm lengths) and don't look down on the pt (e.g., if the pt is in bed, seat yourself rather than stand and look down).

Allow sufficient time for the interview: A cooperative pt with a simple hx may require 30 min or less; a geriatric pt with a long or complex hx may require 90 min or more. It may be necessary to schedule a follow-up interview in some cases.

Violent pts may require a modified setting, as discussed below under "The Difficult Interview."

ESTABLISHING RAPPORT

Establish rapport and maintain it throughout.

First impressions count. Within the first minute, or even the first few seconds, the pt generally forms an impression of you. If the pt sees you as benevolent and trustworthy, all may be well; if not, the pt's attitude may be less than cooperative, and the data gathered in the interview may be unreliable.

Introduce yourself: "Hi Mr. Phillips, I'm Dr. Jones," and offer to shake hands. "I'm going to be your doctor here" (or "Your internist asked me to see you" or "I'm the admitting doctor today") and "I'd like to talk with you and ask a few questions. Would that be O.K.?" If you are a medical student, introduce yourself as such, or as a "student doctor" but not as a doctor. Thus: "Hi Mr. Phillips, I'm Mr. Smith. I'm the medical student working with Dr. Jones, and I'd like to talk with you and ask a few questions. Would that be O.K.?"

Courtesy and respect must be practiced and maintained. Case in point: Unless interviewing children or adolescents, address the pt as either Mr. or Ms., or by title (Reverend, Dr.). If women wish to be called Mrs. or Miss, they'll tell you, and the same goes for first names.

Dress conservatively and wear the white coat.

Listen and pay attention. Every pt has a story to tell, and if *you* provide a proper forum in the interview, the *pt* will provide you with the hx you require to make the dx. If you're distracted or seem uninterested, you're not going to get the history.

ESTABLISHING THE CHIEF COMPLAINT

The chief complaint (CC) is the epitome of the pt's illness and must be clearly established at the *start* of the interview, or the interview will lack proper focus and may fail to provide the necessary dx information.

Open the interview with a request for the CC: "I'd like to start by asking you what led to your coming to the hospital" (or "making the appointment to come here today"). Don't begin with an invitation to digress, such as, "Tell me about yourself," or "What kind of problems have you been having?" (Although the CC may be one of the problems the pt has been having, it may be only one among many, and if the pt is at all reluctant to speak about it, one of the other problems may be offered for discussion.)

Never accept a diagnosis at face value. A pt who announces "I'm bipolar" may or may not be making an accurate statement. The dx, if made by a previous physician, may be incorrect, or the pt may have made it based on a "self-help" book. An appropriate response might be, "Well, O.K. bipolar disorder shows up differently in different people's lives; how does it show up in your life?" Similarly, if the pt uses a vague or poorly defined term (e.g., "I had a nervous breakdown"), don't let it pass, but ask for a clarification.

Look for the pathology, and don't be satisfied until you see it. If a pt responds with something like, "I was having trouble at the office," recognize that that by itself does not constitute pathology. Ask for clarification: "O.K. What kind of trouble were you having?" and keep gently probing until the pt describes some "juicy" pathology. A response such as, "Well, the boss and I weren't getting along" may be closer but is still not good enough. Pursue it: "Well, Mr. Phillips, a lot of people don't get along with their boss but that doesn't bring them to the hospital. So tell me more about what happened." With a response like, "Well, I couldn't take it anymore, so I told him that I knew he'd been putting poison in the coffee, and that if he didn't stop I'd make him stop. So, I guess he thought I was threatening him and he called the cops and they gave me a choice: Either go with them down to the hospital or go to jail. So I came here," *you* can relax, as you've discovered something pathologic enough to constitute a CC.

Occasionally, pts are unable to provide a CC. Delirious, demented, or floridly psychotic pts may lack the ability to articulate one, and other pts (e.g., suspicious pts with delusions of persecution) may distrust the physician and simply be unwilling to offer a CC. Probing for the CC should remain gentle. If the pt starts becoming annoyed, change the subject, and hope that the CC may "leak out" later in the interview. For example, if Mr. Phillips had not been forthcoming, consider something like, "Well, Mr. Phillips, I'd like to switch gears here and instead of asking more about your relationship with your boss, I'd like to hear more about the office in general. What's it like working there?"

If you're unable to establish a CC, proceed to the directive portion of the interview, and plan on securing the CC during your conversation with collateral sources.

CONDUCTING THE NONDIRECTIVE PORTION OF THE INTERVIEW

As soon as a CC is established, adopt a *nondirective* approach that invites the pt to relate the hx behind the CC: "He put poison in the coffee? Tell me more about that." Most pts, with only gentle shepherding, will subsequently touch on the basic elements of the hx: the onset of the illness (including approximate date, mode of onset (acute, gradual, insidious), and any precipitating factors); the evolution of signs and symptoms; any aggravating or alleviating factors; any treatment efforts and their results; pertinent positives and negatives; and any hx of similar sx in the past. "Open-ended" statements such as "Tell me more about that" invite the pt to talk and give full responses, whereas "closed-ended" directive questions (e.g., those with "yes" or "no" answers) may have the opposite effect: "Are you sure he put poison in the coffee?" Setting up a "question and answer" format may seriously limit your ability to gather information. The pt may now simply wait for questions and if you don't ask the right ones, you may not find out what you need to know.

During the nondirective portion of the interview, the pt may at times digress, and some gentle redirection may be required: "O.K., I see how you got your job to begin with, but I'd like to go back to your boss again, and his doing things like poisoning the coffee. Tell me more about that."

Clarifying questions, provided they don't derail the conversation, may be appropriate. For example, "So, that's how you found out about the poisoned coffee. About when was that?" With the answer in hand, then immediately reestablish the nondirective format: "O.K., you found out about a half year ago. Tell me what happened then."

Once you have the basic elements of the hx in hand, it may be appropriate to briefly summarize them: "O.K., let me see if I have this straight. Things were O.K. at the office until about a half year ago when you noticed a strange taste in the coffee and felt sick the next day. You weren't sure it was poison, but a little later on you discovered that your phone was bugged and realized that people were following you. Nothing you did made anything better, and you've never had anything like this happen to you before. Finally you couldn't take it anymore and you confronted your boss who called the police. Is that about right?"

Corrections, if any, by the pt are noted, and if these require elaboration, they are followed up by nondirective questions.

Once the hx is complete, make the transition to the *directive* portion of the interview.

CONDUCTING THE DIRECTIVE PORTION OF THE INTERVIEW

Introduce the directive portion of the interview: "Now I'd like to ask you some routine questions about any other health problems you may have had." Direct questions are generally more closed-ended and deal with medications, allergies, the past medical history (PMH), review of systems (ROS), family history (fhx), and the mental status examination (MSE). Pertinent positive responses should generally be followed by open-ended probes to flush out the important details.

If not already touched on in the nondirective portion of the interview, ask about alcohol and drug use. Don't ask, "Do you drink?"; rather ask, "How much do you drink?" Drinking in the USA is almost ubiquitous; teetotalers won't be offended, and problem drinkers won't be able to exercise their denial as readily. Regarding drugs, ask, "Have you ever used drugs, like marijuana, cocaine, or LSD?" Follow up positive answers with open-ended questions. Although pts tend to hide alcoholism or drug addiction, some will be remarkably forthcoming if questioned in a calm, nonjudgmental way.

Suicidal ideation, if not already covered, must be sought. Suicidal ideation is very common in psychiatric illnesses, and in some illnesses, such as depression, you can assume it's there. Pts are not offended at this question; if they don't have suicidal ideation, they'll tell you, and if they do, they may be relieved to answer a question like, "Since all this started, have you ever felt like hurting yourself?" A positive response is followed by a nondirective approach, during which you should be sure to find out what they were planning to do, where they were planning to do it, how close they've come to doing it, and whether they've ever hurt themselves in the past.

Homicidal ideation, if not already covered, must also be sought: "Since all this started, have you ever felt like hurting someone else?" A positive response also merits a nondirective approach, during which you should be sure to find out who the pt was planning to hurt, what the pt intended to do to the victim, how close the pt came to doing it, and whether the pt has ever hurt someone in the past.

The MSE is saved for last, and those items evident to inspection, or that were already covered (such as Mr. Phillips's delusion of persecution regarding his boss), need not be covered again.

Questions about hallucinations should be simple and direct: "Have you ever heard voices?" or "Have you ever seen things other people don't see, like visions?"

Questions about delusions must be carefully phrased to avoid alerting the pt that you might find such beliefs unusual or "sick." For example, in looking for delusions of persecution, rather than ask, "Do you ever think that people are out to get you?," ask, "Do people in the neighborhood (or office, school, etc.) ever hassle you or give you a hard way to go?"

Introduce the *cognitive portion* of the MSE with a statement like, "Now I'd like to ask you some routine questions to check on memory, arithmetic, and things like that."

Start with memory: "First I'm going to check on memory by giving you 3 words to remember, because in a few minutes I'll ask you to recall them, O.K.? The three words are 'rock, car, and pencil.' Say those once so I know you have them, O.K.?" Assuming the pt has them, check your watch and plan to return to this in 5 min. In the meantime, proceed with the rest of the cognitive portion, and if that doesn't take 5 min, ask some other questions (e.g., ROS questions you may have forgotten earlier), but be sure to avoid any topics likely to stir the pt up emotionally, as this may falsely decrease the pt's ability to recall.

Proceed to the digit span tests, both forward and backward.

Next come calculations. Depending on your estimate of the pt's intelligence, based on vocabulary and evidence of abstract thought earlier in the interview, you may start with serial 7s or try something easier first, such as, "If you take 8 away from 12, what do you have left over?" Introduce serial 7s with, "If you take 7 away from 100 what do you have?" After the pt responds, follow up with, "Now take 7 from that number and keep on subtracting 7 each time until you can't go any further." If the pt has trouble with calculations, ask, "You seemed to have trouble with that. Did you have any trouble with it in school?" It is essential to determine whether the poor calculating ability represents a decrement from a prior higher ability, or simply the fact that the pt never learned in the first place.

Proverbs testing is introduced with a statement like, "Now I'm going to mention an old saying, and I'd like you to tell me what it means to you, in your own words. There's no right or wrong answer; I'm just interested in what it means to you, O.K.? So, 'Don't cry over spilled milk.' What does that mean to you?"

Orientation is checked with direct questions: "O.K., now I'd like you to tell me what today's date is: the month, date, and year," with the pt's response followed by, "And now I'd like you to tell me the name of the building we're in now," followed by, "and the name of the town (or city)." If these questions are simply put, without apology or embarrassment, pts are not offended by them.

When 5 min has passed, ask, "Now I'd like you to recall those 3 words I gave you a few minutes ago. What were they?"

CONCLUDING THE INTERVIEW

After finishing the directive portion of the interview, and before your concluding comments, allow room for some last words: "O.K., that about does it for now. I've asked you a lot of questions and you've told me a lot, but I'm wondering if there's anything I haven't asked about or that you haven't mentioned that's important or that's related to what we've talked about?" After investigating any pertinent responses, invite the pt to ask questions: "O.K., and now I'd like to ask whether you have any questions for me?" Last words or questions may be very revealing, and indeed critical to the dx.

Now ask, if you haven't already, whether it would be all right to speak with a collateral source: "O.K., before we talk about where we go from here, I'd like to ask if it would be O.K. if I spoke with someone who has known you since this all started. I need all the information I can get to help you the most, so it's very important for me to talk with someone else." If the pt agrees, find out who an acceptable source might be; if not, then proceed as in "Collateral Information," below.

Conclude the interview with appropriate comments about dx impression, proposed Rx, and probable length of stay. Tact is critical here, especially when discussing the dx. What is important is for the pt to get well, and if telling the unvarnished truth would hinder that, then some diplomacy is called for. For example, although most depressed pts will accept a dx of major depression without being offended or unduly upset, a fair minority of pts with schizophrenia may be so disturbed at hearing this dx that they reject it out of hand, thus jeopardizing compliance with treatment. In such cases it may be more appropriate to tell pts that they are having a "kind of nervous breakdown"; most pts accept this, and after they improve with treatment and are open to reasonable discussion, you may then turn to the actual dx.

PHYSICAL EXAMINATION

A pertinent physical examination (PE) should be performed on all pts. Inpatients merit a general PE and a detailed neurologic examination. Outpatients are often referred to an appropriate internist or family practitioner; however, even with outpatients a neurologic examination, with practice, can be accomplished in 5 min or less.

For pts in whom the hx and MSE leave you with a ddx that can only be resolved with a PE, then the PE is done before concluding the interview; in other pts, it may follow: "O.K., now that we're done with the interview, I'd like to go ahead and do a physical exam, just to make sure everything is O.K. Would that be O.K.?"

COLLATERAL INFORMATION

Whenever you have any significant doubt about the reliability of the hx from the pt, interview someone who has known the pt over time, such as a friend, family member, or "significant other." Generally this can be done by telephone. The information may either confirm your dx impression or radically alter it. Most "collateral" sources respond well to an approach like, "Hi. I'm Dr. Jones and I'm Peter Phillips's doctor here at the hospital. He mentioned that you knew he was here (or I understand that you were with him when he came to the emergency room) and I'd like to touch base and ask a few questions. Would that be O.K.?"

At this point, the next step depends on whether or not the pt has authorized you to reveal anything found out in the interview or during the PE. If you have been authorized, begin with a summary of the CC: "My understanding is that he came here rather than go to jail after his boss called the police. Is that about right?" Then take the interview from there, first nondirectively, then directively.

If you have not been authorized, you may still, without breaching confidentiality, proceed, providing that the person you are calling already knows the pt is here and that you reveal nothing that the collateral source doesn't already know. Thus: "O.K., I'd like to hear from you what led to his coming to the hospital," followed, if appropriate, by a comment such as, "I've already spoken to him but often pts leave things out, or forget about them, and it's important that I get as full a picture as possible of what happened."

THE DIFFICULT INTERVIEW

Certain conditions make pts difficult to interview; however, certain maneuvers may facilitate the task.

Depression may leave pts so fatigued and hopeless that they either cannot participate or simply give up trying. Empathic encouragement often helps: "I know this is hard for you, but please keep trying—it's very important."

Mania, with its pressured speech and flight of ideas, may propel the conversation down multiple tangential sidetracks before the interviewer even knows what's happened. Active shepherding is often indispensable, and keeping the conversation on track typically requires frequent redirection.

An irritable, impulsive, or potentially violent pt at times is struggling to maintain control, and the presence of a physician who is calm in voice, manner, and posture may serve to shore up the pt's internal controls; conversely, any sign of fear or anxiety may be followed by a rapid unraveling of whatever internal controls the pt had. Practice this calm attitude: Sit in a chair and relax your body; don't sag, but leave yourself free of any muscular tension. Do the same with your voice until you can speak calmly, without fear, tension, anger, haughtiness, or superciliousness. Try this approach with an "easy" pt, and keep trying it until you've mastered it—the results can be dramatic.

In such situations the interview setting should be modified somewhat: If an interview room is used, make sure the door is not blocked, so that the pt doesn't feel trapped (in some cases, leaving the door open may be necessary to reassure the pt).

Of course, some pts are already "unraveled," and with them the setting must be further modified. External controls are necessary: Sometimes a uniformed guard will suffice; at other times leather restraints may be required.

Delusions and hallucinations may constitute stumbling blocks to the maintenance of rapport when the pt asks, as often happens, whether the physician agrees. The pt with delusions of persecution may ask accusingly, "You don't believe me, do you? You think I'm just making this up," and those with voices may inquire, "You hear them too, don't you?". At this point it is critical to *not* cast doubt on the pt's experience or try and argue the pt out of it, as this may lead to an end of the interview. Rather, it is appropriate to sidestep the question with a thoroughly honest response: "It isn't important whether I agree with you or not (or, whether I hear them or not). What I'm interested in, what I want to find out about, is your experience of the world—that's what's important. So I'd like to find out what happened between you and your boss (or, I'd like to hear more about what the voices say)." This is a truthful response, for the diagnostician does indeed have a fundamental interest in the pt's experience of the world; it is precisely this experience that, in large measure, constitutes the illness.

The delirious, demented, or retarded pt, although limited by cognitive deficits, should be interviewed as far as possible. Although the demented pt may not be able to give a reliable account of the past few months, he or she may, in response to direct questioning, recall things unknown to collateral sources, such as a hx of head trauma in the distant past.

Successfully interviewing a difficult pt is only possible if the physician refrains from impatience, anger, and critical or derogatory remarks. Cultivate equanimity, and maintain a benevolent attitude.

1.2 FORMAT FOR REPORTING THE PSYCHIATRIC EVALUATION

Hosp Community Psychiatry 1990;41:49. J Psychiatr Educ 1979;3:99. American Psychiatric Association, Diagnostic and statistical manual of mental disorders, ed 4, American Psychiatric Association, Washington, D.C., 1994.

Introduction: Age, race (if pertinent), marital status, employment status, sex, residence situation (e.g., "lives with a sister in an apt. in the city"), referral source.

CC: See above, in 1.1, for a method of establishing the CC. This may or may not be in the pts own words, depending on the pt's ability to accurately relay the reason for hospitalization.

Source: Note the source of the hx, including the pt, collateral sources, and old records, with comments, if appropriate, regarding the reliability of the source.

Hx of the Present Illness: The following basic elements must be covered:
- *Onset,* noting the approximate date, the mode of onset (acute, gradual, insidious), and any precipitating factors
- *Evolution of signs and symptoms*
- *Aggravating or alleviating factors*
- *Treatment efforts* and their results, with particular attention to dosage and duration of Rx, compliance, and any SEs
- *Pertinent positives and negatives,* e.g., in a pt with chronic psychotic sx, whether or not there were ever any sustained episodes of mood disturbance
- *History of similar sx* in the past, with particular emphasis on any Rx and response

Medications: Include *all* medications (including OTC medications), with generic name and dosage.

Allergies: Be sure to avoid listing *nonallergic* SEs here: Many pts will say, "I'm allergic to" such and such a medicine. However, with close review, it appears that they merely had a nonallergic SE.

PMH: Consider hospitalizations for any reason, surgeries, accidents, or injuries; the level of detail is determined by the pertinence of the event to the present illness. Some authors insist that past psychiatric illnesses be listed under a separate category, e.g., "Past Psychiatric Illness," but this seems inappropriate. Any past psychiatric illness similar or pertinent to the present one is included in the hx of the present illness (HPI), and anything else (e.g., a history of alcoholism in a pt who has been sober for 10 yr and now has a dementia of recent onset) belong with any other PMH items.

Review of Sx:

Fhx: Only the pertinent aspects of the fhx are reported. For example, in a young pt with a mood disorder, the fact that a maternal grandfather died of a "heart attack" is irrelevant, whereas the hospitalization of a paternal aunt for depression, successfully treated with ECT is *very* pertinent.

Personal and Social Hx: *Only* pertinent aspects that bear on the pt's hospitalization and proposed Rx should be included. Thus, if the pt is married and had a similar illness in the past, it's appropriate to comment on whether the spouse was supportive or not; or if the pt had difficulty with calculations on the MSE, or any evidence of alexia or agraphia on the neurologic examination, note the highest academic level and whether or not "special classes" were attended. On the other hand, with an elderly pt with a dementia, a developmental history of childhood and adolescence is basically irrelevant.

MSE: At a minimum the following (various sx are described in 1.3) should be included:

- *Grooming and dress*
- *General description*

    Style of relatedness: e.g., guarded or suspicious; aloof or eccentric; bizarre; manipulative; apathetic or abulic; disinhibited; seductive

    Central themes of pt's conversation

    Pertinent positives and negatives: psychomotor retardation or agitation; hyperactivity (if present, note whether purposeful or not and whether engaged with interviewer or not); distractibility; mannerisms; stereotypies; catatonic symptoms (negativism, automatic obedience, echolalia or echopraxia, posturing)

- *Affect:* type and range

    Pertinent positives and negatives: lability; flattening; inappropriateness; bizarreness; emotional incontinence

- *Mood:* euthymic, depressed, irritable, euphoric (if irritable or euphoric note whether mood is heightened or not), anxious
- *Form of thought and speech:* coherent or not; pertinent positives and negatives: flight of ideas, pressure; circumstantiality, tangen-

tiality; looseness of associations; poverty of thought, poverty of speech; thought blocking; neologisms; obsessions, compulsions

- *Hallucinations:* present or absent; auditory, visual, tactile, olfactory or gustatory. If voices are present, note especially if Schneiderian First Rank symptoms (i.e., voices arguing, voices commenting, voices echoing what the pt thinks) are present. Also note whether command hallucinations are present.
- *Delusions:* present or absent; persecutory, grandiose, referential, of jealousy, of sin, of poverty, nihilistic, erotomanic, somatic, and "pseudomemories." Note especially whether any Schneiderian First Rank symptoms, such as thought withdrawal, thought insertion, thought broadcasting, and delusions of passivity, control, or influence (i.e., "made" thoughts, "made" feelings, "made" actions), are present.
- *Level of consciousness:* alert or not. If not, note how easily aroused.
- *Confusion:* present or absent
- *Orientation*
    Person
    Place
    Time (month, day, year)
- *Memory*
    Immediate (digit span, forward and backward)
    Short term (recall of 3 words after 5 min)
    Long term (recall of events leading up to admission and of significant events of distant past, e.g., autobiographic details (e.g., schools attended), famous public events or figures (e.g., recent wars))
- *Abstracting ability:* proverbs interpretation either abstract or concrete (at times responses may be bizarre)
- *Calculating ability:* serial 7s, and if abnormal, ability to do simple 2-digit or 1-digit subtraction or addition
- *Suicidal and homicidal ideation* (if not already covered in the HPI)
- *Judgment:* traditionally, assess judgment with "sample" situations such as, "What would you do if you found a wallet?" This approach is far less useful than demonstrations of the pt's judgment in life situations in which the pt is likely to find himself or herself. In many instances, this will have become apparent in the nondirective portion of the interview (e.g., a manic pt who

invests enormous sums in obviously bogus enterprises); however, in some cases a "test" question may be needed. Thus, for a security guard with delusions of persecution, you might ask what the pt felt about carrying his concealed weapon into a theater.

- *Insight:* does *not* refer to the degree of "insight" that the pt may or may not have into his or her motivations and the genesis of those motivations; rather it refers simply to whether the pt has any "insight" into the fact that he or she is ill. For example, most pts with mania have no insight, and in fact often think that it is others who are not doing well, whereas most pts with a depressive episode are painfully aware that something is "wrong" with the way they are feeling.

PE: In addition to the general PE, a detailed neurologic examination is necessary, and should include, at a minimum, the following:

- *Handedness*
- *Head,* noting whether the head is normocephalic or of abnormal shape, and noting the presence or absence of any dysmorphic features
- *Pupils,* noting shape, equality, diameter, and reactivity to light (both to direct and to consensual illumination) and to convergence testing
- *Funduscopic exam:* presence or absence of hemorrhages or exudates; position of the optic disk (flat, elevated, deeply cupped), and distinctness of its margins; presence or absence of venous pulsations
- *Cranial nerves*
    II: visual acuity for each eye; visual fields to confrontation
    III, IV, VI: extraocular movements in all 4 directions of gaze, noting presence or absence of disconjugate gaze, nystagmus, or ptosis
    V: masseter strength; sensation to pinprick and light touch in all 3 divisions; corneal reflex on each side
    VII: brow wrinkling and facial movements upon smiling, both voluntarily and involuntarily (i.e., to command "Smile for me," and to a joke, perhaps told at some informal part of the interview, or if the physician is not a humorist, observe for smiling as the pt relates some amusing anecdote)
    VIII: hearing to ticking watch; if abnormal, Weber and Rinne testing
    IX, X: elevation of palate and gag reflex

XI: shoulder shrug, lateral motion of jaw against resistance
XII: tongue protrusion

- *Elementary sensation:* light touch, pinprick, and vibration (testing each of these, at a minimum, on both hands and both feet, noting particularly any asymmetry) and position sense (at the index fingers and great toes)
- *Cerebellar testing:* finger-to-nose; heel-to-knee-to-shin; rapid alternating movements of the hands; presence or absence of dysarthria
- *Station and gait*
    Station: posture, presence or absence of retropulsion
    Gait: on routine testing, presence or absence of festination, decreased associated arm movements, akinesia, foot dragging or circumduction, ataxia; on special testing with the pt walking on the lateral aspects of the feet ("like a bow-legged cowboy"), presence or absence of any dystonic or hemiplegic posturing of the upper extremities
- *Strength:* grade: 0 = no movement; 1+ = visible contraction but no movement of the limb; 2+ = limb movement present but not against gravity; 3+ = limb movement present against gravity but not against resistance; 4+ = limb movement against some resistance; 5+ = full strength (at a minimum, check strength of hand grasp)
- *Atrophy, fasciculations, myotonia:* absence or presence (and, if present, their location)
- *Tremor:* amplitude (fine or coarse); approximate frequency; whether rest, postural, or intention; location; and any other pertinent characteristic (e.g., pill rolling, flapping, dyskinetic)
- *Drift:* presence or absence
- *Rigidity:* absence or presence. If present, note whether spastic, lead pipe, cogwheel, or cataleptic ("waxy flexibility") and note location (at a minimum, test for rigidity at the elbow, wrist, knee, and ankle joints).
- *Gegenhalten:* presence or absence (at a minimum test at elbow joint)
- *Abnormal involuntary movements:* myoclonus, asterixis, dystonia, athetosis, chorea, ballismus, tics
- *DTRs:* grade: 0 = absent; 1+ = present but diminished; 2+ = normal; 3+ = increased; 4+ = greatly increased
    Check at biceps, triceps, brachioradialis, knee, and ankle, and record using a "stick figure" diagram

1.2 Format for Reporting the Psychiatric Evaluation **15**

- *Abnormal reflexes:* flexor or extensor plantar response (Babinski sign); also jaw jerk, snout, suck, palmomental, and grasp reflexes
- *Neglect:* extinction test to double simultaneous visual and tactile stimulation; line bisection test; line cancellation test; drawing a clock and a daisy
- *Apraxia:* at a minimum:
  Constructional apraxia (e.g., draw a house, copy geometric forms)
  Ideational and ideomotor apraxia (first ask pt to pantomime using an object, say a comb or pair of scissors; if pt is unable to do so, then supply actual tool and observe performance with this)
- *Aphasia:* ability to follow complex 3-step commands presented orally; to repeat phrases presented orally; and to express self orally (if any abnormality in expression, note whether effortful or fluent, note also presence or absence of telegraphic speech, paraphasias, incoherence)
- *Alexia and agraphia:* ability to follow complex 3-step commands presented in writing; ability to express self in writing
- *Aprosodia:* ability to respond appropriately to tone of voice and facial expression of others; presence of properly modulated tone of voice and facial expression when speaking
- *Agnosia:* at a minimum:
  Tactile agnosia (i.e., ability to recognize objects by palpation, assuming that elementary sensation is intact)
  Visual agnosia (ability to name common objects upon viewing them)
  Color agnosia (ability to name common colors, perhaps the colors of the common objects used in testing for visual agnosia)
  Anosognosia (i.e., if there are any neurologic deficits, such as hemiplegia, ability to recognize the existence of the problem)

1.3 COMMON PSYCHIATRIC SYMPTOMS AND SIGNS

Arch Gen Psychiatry 1979;36:1315. Bleuler E, Textbook of psychiatry, Arno Press, New York, 1976. Kraepelin E, Clinical psychiatry, Scholar's Facsimiles and Reprints, Delmar, New York, 1981. Schneider K, Clinical psychopathology, The Classics of Psychiatry and Behavioral Sciences Library, New York, 1993.

PSYCHOMOTOR RETARDATION

This is characterized by a more or less profound slowing of thought and activity.

Thought becomes sluggish and effortful; pts may complain that they "can't think" or that the thoughts simply "won't come," and there may be a sense of oppression.

Motor activity is likewise slowed. Pts may sit for long periods, motionless, and when they do engage in movements, they are slow and made only with great effort. Speech is also slow, as if the words were simply too heavy to be moved forward in speech.

PSYCHOMOTOR AGITATION

This is characterized by a dysphoric restlessness of speech and motor behavior.

Depressed pts with psychomotor agitation may pace about, wailing, pleading for help, and wringing their hands.

Impulsive or irritable pts with psychomotor agitation may look like they're "about to blow."

HYPERACTIVITY

This is characterized by an increased rate of motor behavior, and should be qualified as to whether or not the behavior is purposeful and whether or not the hyperactive pt is engaged with the interviewer.

Manic hyperactivity flows from an overabundance of energy. There is evidence of purposefulness (which, at times, due to an abundance of separate purposes, may appear fragmented), and pts are very definitely involved and engaged with those around them.

Catatonic hyperactivity is frenzied, bizarre, and purposeless. Pts tend to keep to themselves and avoid contact with others. They may march in place in a corner, or crawl under the bed where they gesticulate wildly.

Attention-deficit/hyperactivity disorder is typically accompanied by hyperactivity, which manifests in a "fidgety" kind of restlessness, making it hard for pts to remain seated, as for example in the classroom.

STEREOTYPIES

These consist of repeated, generally purposeless, and often bizarre behaviors.

MANNERISMS

Mannerisms are normal movements, such as movements of facial expression, hand movements, or walking, that have undergone a bizarre transformation to become variously stilted, affected, or distorted. A smile may become a bizarre grimace, with everted lips and flaring of the nasal alae; when a handshake is offered, the hand may be held stiffly, with the fingers splayed out and curved back; while walking, the pt may curiously raise the legs as a stork might.

CATATONIC SYMPTOMS

Posturing is characterized by the spontaneous assumption of unnatural and often bizarre postures. One pt slowly assumed a position of crucifixion, and then maintained it for many minutes.

Negativism is characterized by an automatic and almost instinctual resistance to either requests or commands; may be either "passive" or "active." Passively negativistic pts simply do not comply; e.g., pts brought to the dinner table may sit, but neither pick up utensils nor eat, even though they are probably hungry. Actively negativistic pts do the opposite of whatever is requested or expected of them; e.g., asked to open their eyes, they may clamp them shut; asked to finish dressing, they may completely undress. Importantly, this negativism is *not* voluntary. One pt, warned to let the coffee cool before drinking it, abruptly swallowed the entire cup, burning his mouth and esophagus.

Automatic obedience is characterized by a blind, robotic, and stilted compliance with whatever is requested.

Echolalia and echopraxia are characterized by an automatic repetition or mirroring by pts of whatever is said or done by the examiner, or anyone else in immediate view. Echolalic pts repeat what is said, and if asked a question, may simply repeat it back; echopraxic pts repeat whatever is done, and if the examiner makes a gesture, the pt will do the same.

Immobility is common, and pts may retain the same position, with no evidence of movement, for hours or longer; in some cases, bedsores or contractures may result.

Muteness typically accompanies immobility, and this may at times be only partial with pts occasionally muttering incomprehensible phrases.

Rigidity is of the "lead pipe" type, and is often accompanied by catalepsy ("waxy flexibility"), wherein one may place the pt's body or limbs into virtually almost any position and the pt, without being asked to, will retain that position, no matter how uncomfortable, for long periods.

DISTURBANCES OF AFFECT

Lability of affect involves rapid changes in affect; although such lability is normal in 3- or 4-yr-olds, it is not in adults.

Flattening of affect indicates a virtual absence of all feeling and emotional display; lighter degrees of this phenomenon are often termed "blunting" of affect. Such pts are not depressed, rather they simply lack any feeling at all.

Inappropriate affect refers *not* to an affect that is "socially" inappropriate but to an affect that is *incongruent* with the emotion the pt is feeling. For example, although someone who smiled with relief at the funeral of a hated rival might be having a socially inappropriate affect, it would not be considered pathologic, as the affect was con-

gruent with the relief that the individual was feeling. By contrast,
consider the pt with a bizarre smile who reported feeling deeply
depressed; here, the incongruency of the emotion with the affect indicates pathology.

Bizarre affect comes in various forms of grimacing, sneering, pouting,
etc.

Emotional incontinence is characterized by an involuntary and uncontrollable display of emotion (e.g., weeping or laughing) that pts
report is at variance with the way they are feeling. This differs
from inappropriate affect in several respects: First, the affective
display in emotional incontinence is usually not bizarre; second, the
pt with emotional incontinence recognizes that something is wrong,
whereas the pt with inappropriate affect does not; and finally, the
pt with emotional incontinence is unable to stop the affective display, in contrast to the pt with inappropriate affect, who usually
can.

DISTURBANCES OF MOOD

Disturbances of mood represent departures from normal "euthymia."

Depressed mood may be variously described as "down," "blue,"
unhappy, or simply sad.

Irritable mood may manifest with querulousness, argumentativeness, or
hostility.

Euphoria or elation may have different effects on the interviewer,
depending on the cause. For example, in mania, the euphoric mood is
often "infectious" and interviewers, despite their efforts, often find
themselves uncontrollably laughing with the pt. By contrast, the
euphoria seen in an illness like schizophrenia often has a bizarre tinge
to it, and typically leaves the interviewer cold.

Heightening of mood may be seen with either irritability or euphoria.
Here the mood is strongly felt, voluminous, and of such sustained
intensity that pts are carried away by it, whether they want to be or
not. In the face of such turbulence, most examiners find themselves,
unconsciously, moving away (or wishing they could) to put a little
distance between themselves and the breaking storm of emotions.

DISTURBANCES IN THE FORM OF THOUGHT AND SPEECH

Incoherence is a global term indicating a disturbance of syntax such that phrases or sentences fail to "hang together" or cohere into a meaningful whole.

Flight of ideas is characterized by a repetitive, abrupt changing of the subject: a kind of "flightiness" of thought, with the speaker touching on varied subjects, like a bumblebee haphazardly going from subject to subject. Although flight of ideas is usually rapid, and coupled with pressure of speech, it need not be so.

Pressure of speech is characterized by a torrent of words, rapidly spoken, that almost inundates the listener who, in turn, can barely "get a word in edgewise."

Circumstantiality is characterized by a roundabout, circumferential approach to the "point," and examiners may become impatient as they wait for pts to "get to the point."

Tangentiality is characterized by a train of thought that strikes off on a tangent such that pts never get to the "point."

Looseness of associations is a kind of incoherence in which thought, rather than being "goal directed," has broken down into words, phrases, or sentences that seem only accidentally associated. In severe cases, there may be a "word salad" in which the individual words seem grouped at random, with no discernible thread at all.

Poverty of thought indicates a simple lack of thoughts. Pts say few words, because nothing comes to mind to say.

Poverty of speech indicates a lack of content or meaning despite a normal amount of verbiage. Typically, pts are vague, use stock phrases, and tend to repeat themselves.

Thought blocking is evident by a sudden, inexplicable stoppage of speech, often in the middle of a sentence or phrase. When asked, pts respond that their thoughts were suddenly blocked or inexplicably removed. The Schneiderian First Rank symptom of thought withdrawal (see under "Delusions," below) often accompanies this.

Neologisms are invented words, with meanings private to the pts using them. Pts use these words as readily in their speech as they do words of the common language. Importantly, if asked what they mean, most pts make little or no effort to offer a definition.

Obsessions are unwanted thoughts or images that occur involuntarily and repeatedly, despite pts' attempts to not have them. In most cases, pts view them as absurd.

Compulsions are repetitively experienced strong urges to do something, typically in response to an obsessional thought or image. For example, pts who feel compelled to repeatedly go back and check to see if the gas burners are turned off do so in response to the recurrent obsessional doubt that maybe they didn't turn them off, and that the house might burn.

HALLUCINATIONS

Auditory hallucinations may range from simple sounds (bells, laughter) to "voices," which in turn may be indistinct ("mumblings") or quite clear, even overpowering. Voices may condemn, accuse, berate, extol, or magnify pts. In some cases, voices may "command" pts to engage in 1 activity or another. Three specific kinds of voices constitute 3 of the 9 Schneiderian First Rank symptoms, and are very common in schizophrenics: voices arguing with each other, often about the pt; voices commenting on what the pt is doing ("He's combing his hair now; he's thinking foul thoughts; the coward, there he goes"); and voices that echo what the pt is thinking (pts assume that these "audible thoughts" can be heard by others).

Visual hallucinations range in complexity from simple forms of light or shadow to vivid and detailed scenes. Pts may see demons, disembodied heads, angels, etc.

Tactile (or "haptic") hallucinations may be experienced as prickings, stabbings, caresses, or the classic "formication," with a sensation of bugs crawling on or beneath the skin.

Olfactory hallucinations may be of foul, or less commonly, pleasant smells.

Gustatory hallucinations, likewise, may be pleasant or disgusting. Some pts can taste the "poison."

DELUSIONS

Delusions are false beliefs that cannot be accounted for on the basis of the pt's upbringing, religion, or culture. Delusions may be "systematized" in that they have a certain internal coherence and "make sense" as long as one or more basic delusional premises are accepted; or "nonsystematized" wherein the various delusions either have little connection or often stand in contradiction.

Persecutory delusions may involve various different kinds of "persecution": being followed, the phones being tapped, a conspiracy. Often pts believe that large organizations (the Mafia, CIA, FBI, etc.) are involved.

Grandiose delusions may involve wealth, political standing, selection by God or angels, etc.

Referential delusions involve the belief that actual events in some way pertain or refer to the pt: A car horn on a busy street is a signal for the conspirators to act; a newspaper headline hints at the pt's secret governmental involvement; a song played on the radio carries a special message intended specifically for the pt; etc.

Delusions of jealousy are beliefs that pt's significant other is being unfaithful, and are typically buttressed by reference to trivial events, such as the other person being a few minutes late, or a "hang-up" phone call.

Delusions of sin are convictions by pts that they have sinned, often in some monstrous way, or that some past misconduct was far worse than, in fact, it was.

Delusions of poverty, that one's financial resources are depleted, are often unshakable. Showing a "healthy" balance in a checkbook to a pt might prompt only a comment that ruinous bills are about to come due.

Nihilistic delusions involve the belief that some, or all, living things have become dead and lifeless. Some pts believe that *they* are dead; others, that everyone around them is and that the bodies only continue to move by virtue of some machines or magical influence.

Erotomanic delusions refer to pts' beliefs that someone else, typically someone famous, is secretly in love with them.

Somatic delusions are beliefs about the body, that it is somehow changed, misshapen, deformed, or diseased.

Pseudomemories are false beliefs about the past, and often serve to buttress delusions about the present. Pts with delusions of grandeur may report that their parents hid caches of fabulous gems for them; pts with delusions of persecution may report that they are pursued by the FBI because they were present at an assassination and know the "truth."

Schneiderian First Rank symptoms, in addition to the 3 auditory hallucinations noted above, also include 6 delusions: thought withdrawal (the experience that thoughts are somehow withdrawn from the mind, as if by some outside force); thought insertion (that thoughts, not the pt's own, are somehow inserted into the pt's mind, again as if by some outside force or agency); thought broadcasting (that pt's thoughts are picked up and broadcast over the radio, on the TV, etc.); and delusions of passivity, control, or influence: "made" thoughts, that pts' thoughts, although definitely their own, are somehow controlled or directed by some outside force; "made" feelings, that feelings are similarly controlled or manufactured; and "made" actions wherein pts feel as if they were robots, or automatons, perhaps elaborate, grotesque marionettes, with all movement under the control of outside forces.

2. Early Onset Disorders

2.1 MENTAL RETARDATION

Acta Psychiatr Scand 1985;71(Suppl 318):1. Am J Psychiatry 1975;132: 1265. Am J Psychiatry 1982;139:1297.

Epidem: Lifetime prevalence ~1%; of those with mental retardation (MR), 80%–85% have mild, 10%–12% moderate, 3%–7% severe, and 1% profound.

Sx: Onset is in infancy; however, some pts, e.g., esp those with mild MR, may not come to attention until late childhood.

Table 2.1-1 describes the various grades of MR:

- *Mildly* retarded pts often fail to grasp social nuances, and may appear "immature." Affects tend to be broad and lack shading. In tranquil settings, pts may be able to live independently and do simple work; judgment, however, is often poor, and pts often require supervision during times of stress.
- *Moderately* retarded pts have great difficulty in understanding social conventions and often have difficulty in getting along with others. They may be able to survive in group homes and do very simple work, but always with supervision.
- *Severely* retarded pts require ongoing, direct supervision, and may or may not be able to survive in even tightly organized group homes.
- *Profoundly* retarded pts may be unable to stand or sit and generally require institutionalization.

Associated features, seen with all grades, include a low frustration tolerance, impulsivity, and aggressiveness. Those with moderate or higher grades of MR often have stereotypies and self-injurious behaviors. Those with severe or profound degrees may engage in rectal digging or coprophagia.

Table 2.1-1. Grades of Mental Retardation

	Mild	Moderate	Severe	Profound
IQ	50–55 to 65–75	35–40 to 50–55	20–25 to 35–40	<20–25
Maximum developmental age (yr)	7–11	3–7	1–3	<1
Maximum grade level	4–6	2	Preschool	—
Maximum cognitive level	Simple reading, writing, arithmetic	Very limited reading, writing, arithmetic	Few spoken words	No speech
Associated malformations and seizures	Occasional	Occasional	Common	Very common

MR is accompanied by other psychiatric disorders to a greater degree than expected by chance, and the expression of these disorders is typically altered by the MR itself. Depressive episodes of major depression or bipolar disorder may present only with withdrawal, weight loss, insomnia, and psychomotor change. Mania, as in bipolar disorder, may present only with a lack of sleep, irritability, and hyperactivity. Schizophrenia may present with a bizarre deterioration in overall functioning. In all these instances, given the difficulty that MR pts have in reporting sx, it is appropriate to rely on signs.

Lab: Reflects etiology.

Crs: Chronic, and with the exception of certain progressive diseases (e.g., storage diseases such as Tay-Sachs disease), static.

Cmplc: In addition to the difficulty in achieving academic and occupational goals, pts may be subjected to considerable ridicule from other children.

Etiol: In ~50% of pts, a specific etiology may be determined (see Table 2.1-2 for common etiologies); in the remainder, unknown genetic factors appear responsible.

Ddx: Certain developmental disorders, esp a mixed expressive-receptive language disorder, may profoundly impair academic progress; however, here one sees evidence of "native" intelligence especially in the pt's ability to respond to subtle social cues.

Profound deprivation, as may be seen with child abuse or in certain

Table 2.1-2. Etiologies of Mental Retardation

Specific Chromosomal and Genetic Defects

Tuberous sclerosis
Neurofibromatosis (von Recklinghausen's disease)
Lesch-Nyhan syndrome
Prader-Willi syndrome
Laurence-Moon-Biedl syndrome
Aminoacidurias (e.g., phenylketonuria)
Storage diseases (e.g., Tay-Sachs disease)
Down's syndrome
Fragile X syndrome
Klinefelter's syndrome

Intrauterine Insults

Fetal alcohol syndrome
Radiation
Infections (rubella, toxoplasmosis)
Hypothyroidism
Hyperparathyroidism

Perinatal and Postnatal Factors

Perinatal anoxia
Erythroblastosis fetalis
Severe malnutrition

orphanages, may produce a picture similar to severe or lesser degrees of MR, but is distinguished by the pt's ability to gradually "catch up" when placed in a better environment.

Schizophrenia of childhood onset is distinguished by hallucinations and delusions.

Dementia is distinguished by the course of the syndrome. In dementia there is a definite decrement or falling off of intellectual abilities relative to the premorbid level, whereas in MR the course is characterized more by an intellectual development that plateaus or "stalls out" at a certain level, after which it remains static.

Rx: Special education and well-organized group homes are essential.
Behavior modification programs are often effective for the associated features noted above.

Neuroleptics (e.g., thioridazine, haloperidol) may reduce impulsivity, aggressiveness, and stereotypies, and lithium may be effective for aggression and impulsivity.

2.2 READING DISORDER (DEVELOPMENTAL DYSLEXIA)

Ann Neurol 1994;35:732. Arch Neurol 1986;43:1045. JAMA 1992;268: 912.

Epidem: ~4% of school-age children; more common in boys.

Sx: The failure to develop adequate reading skills usually becomes apparent between the ages of 6 and 9 (1st–4th grades).

Although able to understand the spoken word, and to speak adequately themselves, these pts have significant difficulty reading words or comprehending written phrases or passages. When reading out loud, pts often skip over words or misread the words, often supplying a word that is subtly different, either in that a letter is missing or substituted or that there has been a reversal, either of letters or of the whole word; e.g., "gary" may be read for "gray," "lad" for "lab," or "top" for "pot." Even when pts are able to read each word in a passage, comprehension is poor, and pts, when asked, have great trouble in putting what they read into their "own words." Remarkably, though, if the same passage is read aloud to them, they may have little trouble in paraphrasing it.

Writing difficulties typically accompany the reading difficulty. Pts may write "pat" for "tap," or entire sentences may be reversed, with the pt writing from left to right. Importantly, if pts are shown their written work, they find nothing amiss with it.

Associated disorders include attention-deficit/hyperactivity disorder and mathematics disorder.

Lab: NC.

Crs: If pts persist in attempting to learn to read, gradual improvement is seen into adult years.

Cmplc: Frustration and embarrassment may lead to school failure and truancy.

Etiol: Inherited factors important.

MRI suggests a lack of the normal asymmetry of the plana temporalia, with both plana being approximately equal in size. Autopsy studies have revealed ectopic neurons and focal areas of cortical dysplasia.

Ddx: Inadequate schooling during elementary school years, even with children who *are* capable of learning to read, may leave children so embarrassed over their inability to read that they never learn.

Partial blindness should be checked for in all pts.

MR is distinguished by an equal decrement in all cognitive abilities.

Acquired aphasia of the "pure word blindness" type is very rare in children, and is suggested by a loss of whatever prior ability to read that the pt had.

Rx: Remedial education, with a strict focus on reading, is effective. Piracetam, not available yet in the USA, is also helpful.

2.3 MATHEMATICS DISORDER (DEVELOPMENTAL DYSCALCULIA)

Arch Dis Child 1993;68:510. Ped Ann 1987;16:159. Psychol Med 1971; 1:292.

Epidem: 1%–6% of school-age children; may be more common in girls.

Sx: The failure to develop adequate mathematical skills usually becomes apparent between the ages of 6 and 10, in most cases by the 3rd grade.

A range of difficulties: recognizing numerals or writing them; counting to 10; understanding the concept of addition, subtraction, multiplication, or division.

Associated disorders include reading disorder or disorder of written expression.

Lab: NC.

Crs: Varies from chronic to gradual partial (or even full) remission.

Cmplc: Frustration and embarrassment may further impair the child's attempts at learning.

Etiol: Some cases associated with the fragile X syndrome; in the majority the etiology is unknown.

Ddx: Inadequate schooling during elementary school years is very important, as the acquisition of mathematics skills is highly dependent on formal instruction.

MR is distinguished by an equal decrement in all cognitive abilities.

Acquired dyscalculia is very rare, but may be seen with lesions of the left parietal lobe or left striatum.

Rx: Remedial education, focused on mathematics.

2.4 DISORDER OF WRITTEN EXPRESSION (DEVELOPMENTAL DYSGRAPHIA)

J Child Neurol 1995;10(Suppl 1):56. J Learning Disabilities 1991;24: 578. Q J Exp Psychol 1986;38:77.

Epidem: Uncertain; probably rare.

Sx: The failure to develop adequate writing skills usually becomes apparent between the ages of 7 and 10 (3rd–4th grades).

Although able to adequately express their ideas with the spoken words, these pts experience a range of difficulties in writing: Paragraphs are short and poorly organized; sentences display poor syntax and grammar and may be "run-on"; and words are often misspelled.

Mathematics disorder is often present.

Lab: NC.

Crs: Probably chronic.

Cmplc: Embarrassment and shame may lead to defeatism and absenteeism.

Etiol: Uncertain.

Ddx: Poor penmanship is distinguished by a close inspection of the pt's work, which reveals proper syntax, grammar, punctuation, etc.

Isolated poor spelling is not uncommon and is distinguished by the presence of adequate syntax, grammar, punctuation, etc.

Acquired pure dysgraphia due to lesions of Exner's area in the posterior portion of the nondominant inferior frontal gyrus is a rare disorder. A loss of a previously acquired ability to write is suggestive.

Rx: Remedial education.

2.5 DEVELOPMENTAL COORDINATION DISORDER (DEVELOPMENTAL CLUMSINESS, CLUMSY CHILD SYNDROME)

Brain 1962;85:603. Brain 1965;88:295. Pediatr Rev 1989;10:247.

Epidem: 5%–6% of school-age children; more common in boys.

Sx: Clumsiness, depending on the severity, may become apparent anywhere from infancy to the age of 5 or 6.

Infants may have trouble sitting or crawling; toddlers may excessively stumble; preschoolers may often trip and fall, especially when playing games; and early school-age children may fumble at tying shoes, pulling up zippers, or fastening buttons. In later school years, sports are particularly frustrating.

Associated disorders include reading disorder and any of the language disorders.

Lab: NC.

Crs: Probably chronic.

Cmplc: Gym classes are particularly embarrassing; pts may withdraw from neighborhood social contacts into fantasy.

Etiol: Uncertain.

Ddx: MR distinguished by an accompanying decrement in cognitive abilities.

Attention-deficit/hyperactivity disorder distinguished by collisions and fumbles that result from impulsivity and rushing, rather than clumsiness.

Muscular dystrophy, cerebral palsy, Friedreich's ataxia, cerebellar tumors, and ataxia telangiectasia must all be considered.

Rx: Remedial gym classes may be helpful.

2.6 EXPRESSIVE LANGUAGE DISORDER (DEVELOPMENTAL EXPRESSIVE APHASIA)

Ann Neurol 1989;25:567. J Am Acad Child Psychiatry 1979;4:604. J Am Acad Child Psychiatry 1983;22:525.

Epidem: Isolated expressive language disorder is rare; probably more common in boys.

Sx: Difficulty speaking may become apparent by age 3 in severe cases, or in early adolescence in very mild cases.

Although able to follow spoken directions, even complex ones, pts, frustrated at their inability to express their thoughts in speech, may have temper tantrums.

Associated disorders include phonologic disorder, developmental coordination disorder, and attention-deficit/hyperactivity disorder.

Lab: NC.

Crs: Approximately one-half of pts achieve full remission by midadolescence; in the other half speech improves but subtle deficits remain.

Cmplc: Frustration may lead to withdrawal from academic or social activities.

Etiol: Uncertain.

Ddx: Acquired expressive aphasia must be distinguished from the developmental variety. In the acquired type one sees a decrement in the pt's prior ability to speak, whereas in the developmental type there is not so much a loss as there is a failure to acquire the ability "on time." Lesions of various sorts in the dominant frontal lobe must be considered.

MR is distinguished by a decrement in all cognitive abilities.

Autism is distinguished by the disturbance in social contact. Whereas pts with expressive language disorder retain the capacity for affectionate contact, autistic children do not.

Selective mutism is distinguished by the child's ability to speak normally at home or with close friends.

Phonologic disorder, when isolated and severe, may be confused with expressive language disorder; however, close inspection of transcripts will reveal normal syntax.

Mixed expressive-receptive language disorder is distinguished by the difficulty in following complex spoken commands.

Rx: Although there has been some debate, it appears that remedial education is appropriate.

2.7 MIXED RECEPTIVE-EXPRESSIVE LANGUAGE DISORDER (DEVELOPMENTAL SENSORY APHASIA)

Ann Neurol 1989;25:567. J Am Acad Child Psychiatry 1979;4:604. J Am Acad Child Psychiatry 1983;22:525.

Epidem: Mild forms may occur in ~3% of school-age children; severe forms are rare, seen in <0.1%; more common in boys than girls.

Sx: Difficulty understanding spoken language may become apparent by age 2 in severe cases to late childhood in very mild cases.

In severe cases, pts seem unaffected by the content of what is said to them: They may respond to tone of voice, but are unable to follow even the simplest of spoken instructions. In less severe cases, they may understand simple words and be able to follow very simple commands. In mild cases, the difficulty may become apparent when pts appear confused or befuddled when given complex commands, and this is particularly evident when conditional or concessive statements are involved. The difficulty in comprehending spoken language is paralleled by a difficulty in speaking, similar to that seen in developmental expressive language disorder: Simple vocabulary and syntax are favored, and sentences are short and telegraphic at best.

Attention-deficit/hyperactivity disorder is commonly present.

Lab: NC.

Crs: Generally chronic, with little spontaneous improvement.

Cmplc: Academic and social failure are common.

Etiol: Familial; MRI and SPECT suggest dysfunction in the left temporo-parietal area.

> **Ddx:** Acquired mixed receptive-expressive dysphasia is distinguished by the course. In contrast to the developmental kind, wherein there is simply a failure to acquire language skills, in the acquired kind, pts lose some skills already gained. Infarctions, tumors, and encephalitides may be at fault. A common cause is the Landau-Kleffner syndrome, wherein seizures and dysphasia appear in late childhood.

MR is distinguished by the global nature of the deficit. Although pts with mixed receptive-expressive language disorder may not be able to communicate, they may well display a grasp of complex visuospatial problems in their play with games and blocks.

Autism is distinguished by the lack of affective rapport. By contrast, mute pts with mixed receptive-expressive language disorder may "warm up" to the interviewer.

Deafness should always be checked for.

Rx: Remedial education is encouraged.

2.8 PHONOLOGIC DISORDER (DEVELOPMENTAL ARTICULATION DISORDER, DEVELOPMENTAL DYSARTICULATION)

BMJ 1954;1:8. J Speech Hear Disord 1988;53:144. Netsell R, A neurobiologic review of speech production and the dysarthrias, College Hill Press, San Diego, 1968.

Epidem: Anywhere from 2% to 15% of children <8 yr old have some degree of dysarticulation.

Sx: Difficulty with articulation may become apparent by the age of 2 yr in severe cases to age 6 in mild cases.

Characteristic substitutions, omissions, and distortions are seen in speech:

- *Substitutions* typically involve consonants: "wabbit" for "rabbit" (as in Elmer Fudd's "wascally wabbit!").
- *Omissions* also typically involve consonants: "ollipop" for "lollipop."
- *Distortions* show up as lisping, or the misarticulation of sibilants: "thilly boy" for "silly boy."

The overall effect is of a child using "baby talk," and in severe cases, speech may be almost unintelligible.

Associated disorders include developmental coordination disorder and developmental language disorders.

Lab: NC.

Crs: In the vast majority there is a spontaneous remission by age 8; sx persisting past age 8 tend to indicate a chronic course.

Cmplc: Mild cases may bring only shame and embarrassment; severe cases may preclude academic or social success.

Etiol: Familial, probably due to genetic factors.

Ddx: Dysarticulation may be seen with cleft palate or dental malocclusion, and may also occur as part of cerebral palsy.

MR is distinguished by the global cognitive deficits.

Autism may be accompanied by dysmelodic speech but is distinguished by social aloofness.

Deafness, as it is typically accompanied by dysarticulate speech, should always be checked for.

Expressive language disorder or mixed receptive-expressive language disorder is distinguished by disturbances in syntax.

Dialects, to the uninitiated, may sound "dysarticulate." Referring to a "car" as a "ka" might be abnormal in Memphis but quite normal in Boston.

Rx: Speech therapy is effective.

2.9 STUTTERING

Am J Psychiatry 1976;133:331. J Clin Psychiatry 1995;56:238. J Speech Hear Disord 1990;55:370.

Epidem: Stuttering, or stammering, seen in anywhere from 1% to 4% of young children; male-female ratio 3–4:1.

Sx: Onset is insidious, generally over several months, usually between the ages of 2 and 7; it is very rare to see stuttering appear after the age of 10.

Although stuttering may occur with almost any word, it is particularly common in front of words beginning with B, D, K, P, or T. Although pts know what they want to say, they experience a "block" as they attempt to speak, which is typically followed by repetitive and ever more forceful repronounciations of the blocking letter or syllable until it is finally overcome. These efforts are often accompanied by simultaneous grimacing, blinking, or forceful movements of the head and neck. After the stumbling block is breached, there often follows a cascade of normally pronounced words, which may continue until the next block arises.

Stuttering is worse when pts are rushed, under pressure, anxious, or speaking in front of a group. Importantly, pts are often free of stuttering if they are alone, reading aloud, or singing.

Associated disorders include phonologic disorder and expressive language disorder.

Lab: NC.

Crs: By age 16, spontaneous full remission in ~60%, with another ~20% experiencing a partial remission.

Cmplc: Embarrassment, shame, and ridicule are encountered by most, and some may withdraw from social or academic areas to avoid these.

Etiol: Polygenic inheritance most likely.

Ddx: Other causes of stuttering must be ruled out, and these include lesions (infarcts, tumors) in the nondominant frontal lobe, caudate nucleus, or thalamus; medications such as tricyclics, SSRIs, and neuroleptics; and parkinsonian conditions such as Parkinson's disease and progressive supranuclear palsy. Stuttering due to these other causes is distinguished by any of the following: onset >10 yr, acute onset, a lack of forceful repetition of the letter or sound stuttered, a lack of associated facial movements, and a lack of a "cascade" of normally pronounced words following the stutter.

Rx: Speech therapy often successful.

Clomipramine (Anafranil), in doses of 150 mg for adults, is effective; in resistant cases, consideration may be given to low-dose haloperidol (Haldol).

2.10 AUTISM (AUTISTIC DISORDER)

Am J Psychiatry 1984;141:1195. Am J Psychiatry 1990;147:1614. Arch Gen Psychiatry 1993;50:441. J Clin Psychiatry 1992;53:77.

Epidem: Lifetime prevalence 0.02%–0.1%; male-female ratio 3–4:1.

Sx: Onset ranges from earliest infancy up to age 3 yr.

Most distinctive clinical picture seen in middle childhood. Pts typically relate to others as if others were machines, or inanimate objects; rather than playing with other children, pts either keep to themselves or treat others as if they were mere mechanical props. Emotional contact is lacking and some pts may exhibit gaze avoidance or simply stare "through" others. Language and speech are generally disturbed: Pts may have their own idiosyncratic vocabulary, or may be mute; often prosody is disturbed, and speech may exhibit peculiar inflections, or have a "sing-song" character. The overall behavior of these children often appears bizarre: Perseveration and stereotypies (esp arm or hand flapping) are common, and pts often exhibit "fascinations" with various inanimate objects, such as jewelry, bits of cloth, or classically, spinning tops. An "insistence on sameness" is common, and pts may become catastrophically anxious if familiar routines or regimens are transgressed: The same route must be taken to school; the aisles of the grocery store must be traversed in the same order; family members must sit at the same places at the dinner table.

MR, generally of moderate degree, is seen in ~75% of pts, and is often characterized by an "uneven" profile of cognitive abilities with, at times, "islets" of normal or even superior functioning preserved. Some otherwise retarded autistic pts are capable of extraordinary musical performances or feats of memory (e.g., memorizing timetables or phone books).

Table 2.10-1. Secondary Causes of Autism

Fragile X syndrome
Down's syndrome
Tuberous sclerosis
Rett's syndrome
Neurofibromatosis (von Recklinghausen's disease)
Phenylketonuria
Hurler's syndrome
Maternal rubella
Galactosemia
Congenital hypothyroidism

Seizures (grand mal or complex partial) seen in ~20%, and are as
likely to occur in autistic pts of normal intelligence as in those
with MR.

Lab: In some pts MRI reveals cerebellar vermal atrophy; in others a
degree of atrophy of medial temporal structures may also be seen.
These are often subtle, and are not useful for dx purposes.

Crs: Although autism is chronic, most pts experience some diminution
of sx through teenage years, eventually leaving a stable pattern
during adulthood. Two-thirds of pts require some degree of supervision; some, however, are capable of independent living, and may
at times excel in some occupations, often those involving machines
or computers. In all pts, however, some distinctive features persist,
and high-functioning autistic adults generally display some aloofness or awkwardness in social settings, along with some dys-
prosody and stereotyped behavior.

Cmplc: As above, most are incapable of independent living.

Etiol: There are probably 2 different types of autism: primary or idiopathic; and secondary. Autism has been noted in a variety of other
conditions, listed in Table 2.10-1; of these, the fragile X syndrome
is by far the most common.

Primary or idiopathic autism is almost certainly an inherited disease.
Concordance for siblings is ~2.5%–3%, for DZ twins figures
range up to ~20%, and for MZ twins figures range from ~30%
up to 95%.

MRI findings as noted above, under Lab; autopsy studies reveal a
reduced number of cerebellar granule and Purkinje cells, and
in the hippocampus cells are smaller than normal, and more
densely packed. In some pts, classic evidence of neuronal migra-

tion defect is seen, such as areas of polymicrogyria or focal cortical dysplasia.

Biochemical abnormalities include hyperserotonemia in approximately one-third, and in some, elevated CSF endorphin levels.

Ddx: Schizophrenia of childhood onset is distinguished by age at onset (>6 yr) and by the presence of hallucinations and delusions, sx not seen in autism.

Children with deafness, blindness, or a mixed receptive-expressive language disorder, at first glance, may appear similar but are readily distinguished by the preserved, and often obvious, desire for social contact: A deaf child may not be able to communicate, but will respond warmly to human contact.

MR not associated with autism is likewise distinguished by the desire for social contact.

Rx: Rx of children and adolescents with autism is a major task involving behavior modification, special education, and family counseling. A variety of medications may also be useful. It is unclear which of these measures may also be helpful with autistic adults.

Haloperidol (Haldol) (and perhaps risperidone (Risperdal) or olanzapine (Zyprexa)), in low doses, reduces withdrawal and stereotyped behavior, and may facilitate language acquisition in children. Tardive dyskinesia poses a significant risk that must be balanced against these benefits.

Clomipramine (Anafranil), in doses of 3–4 mg/kg/d also reduces social withdrawal and stereotyped behaviors, and appears to facilitate social interaction.

Naltrexone (ReVia), 0.5–1.0 mg/kg/d, or clonidine (Catapres) (transdermal, 0.005 mg/kg/d) causes a modest reduction in restlessness and hyperactivity.

Lithium (Eskalith, Lithobid) may reduce explosiveness and aggressiveness.

2.11 RETT'S SYNDROME (RETT'S DISORDER)

Acta Pediatr 1995;84:971. Ann Neurol 1983;14:471. Ann Neurol 1988; 23:425.

Epidem: Very rare (e.g., <1/150 000); probably exclusively in females.

Sx: The first 5 mo or more of life are normal: There are no perinatal or postnatal problems, and head growth is initially normal. Subsequently, stage I of the illness appears.

Rett's syndrome is best considered in terms of its 4 stages:

- *Stage I,* appearing around the age of 10 mo, is characterized by a slowing of normal development: weight gain may slow, and pts may not learn to crawl.
- *Stage II,* appearing around the age of 18 mo, is characterized by a loss of previously acquired abilities: Pts withdraw from their surroundings and begin to display autistic traits; purposeless midline hand stereotypies appear, often resembling hand wringing or hand washing; head growth decelerates and microcephaly appears along with MR, often severe.
- *Stage III,* appearing around the age of 3 yr, is marked by a partial restitution of abilities lost in stage II; seizures (grand mal, complex partial, or simple partial) if not already present, appear, and eventually affect up to 80% of pts.
- *Stage IV,* which may not appear until adolescence or early adult years, is characterized by the gradual appearance of scoliosis, dystonia, and in some, choreoathetosis.

Lab: MRI may reveal cortical atrophy.

Crs: After reaching stage IV, the course is chronic and generally static for the remainder of the pt's life.

Cmplc: As for MR (see 2.1).

Etiol: Genetic factors strongly suspected (probably X-linked, with male lethality); the MZ concordance is 100%, and the DZ ~0%.

CSF levels of MHPG and HVA are low.

Autopsy studies of children reveal hypoplasia, without gliosis; although the number of cells in the substantia nigra is normal, they lack a normal amount of melanin pigment. Autopsy studies of adults reveal some gliosis; suggesting a 2-stage process.

Ddx: Rett's syndrome is distinguished from other causes of MR and autism by the characteristic course, wherein autistic features and MR become apparent in stage II, but then undergo a partial resolution (esp the autistic features) in stage III; the midline hand stereotypies constitute another valuable clue.

Rx: Habilitative efforts are as discussed for MR in 2.1.

Seizures may be treated with carbamazepine (Tegretol) or divalproex (Depakote).

Bromocriptine (Parlodel) is reported to reduce autistic features, but the effect may not be maintained.

Haloperidol (Haldol), in very low doses (e.g., 0.5–1 mg po) may reduce stereotypies.

Naltrexone (ReVia) should not be given as it appears to exacerbate sx.

2.12 ATTENTION-DEFICIT/ HYPERACTIVITY DISORDER

Am J Psychiatry 1990;147:1018. Arch Gen Psychiatry 1993;50:565. Arch Gen Psychiatry 1995;53:434. Drugs 1993;46:863.

Epidem: Prevalence among school-age children ∼6%; male-female ratio ∼7:1.

Sx: Onset probably in very early childhood; however, may not come to attention until the age of 7 yr.

Classic picture is most evident in school-age children, with hyperactivity, distractibility, and impulsivity. These young pts seem always on the move, unable to sit still in the classroom or at home, always restless and fidgety. Distractibility apparent especially at school, where pts' attention seems to be caught by even trivial stimuli. Impulsivity evident in school as pts blurt out answers, often before thinking about them, or in the neighborhood, as pts disrupt the play of others or commandeer their toys.

Adolescence brings a moderation of sx, and a full remission may be seen in approximately one-third of pts. In the remainder hyperactivity usually manifests with impatience and a sense of restlessness, often with fidgeting and foot tapping; distractibility continues to impair academic progress; and impulsivity may lead to excessive confrontations with authorities.

Adult years find two-thirds of pts or more in remission. In the remainder, sx may be quite mild, relatively speaking. Gross hyperactivity is usually absent, but pts may complain of a sense of restlessness. Distractibility appears more like poor concentration, and impulsivity may manifest with an irritable impatience. Making the dx in an adult may be difficult; the most reliable method involves tracing the current sx back in an unbroken lineage to a typical school-age picture.

Lab: NC.

Crs: As above, with gradual diminution of sx to point of remission in approximately two-thirds of pts by adult years.

Cmplc: Academic failure and repeated conflict with authority are common.

There is a strong link between attention-deficit/hyperactivity disorder in childhood and the presence, in adults or older teens, of antisocial personality disorder (esp in males), somatization disorder (esp in females), alcoholism, and other dependencies on substances, such as cocaine or cannabis. The nature of this link is not clear: These other disorders may be true complications, or, conversely, may represent the adult expression of a diathesis common to them and to attention-deficit/hyperactivity disorder.

Etiol: Strong genetic factor; PET reveals orbitofrontal hypometabolism and CSF levels of HVA, a dopamine metabolite, are low.

Ddx: Two conditions may cause an almost identical clinical picture: low-grade lead encephalopathy, and in a very small number, an inherited resistance to thyroid hormone.

Chaotic homes may lead to a similar condition in children, and sometimes the only way to make the ddx is to observe the child over time in a more benign environment.

Phenobarbital may cause considerable hyperactivity, and should probably not be used in children.

MR children may appear quite hyperactive, but when compared to children of the same *developmental* age, their behavior is typically seen as "age appropriate."

Mania, as in bipolar disorder, is distinguished by the directed pressure of activity, which is in contrast to the undirected restlessness of children with attention-deficit/hyperactivity.

Depression, as in major depression, if accompanied by psychomotor agitation, may produce significant restlessness; however, here one sees despair, fatigue, loss of appetite, etc., sx not seen in attention-deficit/hyperactivity.

Rx: Special classrooms and behavior programs, both at school and at home, may be helpful; however, they are not as effective as pharmacologic treatment.

Pharmacologic Rx is generally indicated. Table 2.12-1 lists the vari-

Table 2.12-1. Medications Useful in Attention-Deficit/Hyperactivity Disorder

Stimulants

Methylphenidate (Ritalin)
Dextroamphetamine (Dexedrine)
Pemoline (Cylert)

Antidepressants

Bupropion (Wellbutrin, Zyban)
Tricyclics (e.g., nortriptyline (Pamelor))
MAOIs (e.g., tranylcypromine (Parnate))

Neuroleptics

Thioridazine (Mellaril)

Other

Clonidine (Catapres)

ous medications found useful. Most pts are treated, at least initially, with either a stimulant or an antidepressant.

Of the stimulants, methylphenidate (Ritalin) is most often used: For children, begin at 5–10 mg qd, increasing by similar increments weekly until sx are controlled, unacceptable SEs occur, or a maximum dose of 60 mg is attained; adults may require higher doses, up to 1 mg/kg/d. The total daily dose is divided into a morning and midday dose. Evening doses may cause insomnia. In some pts time-release preparations may be possible. Using stimulants in adolescents or adults poses certain risks, given their abuse potential, and in such cases an antidepressant may be preferable.

Of the antidepressants, bupropion (Wellbutrin) appears most promising: For adults, it is used as described in 6.1; for children, the total daily dose should be ~3 mg/kg/d. TCAs, though rapidly effective, may lose effectiveness after a few months: Possible cardiotoxicity argues against using desipramine (Norpramin); nortriptyline (Pamelor) may be safest (for adults, use as described in 6.1; for children the total daily dose is ~0.3 mg/kg/d). MAOIs, especially tranylcypromine (Parnate), though consistently effective, are rarely used due to dietary constraints. Neuroleptics are rapidly effective, and may work where other agents fail; however, concerns about tardive dyskinesia constrain their use to short-term emergency: Thioridazine (Mellaril) seems most effective.

2.13 CONDUCT DISORDER

Arch Gen Psychiatry 1984;41:650. J Am Acad Child Adolesc Psychiatry 1995;34:445. J Affect Disord 1988;15:205.

Epidem: Among children and adolescents, present in 2%–9% of females and 6%–16% of males.

Sx: Onset in males in late childhood, in females around puberty.

There is a pattern of repetitive misconduct involving aggressiveness, destruction of property, deceitfulness or theft, and serious violation of rules and regulations.

Aggressiveness may involve bullying, fighting, using weapons, cruelty to animals or people, and rape.

Destruction of property may involve fire setting, vandalism, and wanton destruction of property.

Deceitfulness may involve repeated lying or conning, and theft may be restricted to shoplifting, or advance to purse snatching and breaking and entering.

Serious violation of rules and regulations may involve truancy or running away.

Typically, those with conduct disorder either join a gang, to which they may evince some loyalty, or are "loners," who tend to be more aggressive. Sympathy for others is generally lacking, and although some conduct-disordered youths may feign contrition, true remorse and guilt are generally lacking. Promiscuity and substance abuse or dependence are common.

Lab: NC.

Crs: In approximately two-thirds of pts, misconduct gradually fades, and by adult years conformity to law and custom becomes the rule. In approximately one-third, however, the misconduct is chronic and merges into antisocial personality disorder: This outcome is more likely associated with an onset <10 yr, prominent aggressiveness, and being a "loner."

Cmplc: Academic failure, incarceration.

Etiol: Familial factors: Antisocial personality disorder and alcoholism are common in parents.

Environmental factors: Parents are often in conflict with each other and discipline is typically inconsistent and harsh; some children have been abandoned or removed from the home, and one may find a h/o a string of foster homes or institutional placements.

Attention-deficit/hyperactivity disorder is common in the h/o these conduct-disordered youths, and could easily contribute to their inability to learn rules.

Ddx: Adolescent rebelliousness is distinguished by the rebels' demonstration of loyalty and sympathy to those outside the "authority structure" and by its later onset.

Attention-deficit/hyperactivity disorder, uncomplicated by conduct disorder, is distinguished by the "accidental" nature of the pts' misconduct. The misconduct is clearly related to hyperactivity and impulsiveness rather than to any planning.

Mania, as in bipolar disorder, is distinguished by pressure of speech and activity.

MR may be associated with misconduct, but here the pt is unable to appreciate the rules being transgressed.

Dysthymia or a depressive episode (of major depression or bipolar disorder), by robbing pts of energy, interest, and the ability to concentrate, may lead them to drop out of school and other pursuits and render them "easy prey" for conduct-disordered children or adolescents seeking followers. This is a very important differential, and if there is doubt, a trial of antidepressants may be appropriate.

Rx: Parent training, combined with cognitive behavior therapy for the youth, may be effective. Residential treatment typically fails to generalize.

Medications play a limited role. If attention-deficit/hyperactivity disorder is present, it should be treated; however, stimulants, given the risk of abuse, should probably be second choice. Where aggressiveness is prominent and impulsive, lithium (Eskalith, Lithobid) or haloperidol (Haldol) may be helpful.

2.14 PICA

Arch Int Med 1971;128:472. Br J Psychiatry 1988;152:842. Br J Psychiatry 1992;160:341.

Epidem: Uncertain, but may be common in certain conditions (MR, pregnancy).

Sx: *Pica* is Latin for "magpie," and like the magpie, those with pica eat a variety of nonfood items. Such ingestion of nonfood items is very common in otherwise normal infants and children 3 yr or younger, and is not considered pathologic; eating nonfood items after age 3 yr, however, is pathologic. Among the MR, pica may have an onset at any time from childhood to middle years; in pregnant pts, pica clears either during the pregnancy or in the postpartum period.

Nonretarded children may eat paint, masonry, hair, clothing, dirt, sand, pebbles, plastic cups, or tobacco; retarded individuals, in addition to these items, may also eat trash or feces.

Pica of pregnancy often involves clay or starch.

"Pagophagia," or ice eating, is common with iron deficiency anemia.

Importantly, pts with pica also eat normal food, and weight loss generally does not occur.

Lab: Iron deficiency anemia may be present, and may be either a cause of pica or, as noted below, one of its complications. With lead ingestion (as found in paint chips), "lead lines" may be seen on xray, blood lead levels are high, and erythrocyte protoporphyrin levels are increased.

Crs: In the vast majority of nonretarded children, pica stops by adolescence.

In retarded pts, pica may be chronic.

Pica of pregnancy, as noted, clears as pregnancy ends, and pica secondary to iron deficiency clears with iron Rx.

Cmplc: Constipation or obstruction may occur; hair or cloth bezoars may form; eating contaminated dirt may lead to toxoplasmosis or toxocariasis.

Iron deficiency anemia may occur when clay complexes with dietary iron.

Lead encephalopathy of children is typically the result of pica involving lead-based paint.

Etiol: Among nonretarded children, there is often a h/o lack of parental supervision.

EARLY ONSET DISORDERS

Iron deficiency, as noted, may cause pica; in some pts zinc deficiency may also contribute.

Ddx: In some cultures, eating nonfood items is sanctioned and encouraged.

The following conditions may also be associated with eating nonfood items: schizophrenia, autism, dementia, delirium, the Kleine-Levin syndrome, and the Klüver-Bucy syndrome.

Rx: Iron deficiency anemia should be corrected.

Nonretarded children require close supervision.

Retarded pts may be treated behaviorally with immediate reprimands, very brief restraint, or vigorous tooth brushing, and with individually tailored rewards for abstention from pica.

2.15 RUMINATION DISORDER

Br J Psychiatry 1994;165:303. J Am Acad Child Adolesc Psychiatry 1998;27:300. NEJM 1969;280:802.

Epidem: In nonretarded infants or children, probably rare; among severely or profoundly retarded pts, seen in 3%–10%.

Sx: *Ruminatio* is Latin for "chewing of the cud," which clearly distinguishes rumination from regurgitation or vomiting: The ruminator *rechews* the regurgitated food, whereas the vomiter or the simple regurgitator immediately expels it from the mouth. Occasional rechewing of food is normal in infants up to the age of 3 or 4 mo; past that, it becomes pathologic. Among MR pts rumination typically appears in middle childhood or in adolescence.

Infant ruminators typically lie quietly for a brief period after a feeding; forceful abdominal contractions and arching of the back occur, followed by the regurgitation. These infants then rechew the food, often with a satisfied or blissful countenance; subsequently the food may be either spat out or reswallowed.

Lab: NC.

Crs: Almost all infant ruminators cease rumination by the age of 12 mo; very rarely it may persist, even into adult years.

Rumination in the MR tends to be chronic.

Cmplc: Malnutrition, failure to thrive, and fatalities may occur in a small minority. In children or adults, aspiration pneumonia, caries, and halitosis may occur.

Parents of infant ruminators are often very distressed by the behavior, and this may significantly interfere with the parent-child relationship.

Etiol: Uncertain; in some infants with rumination there appears to be a disturbed mother-infant bond, but in others, no disturbance is seen.

Ddx: Regurgitation or vomiting may occur with pyloric stenosis, hiatal hernia, or a Zenker's diverticulum. In these pts, though, there is no rechewing.

Approximately 10%–20% of pts with bulimia nervosa will engage in rumination; however, this clears with treatment of the bulimia.

Occasional rumination may be seen in MR; however, when the developmental age of the pt is considered, it is usually found to be very low, and in such pts, as with normal infants, occasional rumination is not considered abnormal.

Rx: In some pts, provision of a more nurturant figure during feedings may be effective. In others, aversive techniques (e.g., a drop of bitter lemon on the tongue, or in severe cases, an electric shock to the body, immediately upon regurgitation) are often effective. In some pts, metoclopramide (Reglan) may reduce regurgitation.

2.16 TOURETTE'S DISORDER (GILLES DE LA TOURETTE'S SYNDROME)

Ann Neurol 1980;7:41. JAMA 1995;273:498. Neurology 1977;27:115. Neurology 1986;36:378.

Epidem: Lifetime prevalence ~0.05%; male-female ratio 3:1.

Sx: Average age at onset is 7 yr (ranging from infancy to age 17 yr), usually with a simple motor tic.

Pts eventually have both motor tics and vocal tics, usually within a year. These may be either simple or complex, and examples are given in Table 2.16-1.

Motor tics generally begin on the head or face, and may progress in a rostral-caudal sequence.

Table 2.16-1. Motor and Vocal Tics

	Motor	Vocal
Simple	Blinking, brow wrinkling, grimacing, shoulder shrugging	Snorting, hissing, coughing, sniffing, throat clearing, barking
Complex	Touching, smelling, hopping, throwing, clapping	Words or phrases (which may be perseverated), echolalia, coprolalia (~10%)

Sensory tics, once thought rare, may in fact be common, and consist of 2 types: isolated sensory tics, like tickles or itches, and premonitory urges, which appear just before motor tics.

Approximately one-fourth of pts also experience obsessions or compulsions, usually within 2 yr of the onset of tics; the compulsions often center around symmetry.

Lab: NC.

Crs: In the majority, chronic, with partial remission of sx in early adult years. A minority may experience a full remission; however, tics generally reappear, perhaps after months or years.

Cmplc: Shame, embarrassment, and social ostracism. Frequent motor tics may lead to articular damage, and frequent sensory tics may lead to sufficient scratching to cause excoriations.

Etiol: In many pts, autosomal dominant inheritance, with variable, sex-linked penetrance; in some families a genetic locus has been identified on chromosome 18. Current research suggests that Tourette's disorder and obsessive-compulsive disorder may represent differing phenotypic expressions of the same genotype.

An uncertain percentage of cases may also represent sequelae to Sydenham's chorea.

Ddx: Transient tics, lasting less than a year, or chronic isolated motor or vocal tics probably represent formes frustes of Tourette's disorder. Other causes of tics are listed in Table 2.16-2.

Tardive dyskinesia, rarely, may be characterized by tics; however, these are usually accompanied by chorea, and there is a h/o prolonged neuroleptic exposure.

Stimulant use is an important cause, as many Tourette's pts seen in clinics also have attention-deficit/hyperactivity disorder, and thus may be candidates for stimulant treatment.

Rx: Pharmacologic Rx may involve a neuroleptic, clonidine (Catapres), or clonazepam (Klonopin).

Table 2.16-2. Other Causes of Tics

Tardive dyskinesia ("tardive Tourette's")
Stimulants: methylphenidate (Ritalin), amphetamines (e.g., dextroamphetamine (Dexedrine)), pemoline (Cylert), cocaine
Sydenham's chorea
Neuroacanthocytosis
Postviral encephalitis (encephalitis lethargica, herpes simplex)

Neuroleptics very effective: haloperidol (Haldol) (2–10 mg/d) best studied; risperidone (Risperdal) or olanzapine (Zyprexa) may be viable alternatives. Pimozide (Orap) (1–10 mg/d) often recommended, but possible cardiotoxicity makes it a second choice. Akathisia must be watched for, as it can exacerbate tics.

Clonidine (Catapres) (0.1–1.0 mg/d, in 2 divided doses) somewhat less effective than neuroleptics.

Clonazepam (Klonopin) (0.75–4.0 mg/d, in 2 divided doses) also somewhat less effective than neuroleptics, and poses risk of abuse.

2.17 ENCOPRESIS (FUNCTIONAL ENCOPRESIS)

J Pediatr 1986;108:562. Pediatr Clin North Am 1982;29:315. Pediatrics 1987;80:672.

Epidem: Among children aged 5–12 yr, 1%–1.5%; male-female ratio 4–5:1.

Sx: Normal bowel function with continence generally established before the age of 5 yr; defecation on clothing, in bed, or other places after that is considered pathologic. This continued inappropriate defecation may be "primary" in pts in whom continence was never established, or "secondary" in those in whom bowel function was, for a significant time, normal.

These children are typically constipated, at times impacted, and the soiling represents "overflow incontinence," generally with loose or diarrheal stool (occasionally the stool, rather than being loose, may be well formed). Typically, the soiling is involuntary and a source of great embarrassment; there is controversy, as noted below, as to whether voluntary soiling should be subsumed under the rubric of encopresis.

Lab: NC.

Crs: Frequency of soiling gradually decreases with age, and it is rare to find encopresis in teenagers.

Cmplc: Pts generally experience intense embarrassment and shame, and family conflict over the soiling may be severe.

Etiol: Initial constipation may follow upon anxiety, an acute stress, a change in diet with less fiber, travel with irregular toilet times, or an illness associated with fever or dehydration. Anxiety about defecation may simply follow the constipation, or if there had been a painful bowel movement, may stem from fear of having another one. In any case, when these children experience the urge to have a bowel movement, the anal sphincter, rather than undergoing relaxation, tightens. A vicious cycle then begins with ever-worsening constipation and overflow incontinence.

Ddx: Voluntary soiling, as may be seen in some defiant or oppositional children, is included by some authors under the rubric of encopresis. As these children are generally neither constipated nor subject to overflow incontinence, and as the behavior is quite intentional (with passage of feces in prominent places, often accompanied by smearing of walls or furniture), this seems inappropriate.

Other causes of chronic constipation must be ruled out and include various medications (e.g., antihistamines, anticholinergics), hypothyroidism, partial rectal stenosis, and Hirschsprung's disease.

Occasional soiling past the age of 5 is not abnormal; it is only when the soiling occurs repeatedly, at a frequency of at least once a month, that it is considered pathologic.

Rx: Both the child and parents are educated about the underlying vicious cycle. Catharsis is ensured (with digital disimpaction, if required; otherwise laxatives may be utilized, using the mildest one that is effective), and the child is then placed on a behavioral program to prevent further constipation. Regular toileting times are established, usually 15–20 min after meals (to take advantage of the gastrocolic reflex), and children are rewarded for bowel movements in the toilet (a simple "star chart" may suffice; for others money or small toys may be helpful); children are also expected to place soiled sheets or clothing into the proper hamper (expecting children to actually clean the feces off may be counterproductive). In addition to this behavior program, children should have a high-bran cereal every day, with, in resistant cases, a stool softener (preferably, if the child can swallow it, in capsule form). Once normal bowel function has been established for perhaps a month, the behavioral program may be discontinued; it may be prudent to continue the high-bran diet.

The above approach is effective ~85% of the time; in resistant cases, after confirming the dx, family therapy may be helpful.

2.18 ENURESIS (NOT DUE TO A GENERAL MEDICAL CONDITION, FUNCTIONAL ENURESIS)

Am J Psychiatry 1978;135:1549. Arch Dis Child 1974;49:259. Arch Dis Child 1992;67:182.

Epidem: Prevalence falls with age: at 5 yr, 7% of males and 3% of females; at 10 yr, 3% of males and 2% of females.

Sx: Nighttime dryness usually established by age 5. In most pts with functional enuresis, dryness is simply never established ("primary" enuresis); in a minority (~20%), dryness may be established and persist for a year or more before bed-wetting begins.

Bed-wetting usually occurs in the first third of the night, generally during NREM sleep, and children either sleep through it or awaken shortly after the wetting begins. Bed-wetting may or may not be associated with dreams, which in turn may or may not be about urination.

Lab: NC.

Crs: Spontaneous remission is the rule, with enuresis persisting into late adolescence in only ~1% of pts.

Cmplc: Shame and embarrassment may be intense, and there may be considerable conflict between parents and child.

Etiol: Clearly familial; *not* associated with any particular style of toilet training. Developmental delays are seen in a small minority, and a small percentage of pts will have reduced nocturnal vasopressin secretion.

Ddx: Causes of bed-wetting due to a general medical condition are listed in Table 2.18-1. Dysuria, dribbling, and true polyuria should prompt a thorough investigation; in most cases it is prudent to obtain a screening U/A.

EARLY ONSET DISORDERS

Table 2.18-1. Causes of Bed-wetting due to a General Medical Condition

Urinary Tract Infections

Associated with Polyuria

Diabetes mellitus
Diabetes insipidus

Anatomic Lesions

Bladder outlet obstruction
Urethral valves
Meatal stenosis

Spastic Bladder

Cerebral palsy
Spina bifida

Nocturnal Seizures

Pressure on Bladder

Pelvic masses
Impacted stool (as in encopresis)

Sedating Bedtime Medications

Some authors include daytime, or diurnal, wetting under the rubric of functional enuresis; however, given that these events are generally intentional and found in oppositional or defiant children, this appears inappropriate.

Rx: Behavioral programs generally successful; should they fail, imipramine (Tofranil) or desmopressin (DDAVP) may be tried.

Fluids, except for small amounts for tooth brushing, and ice chips for thirst, are restricted for 1 h or more before bedtime, and the child is asked to urinate just before bedtime. Caffeinated foods and beverages are prohibited. A rubber undersheet is placed on the bed.

Initial behavioral program involves rewarding dry nights with a "star" on a "star chart" coupled with a small amount of money or an appropriate toy. Should the child wet the bed, he or she is expected to strip the sheets and place them in an appropriate hamper, but is not required to wash them. Many children become dry within a month with this program.

A second behavior program, should the initial one fail, involves using an enuresis alarm. These devices sound a bell or buzzer when the sheets are moistened and are effective in up to 85% of children within the first month.

The effective behavior program should be continued for ~3 mo of continuous continence, after which it may be discontinued; should relapse occur, the program is reinstituted, and this may have to be repeated 2 or 3 times before dryness becomes permanent.

Imipramine (Tofranil) is started at about 25 mg hs, and increased at appropriate intervals in 10- or 25-mg increments until dryness or limiting SEs occur, or a maximum dose of ~2.5 mg/kg is reached. The interval between dose increases is set with regard to the frequency of bed-wetting, allowing enough time to see whether or not the dose is effective. It appears that a trough level of 60–80 ng/mL may be required; however, this should only be a rough guide as some children respond at lower levels, and some require much higher levels. If successful, imipramine (Tofranil) should be continued for ~3 mo of continuous dryness, then tapered at about one-third the dose every month, with reinstitution of the previous effective dose if bed-wetting recurs. If bed-wetting recurs after discontinuation, repeat course of treatment may be required before permanent dryness is achieved.

DDAVP, 20–40 mcg hs, by nasal insufflation, is an alternative to imipramine (Tofranil). If effective, it should be continued for ~3 mo of continuous dryness, then discontinued. Recurrences are common, and repeat courses of treatment are the rule. Very rarely, seizures secondary to hyponatremia occur.

Medications work better when combined with a behavioral program.

2.19 SEPARATION ANXIETY DISORDER

Arch Gen Psychiatry 1971;25:204. J Am Acad Child Psychiatry 1986; 25:235. J Am Acad Child Adolesc Psychiatry 1992;31:21.

Epidem: ~4% of school-age children; male-female ratio 1:2–3.
Sx: Onset typically around the age of 6 or 7 yr.

Sx appear upon separation, or the threat of separation, from parents; examples include going to school, or parents going out for the night, and pts may refuse to go to school or insist that parents stay at home. Anxiety may be extreme, and pts may complain of headaches or stomachaches. Sometimes parents simply going to bed may precipitate anxiety, and pts may insist on sleeping with parents, or if refused, may sleep on the floor outside the parental bedroom door.

Pts may be preoccupied with thoughts of loss, danger, or disease, and may have frequent nightmares.

Depressive episodes, as in major depression, are not uncommon.

Lab: NC.

Crs: Sx wax and wane for months or years, but the overall prognosis is good, with spontaneous remission in the vast majority before the end of adolescence.

Cmplc: Absenteeism may lead to academic failure.

Etiol: Familial, but the nature of the familial association is unclear. It does appear that in a substantial minority of pts, separation anxiety disorder is succeeded, in adult years, by panic disorder.

Ddx: Separation anxiety is developmentally normal between ages 8 and 24 mo.

Parental overprotectiveness throughout early childhood may convince children of their inadequacy and leave them anxious over facing any challenge, esp going away to school.

Normal anxiety about going to school may occur in the face of bullying schoolmates or angry teachers.

Panic disorder with agoraphobia is distinguished by the reason behind the school refusal. In panic disorder it is the fear of having an attack, whereas in separation anxiety disorder it is the fear of being separated from parents.

Schizophrenia and autism may be characterized by extreme anxiety upon the departure of parents; however, the other sx of these disorders make the dx.

Haloperidol (Haldol), pimozide (Orap), or propranolol (Inderal) may cause a syndrome similar to separation anxiety disorder.

Rx: Behavior therapy (rewarding progressively longer stays at school) in conjunction with family counseling (esp focusing on any overprotectiveness) is often helpful; if much school has been missed, remedial work at home may be required.

Imipramine (Tofranil) has been found helpful in some studies, but not others. Dosage should probably not exceed 3 mg/kg/d; if effective, continue treatment until pt is asymptomatic for at least 1 mo, then taper gradually over 3 mo until discontinued or until sx reappear, at which point the dose may be increased to the lowest effective dose.

2.20 SELECTIVE MUTISM (ELECTIVE MUTISM)

Acta Psychiatr Scand 1979;59:218. J Am Acad Child Adolesc Psychiatry 1994;33:1000. J Am Acad Child Adolesc Psychiatry 1995;34:836.

Epidem: ~0.04% of school-age children.

Sx: Onset between ages of 3 and 8; may be either insidious or, after an acute emotional trauma, acute.

Although pts speak when alone with family members or close friends, they become mute when others appear, or when at school. Shyness and timidity are common.

Lab: NC.

Crs: Within a few months, most pts begin to speak at school or when strangers are around; rarely the selective muteness persists for years.

Cmplc: School refusal, or a lack of participation in classroom activities may lead to academic failure.

Etiol: Temperamental shyness or maternal overprotectiveness may play a role.

Ddx: ~1% of children will keep quiet during the first month or so of school, after which they engage in normal conversation.

Expressive language disorder is distinguished by inability to speak not only at school or with strangers but also when at home or with friends.

Immigrant children, not yet bilingual, may keep quiet at school, but are able to speak with strangers, provided the strangers can speak the children's native tongue.

Rx: Behavior therapy is generally successful; in some pts, fluoxetine (Prozac) may help.

EARLY ONSET DISORDERS

2.21 REACTIVE ATTACHMENT DISORDER OF INFANCY OR EARLY CHILDHOOD

J Am Acad Child Psychiatry 1972;11:440. J Am Acad Child Psychiatry 1984;22:322. Pediatrics 1984;73:348.

Epidem: Uncertain; probably uncommon.

Sx: Onset in the first few years of life.

As a result of severe abuse or neglect, or of institutionalization in an emotionally sterile environment, pts develop characteristic disturbances in their relations to others.

Infants fail to smile, make eye contact, or follow others with their eyes; if picked up, they fail to reach out and grasp.

Young children are apathetic and listless, and show little interest in the environment.

Children display 1 of 2 characteristic disturbances in their relations with others: either inhibited or disinhibited. The inhibited child remains withdrawn, vigilant, and watchful, and very ambivalent about forming any relationships. The disinhibited child is indiscriminate in forming relationships, and may relate to strangers the same as familiar persons.

Lab: In infants who fail to eat, findings consistent with malnutrition are seen.

Crs: Infants may die from malnutrition; those who survive have chronic difficulty in forming relationships.

Cmplc: An inability to form normal relationships predicts failure in marriage and in any occupation that requires interpersonal contact.

Etiol: Presumably, the normal development and elaboration of relational behaviors require the consistent presence of "good enough" parents, and that without this "stage," these normal relational behaviors never develop.

Ddx: Autism and severe MR are distinguished, in general, by the absence of a h/o severe abuse or neglect; in addition, in autism there may be a lively "relationship" with inanimate objects.

In infants and young children, other causes of failure to thrive must be sought.

Rx: Provision of consistent nurturing adults, if done early enough, is followed by substantial improvement; hospitalization and foster placement are often necessary.

3. Delirium, Dementia, and Related Disorders

3.1 DELIRIUM

JAMA 1987;258:1789. NEJM 1989;320:578. Psychosomatics 1994;35: 374.

Epidem: ~10% of all patients on a general medical-surgery ward; among elderly medical-surgery pts, ~40%.

Sx: Onset generally acute, over hours to days; occasionally sudden (e.g., stroke) or paroxysmal (e.g., complex partial seizure).

Hallmarks are confusions and short-term memory loss.

Confusion ("clouding of sensorium") leaves pts inattentive and unclear about surroundings; digit span ability is reduced.

Short-term memory loss evident in inability to recall 3 of 3 objects after 5 min. Some are unable to even remember being asked to remember. Unable to keep track, pts are often disoriented to time and place.

Circumstantiality and tangentiality are common; incoherence may occur. Hallucinations (visual > auditory) and delusions (often persecutory) are common.

Typically either agitated, or "quiet" and underactive.

Sx typically fluctuate, often worse at night ("sundowning"). Some patients are remarkably "clear" in morning.

Lab: See below, under Etiol.

Crs: Determined by underlying etiology.

Cmplc: "Quiet" deliria may have few direct complications; agitated, or "noisy" delirious pts may refuse care, attempt to escape, pull out lines, etc.

Etiol: See Table 3.1-1: narrow differential accordingly.

Table 3.1-1. Etiologies of Delirium

I. Clear Precipitating Factors

Subdural hematoma
Carbon monoxide poisoning
Dialysis dysequilibrium syndrome
Central pontine myelinolysis (CPM), associated with rapid correction of hyponatremia
Delayed postanoxic delirium

II. Medications

Anticholinergics
Neuroleptics (neuroleptic malignant syndrome, see 15.6)
Serotoninergic drugs (serotonin syndrome, see 15.8)
Dopaminergic drugs (levodopa-carbidopa (Sinemet), bromocriptine (Parlodel), amantadine (Symmetrel))
Others (digoxin (Lanoxin), quinidine, various beta-blockers, prednisone, theophylline, bismuth, podophyllin, baclofen (Lioresal), meperidine (Demerol), lithium (Eskalith, Lithobid), disulfiram (Antabuse))

III. Intoxication and Withdrawal

Methanol intoxication
Cannabis intoxication, when severe (see 4.9)
Phencyclidine intoxication, when severe (see 4.14)
Amphetamine or cocaine intoxication, when severe (see 4.7)
Alcohol or sedative-hypnotic withdrawal (DTs, see 4.4)

IV. Metabolic

Hyperglycemia (thirst, polyuria; glucose 300–600 mg/dL in diabetic ketoacidosis, 600–2000 in nonketotic hyperglycemia)
Hypoglycemia (tremor; glucose <45 mg/dL)
Hypernatremia (Na >160 mEq/L if acute, >170 if gradual)
Hyponatremia (asterixis and myoclonus; Na <120 mEq/L if acute, <110 if chronic)
Hypokalemia (hyporeflexia; K <2.5 mEq/L)
Hypermagnesemia (hyporeflexia; Mg >5 mEq/L)
Hypomagnesemia (myoclonus; Mg <1 mEq/L)
Hypercalcemia (nausea, vomiting, abdominal pain, constipation; Ca >14 mg/dL)
Uremia (asterixis, myoclonus; BUN >100 mg/dL if acute, >200 if chronic)
Hepatic encephalopathy (asterixis; NH_3 >55 mcg/dL: caution, NH_3 may be normal!)
Respiratory failure (asterixis if hypercarbic; PaO_2 <50 mm Hg; PCO_2 >70 mm Hg if acute, >90 if chronic)

V. Encephalitis (MRI, LP)

Viral (e.g., herpes simplex encephalitis)
Bacterial
Postencephalitic

VI. Malnourished Patients (esp Alcoholics)

Wernicke's encephalopathy (nystagmus and ataxia, see 4.6)
Encephalopathic pellagra (rigidity and dysarthria; urine N-methylniacinamide)
Marchiafava-Bignami disease (partial seizures, various focal signs; MRI)

Table 3.1-1. *(Continued)*

VII. AIDS and Other Immunocompromised States (HIV, MRI)

AIDS encephalopathy
TB
Mycoses
Toxoplasmosis
Cytomegalovirus
Progressive multifocal leukoencephalopathy

VIII. Dementing Diseases

Multi-infarct dementia (see 3.4)
Diffuse Lewy body disease (see 3.10)
Alzheimer's disease (see 3.3)

IX. Paroxysmal Onset

Complex partial seizure (EEG, MRI)
Postictal confusion (after complex partial or grand mal seizure)
Petit mal seizure (EEG)
Confusional migraine

X. Specific Clinical Features

Cushing's syndrome (cushingoid habitus with moon facies, "buffalo hump," hirsu-
    tism, hypertension; elevated cortisol levels)
Adrenocortical insufficiency (nausea, vomiting, abdominal pain, constipation or diar-
    rhea, postural dizziness, hypotension; low cortisol levels)
Thyroid storm (tremor, tachycardia, proptosis; increased T7)
Febrile delirium (temperature >105–106°F)
Hypertensive encephalopathy (diastolic >120–140 mm Hg)
Sepsis (fever, tachycardia, tachypnea, leukocytosis)
Rheumatoid arthritis (small joint arthritis; +RF)
Sydenham's chorea (chorea)
Hepatic porphyria (abdominal pain, motor polyneuropathy; increased serum delta-
    aminolevulinic acid)
Pancreatitis (abdominal pain; elevated lipase and amylase)
Systemic lupus erythematosus (constitutional sx, pleurisy, rash, arthritis; +ANA)
Periarteritis nodosa (constitutional sx, rash; leukocytosis, elevated ESR)
Behçet's syndrome (oral or genital ulcers; MRI)

XI. Miscellaneous

Stroke (esp right temporoparietal area; MRI)
Acute hydrocephalus (MRI)
MS (MRI, LP)
Paraneoplastic limbic encephalitis (MRI, antineuronal antibodies)
Hashimoto's encephalopathy (antithyroid antibodies)
Granulomatous angiitis (headache; MRI)
Thrombotic thrombocytopenic purpura (fever, fluctuating sx; thrombocytopenia)
Metal poisoning—lead, thallium, arsenic (nausea, vomiting, abdominal pain; appro-
    priate blood, serum, or urine levels)

I. Clear precipitating factors (e.g., head trauma) readily identifiable.

II. Medications a common cause: Suspect any medication when there is a temporal correlation between starting medicine (or increasing dose) and onset of delirium.

III. Intoxication with illicit substances also a common cause; consider also withdrawal from certain substances (e.g., alcoholic "DTs").

IV. Metabolic etiology very common; asterixis or myoclonus are clues.

V. Encephalitis suggested by headache, fever, or seizures. Always consider herpes simplex, as it is treatable.

VI. Malnourished patients (e.g., alcoholics) prone to thiamine (Wernicke's encephalopathy) or niacin (encephalopathic pellagra) deficiencies.

VII. AIDS deliria may be caused by AIDS encephalopathy or by opportunistic infection.

VIII. Dementing illnesses may be "punctuated" by delirium (e.g., in multi-infarct dementia where each fresh stroke presents with a delirium, which, upon resolution, leaves pt 1 "step" lower into the dementia).

IX. Paroxysmal onset suggestive of a complex partial seizure; "confusional migraine" rare and suggested by severe headache.

X. Specific features ("cushingoid" habitus) immediately suggestive of certain causes.

XI. Miscellaneous causes.

When ddx cannot be narrowed after hx and PE, consider the laboratory "screen" in Table 3.1-2: This will "catch" >90% of causes.

Note that a delirium may have multiple causes (e.g., in an alcoholic, head trauma (subdural hematoma), DTs, and Wernicke's encephalopathy).

Ddx: Dementia is distinguished by the absence of confusion.

Rx: Treat underlying cause.

Environmental measures help pt "stay in touch": large calendars; large digital clocks; familiar items (e.g., family photos); call button in easy reach; a view from a window (critical!); night-lights.

Agitated pts may be given haloperidol (Haldol) 2.5 mg, either q 2 h po, or qh im, until pt is calm, unacceptable SEs occur, or maxi-

Table 3.1-2. Laboratory Screen for Delirium

Na	NH_3
K	Toxicology (serum and urine)
Glucose	CBC
BUN	MRI
Ca	EEG (if paroxysmal onset)
Mg	LP (if encephalitis suspected)
Liver enzymes	ABGs (if respiratory failure suspected)
Bilirubin	

mum dose of 20 mg (higher doses allowed in the young with intact hepatic function) is reached.

1:1 nursing care may be required; leather restraints are at times life-saving.

3.2 DEMENTIA

Acta Neurol Scand 1996;93(Suppl 165):92. Acta Neurol Scand 1996; 94(Suppl 168):39. Am J Psychiatry 1997;154(May Suppl):1. J Clin Psychiatry 1994;55(Suppl 2):13. J Neurol Neurosurg Psychiatry 1994;57:1451. Neurology 1995;45:211.

Epidem: Prevalence rises with age; ~10% >60, ~30% >80 yr.

Sx: Onset ranges from insidious (e.g., Alzheimer's) to acute (e.g., large stroke).

Global decrement in intellectual functioning (decreased memory, abstracting, and calculating abilities), occurring in a "clear sensorium" *without* confusion.

Memory defect is primarily anterograde, with relatively less of a retrograde component. Anterograde defect is evident in inability to recall 3 of 3 words after 5 min, tendency to forget things said or done minutes earlier (often "losing" things); retrograde defect increases as dementia progresses and pts are unable to recall events progressively further in past (job, children, marriage, schooling).

Abstracting defect formally tested with proverbs testing ("People in glass houses shouldn't throw stones."). Demented pts are often concrete ("might break the glass") rather than abstract ("everyone has their faults"). In day-to-day life pts have difficulty mastering new and complex situations.

Calculating ability formally tested with "serial 7s" ("subtract 7 from 100, then subtract 7 from *that* number, and keep on going as far as you can"), keeping in mind whether pt ever learned to subtract. In day-to-day life, this defect may leave pts agitated at check-out counters when they find they've totaled their purchases incorrectly.

Clear sensorium present most of the time in all pts. Exceptions include late Alzheimer's disease (when confusion may become chronic), diffuse Lewy body disease (where episodes of confusion may occur early), and multi-infarct dementia (where each new stroke may be heralded by a temporary confusion).

In addition to global decrement in intellectual functioning, most pts, at some point, also have associated features, such as a personality change, mood changes (usually depression), agitation, and delusions and hallucinations. PE may reveal important associated findings, such as parkinsonism, chorea, "focal" signs (e.g., aphasia, apraxia), etc.

Lab: As for the underlying etiology.

Crs: Determined by underlying cause: Some are progressive (e.g., Alzheimer's); some static (e.g., dementia due to head trauma); some potentially reversible (e.g., B_{12} deficiency).

Cmplc: Inability to work, wandering away; in advanced cases, falls, decubiti, dehydration, etc.

Etiol: See Table 3.2-l; proceed with ddx according to associated features.

If, after hx and PE, ddx cannot be reasonably narrowed, consider a laboratory screen, as in Table 3.2-2. *First screen* items are divided into routine ones, and those indicated only by clinical suspicion; *second screen* items are more or less invasive and should only be used if clinical situation warrants.

Ddx: Amnestic syndromes (see 3.16) are distinguished by lack of global intellectual decrement. Note, however, that some dementing diseases (e.g., Alzheimer's) may present with amnesia.

Delirium is distinguished by presence of "clouding of sensorium" and confusion. Note, however, that some dementias may at times cause confusion, which can be chronic (e.g., late in Alzheimer's) or episodic (e.g., with each fresh stroke in multi-infarct dementia or early in diffuse Lewy body disease).

MR is distinguished by the course. In MR, cognitive development pro-

Table 3.2-1. Etiologies of Dementia

I. Associated with Gradual Onset and Slow Progression

Alzheimer's disease (see 3.3) (MRI)
Binswanger's disease (see 3.6) (MRI)
NPH (ataxia and urinary incontinence; MRI)
Hypothyroidism (myxedematous appearance; thyroid profile)
Neurosyphilis (general paresis of the insane, "GPI") (FTA, note serum VDRL often *normal;* MRI, LP)
Lyme disease (h/o arthritis; MRI, anti-*Borrelia* antibodies)

II. Associated with Parkinsonism

Parkinson's disease (see 3.9)
Diffuse Lewy body disease (see 3.10) (MRI)
Arteriosclerotic parkinsonism (focal deficits; MRI)
Progressive supranuclear palsy (vertical gaze palsy, falls, axial extension; MRI)
Striatonigral variant of MSA (mild ataxia, mild signs of autonomic failure such as impotence, orthostatic dizziness, incontinence; MRI)
Dementia pugilistica (distant h/o repeated head trauma, ataxia; MRI)

III. Associated with Chorea

Huntington's disease (see 3.11) (MRI, genetic testing)
Neuroacanthocytosis (lip biting; 3 "wet preps" for acanthocytes, elevated CPK)
Acquired hepatocerebral degeneration (h/o severe or recurrent hepatic encephalopathy)

IV. Associated with Strokes

Multi-infarct dementia (see 3.4) (MRI)
Lacunar dementia (see 3.5) (MRI)
Cerebral amyloid angiopathy (MRI)

V. Associated with the Frontal Lobe Syndrome (see 3.21)

Pick's disease (see 3.12)
Frontotemporal degeneration (MRI)

VI. Associated with Head Trauma

Dementia due to head trauma (see 3.8)

VII. Associated with Substance Dependence

Alcoholic dementia (see 3.14)
Inhalant-induced dementia (see 3.15)

VIII. Associated with AIDS and Other Immunocompromised States

AIDS dementia (see 3.7) (HIV, MRI)
Opportunistic infections (progressive multifocal leukoencephalopathy, cytomegalovirus encephalitis, toxoplasmosis, mycoses) (MRI)

Table 3.2-1. *(Continued)*

IX. Miscellaneous

Creutzfeldt-Jakob disease (see 3.13) (myoclonus; EEG, MRI, LP (14-3-3 protein))

Brain tumors (MRI)

B_{12} deficiency (macrocytic anemia (caution: may *not* be present), B_{12} level, serum methylmalonic acid and homocysteine levels)

Folate deficiency (RBC folate level; *always* check for concurrent B_{12} deficiency)

Systemic lupus erythematosus (constitutional sx, pleurisy, arthritis; ANA)

MS (MRI, LP)

Wilson's disease (personality change, unusual tremor or chorea, Kayser-Fleischer ring; copper and ceruloplasmin levels)

Postanoxic dementia (MRI)

Postencephalitic dementia (MRI)

Paraneoplastic limbic encephalitis (antineuronal antibodies, MRI)

Subacute sclerosing panencephalitis (myoclonus; EEG, MRI)

Metachromatic leukodystrophy (leukocyte arylsulfatase A level)

Adrenoleukodystrophy (MRI, very-long-chain fatty acid level)

Metal poisoning (arsenic and thallium (often associated with hair loss and polyneuropathy), mercury, lead, manganese; appropriate blood, serum, or urine levels)

Granulomatous angiitis (headache; MRI, angiography, biopsy)

---

ceeds only to a certain point, then "plateaus" or "stalls out" to remain at that level indefinitely; in dementia, however, rather than a "stalling out" there is a definite *decrement* in intellectual functioning.

Depressive episodes, as may be seen in major depression (see 6.1) or bipolar disorder (see 6.6), may at times be dominated by difficulty with concentration and memory to the point where pts become disoriented and unable to do simple calculations or understand proverbs. Dx suggested by a h/o prior episodes of depression and by the dependence of incorrect answers on a tendency to "give up" trying rather than on an absolute inability to answer the question. Often referred to as "pseudodementia" or "dementia syndrome of depression."

Rx: Treat the underlying cause, if possible.

Environmental measures: Maintain familiar surroundings and routines; night-lights, large calendars, large digital clocks, and for wanderers, locked doors and windows. If hospitalized or institutionalized, maintain these measures; also ensure a window with a view (critical!). Financial management should be assumed by others; guardianship may be required.

Table 3.2-2. Laboratory Screen for Dementia

First Screen

Routine:
  MRI
  Thyroid profile
  FTA
  HIV
  EEG
  B$_{12}$ level
  RBC folate level
  ANA
  CBC
  Chem survey
If indicated by clinical suspicion:
  Anti-*Borrelia* antibodies
  Genetic testing for Huntington's disease
  "Wet prep" for acanthocytes
  Copper and ceruloplasmin levels
  Antineuronal antibodies
  Leukocyte arylsulfatase A level
  Very-long-chain fatty acid level
  Metal levels

Second Screen

LP
Angiography
Biopsy

Depression may be treated with antidepressants (e.g., an SSRI such as citalopram (Celexa) 20 mg or a TCA such as nortriptyline (Pamelor) 25–75 mg).

Agitation, if part of depression, treated as above. If not, consider low-dose carbamazepine (Tegretol) (50–200 mg) or a low-potency phenothiazine neuroleptic (e.g., thioridazine (Mellaril) 50–200 mg).

Delusions or hallucinations may be treated with low-dose neuroleptic (e.g., olanzapine (Zyprexa) 5–10 mg, risperidone (Risperdal) 2–6 mg, haloperidol (Haldol) 2.5–5 mg).

Insomnia treated with lorazepam (Ativan) 1–2 mg hs (but, prevent daytime naps!).

3.3 ALZHEIMER'S DISEASE

Arch Neurol 1988;45:1182. Neurology 1996;46:130. Neurology 1997; 48(Suppl 6):2. Neurology 1997;48(Suppl 6):17. Neurology 1998;50: 136. Neurology 1998;50(Suppl 1)2.

Epidem: 5% of those >56 yr; ~20% of those >80 yr.

Sx: Onset gradual and generally >50 yr; typically with either amnesia or personality change; rarely presents with a progressive aphasia.

Amnesia initially primarily anterograde: Pts forget where they put things or what happened earlier in the day; disorientation to time and place common. Retrograde amnesia worsens with progression of disease: Pts forget where they worked, then the names of children, whom they married, where schooled, etc.

Personality change: apathy or coarsening of behavior; elements of a frontal lobe syndrome (see 3.21) may appear.

Global cognitive deficits (see 3.2) eventually appear.

Associated sx include depression (in approximately one-fourth), hallucinations (visual > auditory), and delusions (persecutory most common; "phantom boarder" also occurs).

Most patients eventually gradually develop focal signs such as aphasia and apraxia. Mild parkinsonism may occur, and myoclonus and seizures are seen in a minority.

Lab: MRI reveals widespread cortical atrophy, generally most prominent in temporal and parietal lobes.

Apolipoprotein E (ApoE) genotyping (see below) lacks specificity and is not recommended for dx purposes.

Crs: Progressive, with death within 5–7 yr from intercurrent illness.

Cmplc: See 3.2.

Etiol: Senile plaques and neurofibrillary tangles throughout cortex, also present in some subcortical structures, esp the nucleus basalis of Meynert (nbM). The nbM is the principal source of cholinergic innervation to the cortex, and cell loss there correlates well with degree of amnesia.

Approximately 20% of cases are clearly familial, with mutations on chromosomes 14, 19, and 21. In remainder there is strong association with presence of ApoE epsilon 4 allele.

Ddx: See 3.2.

Binswanger's disease (see 3.6) is suggested by early appearance of focal deficits and by widespread leukoencephalopathy on MRI.

Normal-pressure hydrocephalus (NPH) is suggested by early ataxic-apraxic gait and urinary incontinence.

Rx: For general Rx of dementia, see 3.2.

Estrogen replacement in females and daily NSAID for both sexes may prevent or forestall onset.

Vitamin E or selegiline may retard progression of disease.

Donepezil (Aricept) (5 mg hs, increased to 10 mg hs if no or minimal response at 6 wk) may improve memory in mild to moderate disease, but does not slow progression of disease. If donepezil (Aricept) fails, consider tacrine (Cognex) (not first choice, given hepatotoxicity).

Depression and psychotic symptoms may be treated as in 3.2.

Avoid medications with anticholinergic activity as they may worsen memory.

3.4 MULTI-INFARCT DEMENTIA

Acta Neurol Scand 1989;73:292. J Neurol Neurosurg Psychiatry 1988; 51:1037. Lancet 1974;2:207.

Epidem: Probably third most common cause of dementia, after Alzheimer's disease and diffuse Lewy body disease.

Sx: Onset of first stroke generally in 50s or 60s.

Fully developed clinical picture characterized by global cognitive deficit (see 3.2), depression and lability, and numerous focal signs, reflecting location of infarctions, such as hemiplegia, aphasia, apraxia, aprosodia, and in advanced cases, pseudobulbar palsy.

Lab: MRI reveals multiple cortical or subcortical lesions secondary to infarction or intracerebral hemorrhages.

Crs: Typically downhill in a "stepwise" fashion, with each fresh stroke bringing patient 1 "step" further down into dementia. Exceptions to stepwise course include multiple, closely spaced infarctions, as, e.g., in hypertensive encephalopathy.

In most pts, each fresh stroke is heralded by a delirium, which, upon clearing, reveals the pt to be 1 "step" further down.

Cmplc: See 3.2.

Etiol: Most due to arteriosclerosis; other causes include cerebral amyloid angiopathy, polyarteritis nodosa, vasculitis secondary to cocaine or amphetamines, cranial arteritis, systemic lupus erythematosus, meningovascular syphilis.

Ddx: See 3.2.

Rx: For general Rx of dementia, see 3.2.

Treat the underlying cause; if arteriosclerosis, aspirin 65 mg/d and dipyridamole (Persantine) 75 mg tid.

3.5 LACUNAR DEMENTIA

Arch Neurol 1987;44:1127. Arch Neurol 1990;47:129. Arch Neurol 1994;51:999. Neurology 1986;36:340.

Epidem: Uncommon.

Sx: Onset in 50s or 60s. Depending on size and location, each individual lacunar infarction may or may not bring pt to clinical attention. Eventually, with sufficient accumulation of lacunes, dementia appears.

In addition to global cognitive deficit (see 3.2), there are elements of a frontal lobe syndrome (see 3.21), and pseudobulbar palsy is not uncommon. Most pts also have one or more "lacunar" syndromes, e.g., pure motor hemiplegia, pure sensory stroke, ataxic hemiparesis, or dysarthria-clumsy hand syndrome.

Lab: MRI reveals multiple lacunes (usually >12) bilaterally in subcortical structures, such as thalamus, internal capsule, basal ganglia (note: CT may *miss* lacunes).

Crs: Typically progressive, either with "steps" (as described in 3.4) or more or less smoothly.

Cmplc: See 3.2.

Etiol: Multiple small cystic infarctions, or lacunes, occur in distribution of penetrating arterioles; most pts hypertensive.

Ddx: See 3.2.

Alzheimer's disease is distinguished by absence of lacunar syndromes, and by late appearance, if ever, of pseudobulbar palsy.

Multi-infarct dementia is distinguished by h/o major cortical strokes.

Rx: For general Rx of dementia, see 3.2.

In treating hypertension, avoid hypotension, as this may drop perfusion pressure below critical point in penetrating arterioles, leading to another lacunar infarction. Same caution applies when using neuroleptics or antidepressants.

Aspirin 65 mg qd is prudent.

3.6 BINSWANGER'S DISEASE (SUBCORTICAL ARTERIOSCLEROTIC ENCEPHALOPATHY)

Arch Neurol 1985;42:951. JAMA 1987;258:1782. J Neurol Neurosurg Psychiatry 1990;53:961. Neurology 1978;28:1206.

Epidem: Uncommon.

Sx: Onset gradual in 50s or 60s.

Pts are forgetful, inattentive, concrete, and often depressed. With progression, a global intellectual deficit (see 3.2) appears, often accompanied by focal signs such as aphasia and apraxia; pseudobulbar palsy may occur. Hallucinations (visual > auditory) and delusions, typically of persecution, are common, and agitation may occur.

Lab: MRI reveals widespread, often patchy, leukoencephalopathy in centrum semiovale.

Crs: Progressive over many years.

Cmplc: See 3.2.

Etiol: Widespread arteriolar lipohyalinosis accompanied by demyelinization, at times cystic. Most pts hypertensive, but disease has been seen in normotensive pts.

Ddx: For general ddx of dementia, see 3.2.

Alzheimer's disease is distinguished by late appearance of focal signs, and by absence of leukoencephalopathy on MRI.

MRI may be misleading: Symmetric periventricular hyperintensity on T2-weighted scans and ventricular "capping" are not uncommon in normal persons, and must be distinguished from the patchy, widespread leukoencephalopathy seen with Binswanger's.

Rx: For general treatment of dementia, see 3.2.

Aspirin 65 mg qd is prudent.

3.7 AIDS DEMENTIA

Ann Neurol 1992;32:321. Brain 1988;111:245. Neurology 1993;43: 2230. Q J Med 1992;82:223.

Epidem: >50% of AIDS pts eventually develop AIDS dementia.

Sx: Onset insidious, generally several years after HIV infection; most pts already have other sx of AIDS (thrush, *Pneumocystis carinii* pneumonia, Kaposi's sarcoma, etc.); in a small minority, dementia may be the presenting sx of AIDS.

When fully developed, apathy and psychomotor retardation are often more prominent than a global cognitive deficit (see 3.2); ataxia and long-tract signs may also be present.

Lab: HIV serology positive; MRI reveals cortical atrophy, ventricular dilatation, and widespread, patchy leukoencephalopathy. CSF analysis may reveal mononuclear pleocytosis and increased protein.

Crs: Rapidly progressive, with death in months to a year.

Cmplc: See 3.2.

Etiol: HIV crosses blood-brain barrier either directly or via a "Trojan horse" strategy, hiding within a peripheral monocyte, which, once inside the brain, transforms into a macrophage.

Multinucleated giant cells and microglial nodules widespread throughout brain; myelin pallor is diffuse, with, in some pts, vacuolization.

Ddx: For the general ddx of dementia, see 3.2.

Opportunistic infections: TB, progressive multifocal leukoencephalopathy, cytomegalovirus encephalitis, toxoplasmosis, mycoses.

Neurosyphilis may accompany AIDS; perform serum FTA.

B_{12} deficiency often present with AIDS dementia; measure B_{12} level, and if any doubt, serum methylmalonic acid and homocysteine levels.

Rx: For the general Rx of dementia, see 3.2. Should neuroleptics be required, use olanzapine (Zyprexa) or some other agent unlikely to cause parkinsonism, as these pts are particularly liable to these SEs.

Aggressive triple antiretroviral Rx is essential.

3.8 DEMENTIA DUE TO HEAD TRAUMA

Ann Neurol 1982;12:557. J Neurol Neurosurg Psychiatry 1956;19:163. J Neurol Neurosurg Psychiatry 1989;52:838.

Epidem: Most common in young males where it is associated with motor vehicle accidents.

Sx: Three common sequelae of head trauma: diffuse axonal injury (DAI), with or without "coup" and "contrecoup" injuries; subdural hematoma; and subarachnoid hemorrhage. All 3 may occur in same pt.

DAI occurs secondary to severe acceleration-deceleration, wherein the cranium comes to an abrupt halt (e.g., against a steering wheel). Coma is immediate, and if damage is severe, consciousness is not regained. If consciousness is regained, pts may emerge into a persistent vegetative state, or in less severe cases, be left with a dementia. In addition to a global intellectual deficit (see 3.2), there is often also a personality change characterized by irritability, moodiness, and at times, violent outbursts.

Subdural hematoma may be acute, subacute, or chronic. Acute subdural hematoma, secondary to brisk arterial bleeding, presents a neurosurgical emergency. Subacute and chronic subdural hematomas result from slower venous bleeding, and thus present later, within days to weeks for subacute cases, and months to years for chronic cases. Subacute subdural hematoma may present either with a delirium or with a dementia, and chronic subdural hematoma typically presents with a gradually developing dementia. Importantly, in the elderly, even *trivial* head trauma can cause a chronic subdural hematoma, and some elderly pts may not even recall the trauma.

Subarachnoid hemorrhage may be followed by vasospasm of multiple arteries, leading to a multi-infarct dementia.

Significant head trauma may also cause contusions, lacerations, or intracerebral hemorrhages.

Importantly, there is no correlation between the presence of a skull fracture and any of the above sequelae of head trauma.

Lab: MRI reveals subdural hematomas, infarcts, and intracerebral hemorrhages. In DAI, MRI reveals generalized cortical atrophy and ventricular dilatation; there may also be evidence of widespread petechial hemorrhages.

DELIRIUM, DEMENTIA, AND RELATED DISORDERS

Crs: With DAI there is typically some recovery over the first year, after which the condition is static.

Cmplc: For general complications of dementia, see 3.2.

Personality change often strains relations with others.

Etiol: With acceleration-deceleration, lengthy structures such as axons and arterioles undergo tremendous shearing and torsional strain with subsequent rupture or damage.

Ddx: If, after apparent stabilization, there is a significant worsening of dementia, consider the development of hydrocephalus.

Rx: For the general Rx of dementia, see 3.2.

Subdural hematomas may or may not require evacuation.

In DAI, violent outbursts may respond to high-dose propranolol (Inderal) (e.g., 240–480 mg/d). Irritability and moodiness may respond to an antidepressant, e.g., nortriptyline (Pamelor).

3.9 PARKINSON'S DISEASE

Acta Neurol Scand 1987;75:191. Acta Neurol Scand 1996;94:323. Am J Psychiatry 1992;149:443. Br J Psychiatry 1989;154:596. Neurology 1998;50(Suppl 1):33.

Epidem: Parkinson's disease has a prevalence of 0.25% in general population; approximately one-third eventually develop a dementia.

Sx: The dementia of Parkinson's disease does not appear until years after the motor signs of parkinsonism are well established.

Motor signs usually make an insidious appearance in the 50s or 60s, and include tremor, rigidity, and bradykinesia. Tremor is rhythmic, at a frequency of ~3 cps, and presents at rest; in the hands it produces the typical "pill-rolling" movements. Rigidity is generalized and of the cogwheel type. Bradykinesia represents a generalized slowness of movement (and thought), and its severity is not well correlated with severity of rigidity.

Dementia is generally mild; importantly, focal signs such as aphasia or apraxia are generally absent.

Delusions (generally persecutory) and hallucinations (visual > auditory) often accompany dementia; visual hallucinations may also occur as a SE of dopaminergic treatment.

Depression may be seen in approximately one-fourth of all pts.

Panic attacks occur in a minority, typically during the "off" period when the prior dose of levodopa is losing effect and motor signs are worsening.

Lab: NC.

Crs: Progressive, with severe disability in ~15 yr.

Cmplc: For complications of dementia, see 3.2.

Motor signs eventually disable pt.

Etiol: Both environmental (e.g., exposure to well water) and genetic factors present.

Lewy bodies found in substantia nigra, and cell loss here correlates with severity of motor sx.

With dementia, Lewy bodies also found in nbM or scattered throughout cortex.

With depression, cell loss and Lewy bodies seen in dorsal raphe nucleus of the midbrain.

Ddx: Diffuse Lewy body disease (see 3.10) is distinguished by fact that dementia either *precedes* the onset of motor parkinsonian signs or occurs concurrent with them; furthermore, the motor signs are generally mild.

Arteriosclerotic parkinsonism is distinguished by focal deficits and a h/o strokes.

Progressive supranuclear palsy is distinguished by vertical gaze palsy, falls, and axial extension (in contrast to flexion posture seen in Parkinson's disease).

Striatonigral variant of multiple system atrophy (MSA) is distinguished by presence of mild ataxia and mild autonomic failure (impotence, orthostatic dizziness, incontinence).

Dementia pugilistica distinguished by h/o distant head traumas and presence of ataxia ("punch drunk").

Rx: Selegiline (Eldepryl), 10 mg/d, may retard the progression of the disease (*very* controversial).

Motor signs treated with levodopa-carbidopa (Sinemet). With progression, direct-acting dopaminergic agents (e.g., bromocriptine (Parlodel)) added to "smooth out" control of motor sx. When these fail, consideration may be given to tolcapone (Tasmar); however, hepatotoxicity makes this a "second line" agent.

For general Rx of dementia, see 3.2. If psychotic sx require treatment, use neuroleptics with lowest likelihood of causing parkinsonism, such as olanzapine (Zyprexa) 5–10 mg/d or clozapine

(Clozaril) 6.25–12.5 mg/d (interestingly, Rx with clozapine may also *reduce* severity of motor sx).

Depression responds to antidepressants. Bupropion (Wellbutrin) may cause confusion and dyskinesia and should not be used. SSRIs may worsen motor sx and should be used only with caution. TCAs (e.g., nortriptyline (Pamelor)) are useful; however, if selegiline (Eldepryl) is already in place and the dose is above 10 mg, caution is necessary. Selegiline (Eldepryl) at doses of 10 mg or less is a selective MAO-A inhibitor; however, at doses >10 mg it loses selectivity and also inhibits MAO-B, thus creating possibility of a hypertensive crisis if a TCA is added, or a potentially fatal serotonin syndrome (see 15.8) if SSRI is used concurrently.

ECT is effective for depression, and is also effective for the motor sx *regardless of whether pt is depressed or not.*

Panic attacks may be treated with antidepressants, with above cautions, or high-potency benzodiazepines, alprazolam (Xanax), or clonazepam (Klonopin) (see 7.1).

3.10 DIFFUSE LEWY BODY DISEASE (LEWY BODY DEMENTIA, SENILE DEMENTIA OF THE LEWY BODY TYPE, CORTICAL LEWY BODY DISEASE)

Br J Psychiatry 1994;165:324. Neurology 1996;47:1113. Neurology 1997;48:376.

Epidem: Probably common; autopsy studies suggest that after Alzheimer's disease, it is the second most common cause of dementia in the elderly.

Sx: Onset gradual in 60s or 70s.

Pts present with either dementia or a mild parkinsonism. Dementia, early on, is distinguished by brief episodes of confusion and by unexplained falls; hallucinations (visual ≫ auditory) and delusions (typically of persecution) are very common; and most pts display an unusual sensitivity to neuroleptics, developing severe parkinsonian SEs. With progression, a global intellectual deficit (see 3.2) appears, as do mild focal signs such as apraxia or aphasia.

Lab: MRI shows mild cortical atrophy and ventricular dilatation.

Crs: Rapid progression, with death generally in a few years.

Cmplc: See 3.2.

Etiol: Lewy bodies throughout the cortex and in the nbM and substantia nigra.

Ddx: See discussion of ddx for Parkinson's disease in 3.9.

Rx: For general Rx of dementia, see 3.2.

If neuroleptics are required for psychotic sx, consider olanzapine (Zyprexa) (5–10 mg/d) or low-potency phenothiazine (e.g., thioridazine (Mellaril), 25–100 mg); whether risks of Rx with clozapine (Clozaril) are justified by potential gains is not clear.

Motor parkinsonian sx are mild and generally do not require Rx with levodopa-carbidopa (Sinemet).

3.11 HUNTINGTON'S DISEASE (HUNTINGTON'S CHOREA)

Am J Psychiatry 1983;140:728. Arch Neurol 1993;50:1157; NEJM 1994;330:1401. Psychiatr Clin 1997;20:791.

Epidem: Lifetime prevalence among those of European descent 0.004%– 0.008%; less common in blacks and Japanese.

Sx: Onset gradual and insidious, generally in late 30s; may be with either chorea or dementia.

Dementia usually presents with a personality change characterized by a deterioration in personal care, poor judgment, irritability, and impulsivity, followed by a global intellectual deficit (see 3.2). Delusions (typically persecutory) and hallucinations (visual > auditory) are common; depression may occur but mania is rare.

Chorea typically presents with a certain clumsiness and restlessness; inexplicably dropping things is a common presentation. Unmistakable chorea generally first appears in the face (where it often involves the forehead) or upper extremities, eventually spreading to the lower extremities. Chorea characteristically jumps, lightning like, from one body part to another; lower-extremity involvement may create a "dancing and prancing" gait.

Eventually, all pts develop both dementia and chorea.

Lab: MRI may be normal early in course but eventually shows atrophy of heads of caudate nuclei.

Genetic testing reveals expanded trinucleotide repeat (CAG) on chromosome 4.

Crs: Progressive, with death from intercurrent disease in 10–30 yr.

Cmplc: See 3.2 for complications of dementia.

Chorea eventually is disabling; early on pts may be mistakenly arrested for public intoxication.

Etiol: Autosomal dominant inheritance; cell loss most prominent in caudate nucleus, but also present throughout cortex.

Ddx: Neuroacanthocytosis is distinguished by lip biting, confirmed by finding increased acanthocytes on 3 "wet preps."

Acquired hepatocerebral degeneration suggested by h/o severe or repeated episodes of hepatic encephalopathy; most often found in chronic alcoholics.

Wilson's disease indicated by Kayser-Fleischer rings and by distinctive copper and ceruloplasmin levels.

Tardive dyskinesia (see 15.7) distinguished by the repetitive, stereotyped nature of choreic movements, in contrast to the lightning-like, unpredictable changes seen in Huntington's disease; furthermore, tardive dyskinesia causes neither forehead chorea nor a "dancing and prancing" gait.

Rx: For general Rx of dementia, see 3.2.

Neuroleptics (haloperidol (Haldol) 2.5–10 mg, risperidone (Risperdal) 3–6 mg, olanzapine (Zyprexa) 5–10 mg) diminish severity of chorea and psychotic sx.

Depression, at times, may respond to a neuroleptic; otherwise use an antidepressant such as an SSRI or TCA (e.g., nortriptyline (Pamelor)). Bupropion (Wellbutrin) may worsen chorea and should not be used.

Mania may respond to a neuroleptic; if not, use a mood stabilizer, e.g., divalproex (Depakote).

3.12 PICK'S DISEASE

Ann Neurol 1984;16:467. Neurology 1981;31:1415. Neurology 1993; 43:289.

Epidem: Rare.

Sx: Onset insidious between ages 30 and 60 yr.

Most pts present with a personality change, often of the frontal lobe type (see 3.21); occasionally, elements of the Klüver-Bucy syndrome (see 3.22) occur. Rarely, pts present with amnesia or aphasia. Gradually, a global cognitive deficit (see 3.2) appears, which may be accompanied by an aphasia (typically expressive) or seizures.

Lab: MRI reveals cortical atrophy, most prominent in frontal and temporal lobes. Characteristically, the posterior portion of the superior temporal gyrus is spared.

Crs: Progressive with death from intercurrent disease in 3–10 yr.

Cmplc: See 3.2.

Etiol: In a minority, autosomal dominant inheritance is seen.

Lobar, "knifelike" atrophy is found; microscopically gliosis and neuronal loss are seen; remaining neurons often display characteristic Pick bodies.

Ddx: Alzheimer's disease may present with a frontal lobe syndrome, but rarely with a Klüver-Bucy syndrome; "lobar" atrophy is unusual on MRI in Alzheimer's disease.

Frontotemporal dementia is a poorly defined entity that, in fact, probably includes many pts with Pick's disease; there are, however, some pts with similar presentation to Pick's who lack the typical histopathologic changes of Pick's.

Rx: For the general Rx of dementia, see 3.2.

3.13 CREUTZFELDT-JAKOB DISEASE

Ann Neurol 1986;20:597. Ann Neurol 1994;35:513. Arch Neurol 1993; 50:1129. NEJM 1996;335:924.

Epidem: Yearly incidence of 5/1 000 000.

Sx: Onset gradual or subacute; age at onset varies by type of disease (inherited, transmitted, sporadic; see below).

Pts may present with either dementia or other sx, including myoclonus, parkinsonism, ataxia, cortical blindness or hemianopia, and pyramidal tract signs. Eventually all pts have both dementia and one or more of these other sx.

Dementia may be nonspecific, consisting only of a global intellectual deficit (see 3.2), or may be marked by a personality change or bizarre behavior.

Lab: CT or MRI may reveal progressive cortical atrophy.

EEG eventually abnormal in most, classically with periodic spike–slow wave complexes.

CSF may contain the "14-3-3" protein, which is generally found only in pts with Creutzfeldt-Jakob disease or in pts with *acute* neuronal injury (e.g., recent infarction).

Crs: Progressive, with death in months to a year.

Cmplc: See 3.2.

Etiol: Creutzfeldt-Jakob disease is the most common of the "prion" diseases. Prion proteins are naturally occurring cell membrane proteins; in prion diseases, the prion protein exists in an abnormal isoform that aggregates into the "prion." These prions are widespread, indeed systemic; microscopically, widespread neuronal loss and vacuolization, leading to a "spongiform" appearance of the cortex, are seen.

Inheritance accounts for ~15%, with onset in the 50s.

Transmissible cases appear after a latency of 10–25 yr after infection. Most cases are iatrogenic (corneal transplants, dura mater grafts, stereotaxic electrodes, human growth hormone); recent European cases ("bovine spongiform encephalopathy") raised specter of transmission to humans via infected beef products.

Sporadic cases may have onset anywhere from teenage years to the 80s, with most cases occurring in the 60s.

Ddx: For general ddx of dementia, see 3.2.

Early appearance of myoclonus is fairly distinctive.

Rx: For general Rx of dementia, see 3.2.

Prions are resistant to autoclaving and formalin; thus all contaminated items should be disposed of or washed in hypochlorite bleach. Pins and Wartenberg pinwheels used for sensory testing should *never* be used more than once.

3.14 ALCOHOLIC DEMENTIA (ALCOHOL-INDUCED PERSISTING DEMENTIA)

Alcoholism: Clin Exp Res 1994;18:1330. J Neurol Neurosurg Psychiatry 1985;48:211. Neurology 1981;31:377.

Epidem: Occurs in ~10% of all chronic alcoholics, and accounts for ~20% of all cases of dementia.

Sx: Onset occurs insidiously after many years or decades of chronic alcoholism.

Global intellectual deficit (see 3.2) is often accompanied by a personality change with coarsening and disinhibition; apathy may occur and judgment may be profoundly impaired. Occasionally there may be focal signs (e.g., aphasia or apraxia) of minor degree.

Lab: MRI shows generalized cortical atrophy and ventricular dilatation.

Crs: With continued drinking, progressive; with abstinence there is a gradual, but incomplete, improvement over perhaps a year, with a stable course thereafter.

Cmplc: As described in 3.2.

The dementia often precludes involvement in rehabilitative efforts, e.g., AA.

Etiol: Alcohol is a direct neurotoxin.

Ddx: Subdural hematoma usually is distinguished by prominent focal signs (e.g., hemiplegia); however, as focal signs may be minimal, and head trauma is so common in chronic alcoholics, MRI is always appropriate.

Acquired hepatocerebral degeneration is distinguished by chorea.

Rx: For the general Rx of dementia, see 3.2.

Abstinence is essential; adequate nutrition and vitamin supplementation (esp thiamine) are appropriate.

3.15 INHALANT-INDUCED DEMENTIA

Ann Neurol 1988;23:611. Neurology 1986;36:698. Neurology 1990;40:532.

Epidem: Precise figures not available; may not be rare.

Sx: Onset insidious after years of chronic inhalant use.

Pts develop apathy, dullness, and concrete thinking, all of which evolve into a global intellectual deficit (see 3.2). Cerebellar ataxia may be present.

Lab: MRI reveals global atrophy and widespread increased signal intensity in the centrum semiovale on T2-weighted scans.

Crs: With continued inhalant use, progressive; with abstinence, probably static.

Cmplc: See 3.2.

Etiol: Of the various hydrocarbons found in inhalants, toluene appears most toxic; pathologically there is widespread demyelinization.

Ddx: For a general discussion, see 3.2.

Alcoholic dementia, when accompanied by alcoholic cerebellar degeneration, may present a similar clinical picture, and the ddx rests on the h/o alcoholism.

Hypothyroidism may present with dementia and ataxia; however, it is distinguished by the presence of myxedematous changes, cold sensitivity, constipation, hair loss, etc.

Olivopontocerebellar degeneration may be hereditary or sporadic. Hereditary cases are suggested by fhx; sporadic cases occur as part of MSA and are generally accompanied by mild parkinsonism and mild autonomic failure (impotence, orthostatic dizziness, incontinence).

Rx: For general Rx of dementia, see 3.2.

Abstinence is essential.

3.16 AMNESTIC DISORDERS

Acta Neurol Scand 1974;50:133. Brain 1992;115:749. S Med J 1989;71: 1221.

Epidem: Some forms of amnesia such as "blackouts" (see 4.2) are very common, whereas others such as transient global amnesia (TGA) (see 3.18) are relatively rare.

Sx: Any given amnesia usually has 2 components, anterograde and retrograde, and usually the anterograde component is more prominent. In anterograde amnesia, pts are unable to "lay down" new memories; by contrast, retrograde amnesia pts are unable to recall events that they previously were able to remember.

Formal testing for amnesia involves checking "immediate," "short-term," and "long-term" memory. Immediate memory is checked with digit span, and is usually normal unless pts are confused. Short-term memory is checked by offering pts 3 words (e.g., "rock, car, and pencil"), asking them to memorize them, and then after 5 min, asking that they recall them. Normally, pts can recall

all 3. Long-term memory is checked by asking pts to recall significant events that occurred at successively more distant points in the past. These events either may be autobiographic (e.g., place of work, names of children, marriage, schooling) or involve notable public figures (e.g., names of the last 4 presidents). Normally pts have little trouble recalling such significant autobiographic or public events.

Formal testing reveals different results depending on the kind of amnesia. In chronic amnesias (e.g., Korsakoff's syndrome (see 3.17)), anterograde amnesia is always present, and the extent of retrograde amnesia is variable, with a "blanket" of amnesia covering months to decades of time before the amnesia began. In episodic amnesias (e.g., TGA (see 3.18)), the results are quite different depending on whether pts are tested while *in* the episode or *after* the episode has resolved. When pts are tested while in the episode, there is anterograde amnesia, accompanied by retrograde amnesia of variable extent covering events that occurred before the episode began; in contrast, after the episode has ended, pts can recall the events that preceded the start of the episode, and can also recall all the events that followed upon the termination of the episode; however, and this is critical, pts have no recall of any events they experienced while *in* the episode—it remains as a kind of permanent "island" of amnesia.

Lab: Determined by underlying etiology.

Crs: Determined by underlying etiology.

Cmplc: With chronic amnesias, pts may be completely disabled and require institutionalization. With some episodic amnesias, such as blackouts, others may not even recognize that the pt is in a blackout, whereas with other episodic amnesias, such as TGA, pts may be very agitated.

Etiol: Table 3.16-1 divides the amnesias into chronic and episodic types.

Korsakoff's syndrome, most commonly seen as a sequela to Wernicke's encephalopathy in alcoholics, is the prototype of a chronic amnesia, and is discussed in 3.17.

Paraneoplastic limbic encephalitis may present with an amnesia, but is usually eventually joined by a personality change, seizures, or a dementia.

Prodromes to certain dementias, most notably Alzheimer's disease, may consist of a lengthy amnesia.

Table 3.16-1. Etiologies of Amnesia

Chronic Amnesias

Korsakoff's syndrome (see 3.16)
Paraneoplastic limbic encephalitis (MRI, antineuronal antibodies)
Prodrome to dementia (e.g., as in Alzheimer's disease)

Episodic Amnesias

TGA (see 3.18)
Epileptic amnesia (paroxysmal onset; EEG, MRI)
Blackouts (see 4.2)
Concussion (see 15.9)
TIAs

TGA, most commonly seen in middle-aged men, is the prototypical episodic amnesia, and is discussed in 3.18.

Epileptic amnesia, also known as "pure epileptic amnesia," is distinguished by its paroxysmal onset. Unlike typical complex partial seizures, there is no clouding of consciousness or automatisms (e.g., lip smacking). The amnestic seizure usually lasts from minutes to, exceptionally, hours. Importantly, at other times most pts have other types of seizures, i.e., typical complex partial or grand mal.

Blackouts, as commonly seen in alcoholics, are discussed in 4.2.

TIAs, when involving the temporal lobes or anterior thalamus, may present with an episode of amnesia, lasting perhaps only minutes; these are very rare.

Amnesia associated with concussion is discussed in 15.9.

Ddx: Delirium is distinguished by the presence of confusion.

Dementia is distinguished by the presence of a global intellectual deficit, with, in addition to amnesia, deficits in abstracting and calculating ability. Importantly, as noted above, some dementias may present with a pure amnesia.

Dissociative amnesia, discussed in 9.1, by convention is not grouped with the amnesias listed in Table 3.16-1. Most pts are teenagers or young adults; the episode of amnesia is triggered by a highly emotional event, and pts are eventually able, with psychotherapy, hypnosis, or with the passage of time, to recall events that occurred while the amnesia was present.

Rx: Rx is directed at the underlying cause; Korsakoff's syndrome, TGA, and blackouts are all discussed in their respective chapters.

Paraneoplastic limbic encephalitis is approached by finding and treating the underlying neoplastic process; epileptic amnesia, with anticonvulsants; and TIAs, with aspirin, dipyridamole (Persantine), or clopidogrel.

During an ongoing amnesia, most pts benefit from a degree of supervision.

3.17 KORSAKOFF'S SYNDROME (WHEN OCCURRING SECONDARY TO WERNICKE'S ENCEPHALOPATHY IN ALCOHOLICS, KNOWN AS ALCOHOL-INDUCED PERSISTING AMNESTIC DISORDER)

Br J Psychiatry 1995;166:154. J Neurol Neurosurg Psychiatry 1963;26: 127. J Neurol Neurosurg Psychiatry 1995;59:95.

Epidem: Apparently uncommon, but probably underdiagnosed.

Sx: Pts display a combination of anterograde amnesia and a retrograde amnesia of variable extent (see 3.16); confabulation is a common, but not invariable, feature.

Except for the amnesia, pts are often remarkably clear, and to casual inspection, may not appear ill at all: They are not confused, track well in conversation, and have no difficulty with calculations or abstract concepts. The illness becomes apparent when one asks these pts what happened more than 5 min ago. Pts have no recall of this, and often confabulate a reply. For example, one pt, when asked by the physician whether the 2 of them met together earlier responded that yes, indeed, they'd met at a local bar earlier, had a few drinks, and enjoyed each other's company. The retrograde amnesia is of variable extent, and often becomes "patchy" the further back one goes. Thus, pts may have no recall of the past few years, and then a hazy recall of the few years before that. On formal testing, digit span ability is intact. There is a failure to recall 3 of 3 words after 5 min, and to recall significant autobiographic and public events that occurred for a variable period of time before the onset of the syndrome.

Table 3.17-1. Etiologies of Korsakoff's Syndrome

Sequela to Wernicke's Encephalopathy

Alcoholism
Protracted nausea and vomiting
Parenteral feeding with inadequate thiamine

Focal Lesions in the Circuit of Papez

Hippocampus
  Herpes simplex encephalitis
  Infarction in the area of the posterior cerebral arteries
  Hypoxia (hanging, drowning, carbon monoxide)
  Temporal lobectomy
Fornix
  Tumors
  Surgery
Mammillary bodies
  Tumor (e.g., upward pressure from a craniopharyngioma)
  Surgery
Thalamus (anterior nuclei)
  Infarcts
  Tumors

Aneurysm of the Anterior Communicating Artery

Subsequent either to rupture or to surgical repair

Lab: Determined by underlying cause; MRI diagnostic in most pts.
Crs: In most pts, over long f/u, there is some partial improvement.
Cmplc: Close supervision or institutionalization is often required.
Etiol: See Table 3.17-1.

    Wernicke's encephalopathy, as most commonly seen in alcoholics, is the most common cause of Korsakoff's syndrome. In these cases, after the delirium of Wernicke's encephalopathy clears, pts are left clear-headed but amnestic. In such pts the resulting Korsakoff's syndrome may also be accompanied by some low-level residual sx of Wernicke's encephalopathy, such as nystagmus and ataxia.

    Focal lesions of the circuit of Papez capable of causing amnesia are almost always bilateral. When a unilateral lesion is followed by Korsakoff's syndrome, subsequent investigation shows that the contralateral structure had already been damaged.

    Aneurysms of the anterior communicating artery, subsequent to either rupture or surgical repair, may cause damage to one of the structures of the circuit of Papez, e.g., the nearby columns of the fornix.

Ddx: See 3.16 for a discussion of the ddx of amnesia.

Korsakoff's syndrome is distinguished from the episodic amnesias, ipso facto, by its chronicity.

Korsakoff's syndrome is distinguished from the amnesia of paraneoplastic limbic encephalitis and from the amnestic prodrome to such dementias as Alzheimer's disease, by the h/o Wernicke's encephalopathy immediately preceding the onset of the chronic amnesia.

Rx: Preliminary data suggest that in Korsakoff's syndrome secondary to Wernicke's encephalopathy, fluvoxamine (Luvox) may improve memory.

Most pts require supervision or institutionalization.

3.18 TRANSIENT GLOBAL AMNESIA

Arch Neurol 1982;39:605. Neurology 1980;30:80. Neurology 1987;37:733.

Epidem: Rare.

Sx: TGA is a prototypical example of an episodic amnesia, as discussed in 3.16; the first episode usually occurs in the 50s or 60s.

The onset of the episode is abrupt, and in approximately one-half of pts is preceded by a highly emotional event, such as sexual intercourse or an argument. During the episode, pts are unable to keep track of ongoing events, and are unable to recall 3 of 3 words after 5 min. The retrograde component of the amnesia is generally brief in extent, covering events that occurred in the several hours that preceded the onset. During the episode, pts, though not confused, are often anxious, even agitated, and typically repeatedly ask where they are or what's going on. Importantly, pts, during the episode, are still able to engage in complex activities; e.g., a pianist may continue to play faultlessly. Typically, the episode lasts about 6 h (range, 1–24 h), and then resolves spontaneously. Subsequently, pts are able to keep track again, and are able to remember the events that occurred up to the onset of the episode; in retrospect, however, the episode itself remains an "island" of amnesia, and pts are unable to recall events that occurred during the episode itself.

Lab: NC.

Crs: Most pts have only 1 episode; in a minority, subsequent episodes may appear infrequently, perhaps every 2–3 yr.

Cmplc: Provided pts are supervised during the episode, there are few complications.

Etiol: Unknown; vascular, migrainous, or epileptic mechanisms are suspected.

Ddx: For a general discussion of the ddx of amnesia, see 3.16.

Epileptic amnesia is generally of earlier onset; the episodes are shorter (<1 h) and tend to recur more frequently. Furthermore, most pts, at other times, will have more typical seizures, such as complex partial or grand mal.

Blackouts (see 4.2) are suggested by h/o intoxication.

Concussion is indicated by h/o head trauma.

TIAs are generally briefer, lasting from a few to 15 min.

Dissociative amnesia (see 9.1) may be suggested by the presence of a highly emotional precipitant. Pts with dissociative amnesia, however, are much younger and are able later, with the assistance of psychotherapy, hypnosis, or the passage of time, to recall events that occurred during the episode.

Rx: Supervision is required during the episode.

Given the uncertainty etiology, preventive Rx is uncertain. Some will treat with aspirin, some with a migraine prophylactic agent (e.g., divalproex (Depakote)), and some with an anticonvulsant (e.g., again, divalproex (Depakote)).

3.19 CATATONIA

Acta Psychiatr Scand 1996;93:137. Am J Psychiatry 1986;143:976. Arch Gen Psychiatry 1976;33:579. Arch Gen Psychiatry 1977;34:1223.

Epidem: Uncertain; probably not rare.

Sx: Catatonia exists in 2 forms: stuporous catatonia and excited catatonia; stuporous form far more common.

Stuporous Catatonia: Characterized by varying degrees of immobility, muteness, and rigidity, which may be accompanied by associated sx such as posturing, negativism, automatic obedience, echopraxia, and echolalia.

Immobility may be striking, with pts maintaining the same position for hours to days. Some may stretch out on the floor or a bed, some may lie curled into a ball, others may stand in a corner. The eyes may be rigidly closed or fixed open in a vacant stare.

Muteness may be total or partial. Some pts may occasionally mutter, or declaim senseless phrases.

Rigidity is of the "lead pipe" type, and is often accompanied by catalepsy (or "waxy flexibility") wherein the limbs or body of the pt will remain in whatever position they are placed for minutes to hours, regardless of how uncomfortable and importantly, without the pt being asked to keep the position.

Posturing is said to occur when the pt spontaneously assumes unnatural, and at times bizarre, postures, which are then maintained for long periods. One pt stood, storklike, on 1 leg for hours, another assumed a posture of crucifixion, while yet another sat in a squat, with arms thrust forward.

Negativism represents an automatic, unreasoning, and almost instinctual resistance to either requests or commands, and may be either "passive" or "active." In passive negativism, pts simply do not comply: They may not get out of bed if asked; if brought to dinner, they may sit but not eat; if offered medication, they will not open their mouths. In active negativism, pts do the opposite: If asked to open the eyes wide, they may shut them; if asked to button their robes, they may disrobe.

Automatic obedience is the opposite of negativism. Pts comply with whatever is asked of them, but do it in a robotic and stilted manner.

Echopraxia and echolalia are said to occur when pts repeat or mimic whatever the interviewer does or says, respectively, and do this automatically, and without being asked to. Echopraxic pts may mimic the interviewer's gestures; echolalic pts, upon being asked a question, may simply repeat it.

Excited Catatonia: Characterized by bizarre, at times frenzied, hyperactivity. Pts may loudly declaim, march in place, or gesticulate. Importantly, excited catatonic behavior often has no purpose, and pts, in their hyperactivity, tend to keep to themselves, perhaps by marching in step in a corner, or crawling under their beds where they gesticulate and declaim.

Table 3.19-1. Etiologies of Catatonia

Stuporous Catatonia

Schizophrenia (see 5.1)
Depression (see 6.1)
Mania (during stage III) (see 6.6)
Drug induced
  Neuroleptics (see 15.6)
  Disulfiram
  Phencyclidine intoxication (see 4.14)
Encephalitis
  Paraneoplastic limbic encephalitis
  Viral encephalitis
  Lyme disease
Epileptic
  Complex partial seizure
  Postictal psychosis
  Psychosis of forced normalization
  Chronic interictal psychosis
Focal lesions
  Associated with some right-hemisphere lesions (e.g., infarction)
Other
  Wilson's disease
  Hepatic encephalopathy
  Late-onset Tay-Sachs disease

Excited Catatonia

Schizophrenia (see 5.1)
Mania (during stage III) (see 6.6)
Viral encephalitis

Lab: Determined by the underlying cause.

Crs: Determined by the underlying cause.

Cmplc: Supervision and basic care often required; some stuporous catatonics may require tube feedings.

Excited catatonia may evolve into the potentially fatal Stauder's lethal catatonia, characterized by a fulminant exacerbation of excitation accompanied by fever and hypotension.

Etiol: See Table 3.19-1.

By far, the most common cause of both stuporous and excited catatonia is schizophrenia; at the height of a manic episode (stage III), catatonia not uncommonly appears.

Ddx:

Stuporous Catatonia: Stupor of other causes is distinguished by drowsiness, in contrast with the alertness of catatonia.

Akinetic mutism is distinguished by the response to pinprick: The akinetic mute typically pulls away, or makes some gesture to ward off the pin whereas the stuporous catatonic remains immobile.

Excited Catatonia: Mania (stage I or II) (see 6.6) is distinguished by the purposefulness and other-directedness of the pt's behavior, in contrast with the withdrawal seen in catatonia.

Rx: Treat underlying cause.

Stuporous catatonics must be observed for aspiration, decubiti, and fecal impaction.

Lorazepam (Ativan) 2 mg im often lyses catatonia.

Stauder's lethal catatonia responds to ECT.

3.20 PERSONALITY CHANGE (DUE TO A GENERAL MEDICAL CONDITION)

Arch Gen Psychiatry 1989;46:1126. Brain 1989;112:699. J Neurol Neurosurg Psychiatry 1992;55:475.

Epidem: Uncertain; probably common.

Sx: Onset ranges from acute (e.g., after a stroke) to gradual (e.g., with a slow-growing tumor).

The pt's personality undergoes a significant change relative to its premorbid structure. Minor preexisting personality traits may become quite pronounced, or new, completely uncharacteristic, traits may appear. In either case, others note that the pt is "not himself" anymore.

Specific kinds of personality change may have localizing value. The frontal lobe syndrome (see 3.21) localizes to the frontal lobes or their subcortical connections, and the Klüver-Bucy syndrome (see 3.22) localizes to the temporal lobes. Other changes (e.g., childishness, quarrelsomeness, suspiciousness) have less localizing value.

Lab: Determined by the underlying etiology; MRI often diagnostic.

Crs: Determined by the underlying etiology, and may range from progressive (e.g., with a growing brain tumor) to partially remitting (e.g., after head trauma of the closed head injury type).

Table 3.20-1. Etiologies of Personality Change

Trauma

Closed head injury (see 3.8)
Chronic subdural hematoma

Brain Tumors

Dementing Disease, as Their Prodrome

Alzheimer's disease (see 3.3)
Huntington's disease (see 3.11)
Pick's disease (see 3.12)
Frontotemporal dementia
Wilson's disease

Infectious Conditions

AIDS
Neurosyphilis

Metal Poisoning

Mercury
Manganese
Lead

Other

MS
Paraneoplastic limbic encephalitis
B_{12} deficiency
Interictal personality syndrome (see 3.23)

Cmplc: Work and family relations are strained, and in some cases, there may be legal consequences.

Etiol: See Table 3.20-1.

Ddx: Personality *disorders* (e.g., antisocial personality disorder), in contrast to personality *change,* have their origin in childhood and adolescence and represent not a change, but a coalescence of personality into its lifelong pattern.

Delirium and dementia are distinguished by intellectual deficits. Note, however, that many dementias may present with, or be accompanied by, a personality change.

Schizophrenia may present with a personality change, but the subsequent appearance of psychotic symptoms enables the correct dx.

Rx: The underlying cause is treated, if possible.

Supervision or institutionalization may be required. See 3.21 for the frontal lobe syndrome, 3.22 for the Klüver-Bucy syndrome, and 3.23 for the interictal personality syndrome.

Irritability may respond to a mood stabilizer (e.g., divalproex (Depakote)) and suspiciousness to a neuroleptic (e.g., olanzapine (Zyprexa), risperidone (Risperdal), or haloperidol (Haldol))).

3.21 FRONTAL LOBE SYNDROME

Ann Neurol 1986;19:320. Arch Neurol Psychiatry 1925;81:707. Br J Psychiatry 1971;119:19. JAMA 1952;150:173.

Epidem: One of the most common of the personality changes.

Sx: Pts present with varying combinations of disinhibition, affective changes, abulia, and a lack of foresight and good judgment.

Disinhibition, more common when the orbitofrontal regions are affected, is characterized by an overall coarsening of behavior. Attention to social nuances and morality is lost. Pts may become demanding, profane, and gluttonous; unwelcome sexual advances are not uncommon. Typically, pts are unconcerned with the effect of their disinhibited behavior on others.

Affective changes tend either toward depression (with prominent left frontal lobe involvement) or toward a shallow euphoria (with prominent right frontal lobe involvement). The euphoria is typically silly and not infectious; classically, pts are disposed toward puerile jokes and puns (witzelsucht). Irritability may also occur.

Abulia is characterized by a profound lack of initiative and motivation. Although abulic pts may be able to complete tasks with constant supervision, when left to their own devices, feeling no motivation or ambition, they lapse into quietude.

Lack of foresight and good judgment reflects a general inability to plan and organize complex behavior, and may be more common when the frontal convexity is involved. In extreme cases, pts may display gross perseveration.

Lab: MRI diagnostic in most pts.

Crs: Determined by underlying cause.

Table 3.21-1. Etiologies of the Frontal Lobe Syndrome

Focal Lesions (e.g., Tumors, Infarction, Abscess)	Dementing Conditions
	Alzheimer's disease (see 3.3)
Frontal lobes	Pick's disease (see 3.12)
Anterior portion of corpus callosum	Frontotemporal dementia
Thalamus (dorsomedial nucleus)	Progressive supranuclear palsy
Basal ganglia (caudate or globus pallidus)	Corticobasal ganglionic degeneration
Mesencephalon (ventral tegmental area)	Metachromatic leukodystrophy
	Amyotrophic lateral sclerosis

Cmplc: Work and personal relationships suffer; legal consequences may follow disinhibition or irritability.

Etiol: See Table 3.21-1.

Focal lesions are generally bilateral; occasionally, however, unilateral lesions may cause the syndrome.

Ddx: Major depression (see 6.1) and dysthymia (see 6.2) are distinguished from a depressive frontal lobe syndrome by other frontal lobe sx, such as disinhibition.

Mania is distinguished by the depth and infectiousness of manic euphoria, in contrast to the shallow and noninfectious euphoria of the frontal lobe syndrome.

Rx: Treat the underlying etiology, if possible.

Neuroleptics may reduce disinhibition; antidepressants, depression; euphoria rarely requires Rx. Irritability, if explosive, may respond to propranolol (Inderal) in doses of 240–480 mg/d (if tolerated).

3.22 KLÜVER-BUCY SYNDROME

Neurology 1955;5:373. Neurology 1981;31:1415. Neurology 1983;33: 1141.

Epidem: Rare.

Sx: Full syndrome contains "psychic blindness," "hypermetamorphosis," "hyperorality," and "hypersexuality."

Psychic blindness refers to an indiscriminate interest in whatever

Table 3.22-1. Etiologies of the Klüver-Bucy Syndrome

Herpes simplex encephalitis
Bilateral temporal lobectomies
Bilateral temporal lobe contusions
Pick's disease
Complex partial seizures
Postictal

comes into view. There is absence both of an appreciation of danger and of appropriate fear.

Hypermetamorphosis is characterized by a seemingly compulsive tendency to handle and examine whatever is around, regardless of whether it is useful or not.

Hyperorality is characterized by a strong tendency to put things in the mouth, regardless of their edibility. Some pts may eat enormous amounts of food; others may eat paper clips, toilet paper, or even feces.

Hypersexuality is evident in an indiscriminate sexuality. There may be overt masturbation or crude advances made toward others, regardless of gender.

Lab: With the exception of ictal and postictal etiologies, where EEG is required, MRI is revealing for most of the etiologies noted in Table 3.22-1.

Crs: Determined by the underlying etiology.

Cmplc: Most pts are socially disabled during the syndrome.

Etiol: See Table 3.22-1.

In all pts, there is either bilateral damage to temporal structures or as in seizures, bilateral temporal dysfunction.

Ddx: Paranoid schizophrenia may produce similar behavior; however, this always occurs in the context of psychotic sx more typical for schizophrenia, e.g., auditory hallucinations, persecutory delusions.

Rx: Institutional care may be required.

Anecdotally, neuroleptics (e.g., haloperidol (Haldol), olanzapine (Zyprexa)) may dampen some of the sx.

3.23 INTERICTAL PERSONALITY SYNDROME (GESCHWIND SYNDROME)

Arch Gen Psychiatry 1975;32:1580. Arch Neurol 1977;34:454. Cortex 1979;15:357. J Neurol Neurosurg Psychiatry 1982;45:481. Neurology 1974;24:629.

Epidem: Uncertain; possibly rare.

Sx: Gradual onset of a personality change after many years of repeated complex partial or grand mal seizures.

Classically, pts demonstrate "viscosity" or "stickiness," namely, an abnormal persistence of affect, train of thought, or action. Affects tend to be deep and to persist long beyond the situation that occasioned them. Speech is verbose and circumstantial, and pts may resist any attempt to change the subject. Hypergraphia, perhaps representing the written equivalent of verbose speech, may lead to a stultifying abundance of letters, journals, diary entries, etc.

Coupled with viscosity, there is often also a preoccupation with matters ethical, religious, or philosophical; a global hyposexuality; and a tendency toward quarrelsomeness.

Lab: EEG and MRI results consistent with epilepsy.

Crs: Probably chronic.

Cmplc: Viscosity strains relations at home and work; hyposexuality may strain a marriage.

Etiol: Recurrent seizure activity in the temporal lobes may "kindle" changes in the limbic system.

Ddx: For a general discussion of the ddx of personality change, see 3.20.

Personality change in an epileptic may be due to a slowly growing tumor in the temporal lobe, and thus MRI is appropriate in all pts.

Rx: Best Rx is prevention, and all pts with epilepsy should be aggressively treated to forestall the development of the syndrome.

Anecdotally, effective treatment of epilepsy, e.g., with temporal lobectomy, may be followed by resolution of the syndrome.

4. Substance-Related Disorders

4.1 ALCOHOLISM (ALCOHOL DEPENDENCE)

Am J Psychiatry 1979;136:603. Am J Psychiatry 1993;150:786. Arch Gen Psychiatry 1980;37:561. Arch Gen Psychiatry 1992;49:881.

Epidem: Lifetime prevalence in USA ~10%; male-female ratio 3:1.

Sx: Onset gradual in late teens or 20s, later in females than males; onset >45 yr is unusual.

After a decade or more, the full picture is often evident: Alcoholics persistently become intoxicated, despite serious adverse consequences such as marital discord, legal problems (e.g., DUI), work problems, and health problems (see complications below). Alcoholics eventually also develop tolerance and withdrawal: In tolerance, progressively larger amounts are required to reach the desired intoxication; in withdrawal, pts experience either the "shakes" (see 4.3) or DTs (see 4.4). Importantly, in a minority, tolerance may eventually be lost, at times abruptly: Pts capable of drinking a fifth of whisky with little effect now find themselves hopelessly intoxicated after 2 or 3 drinks.

Almost all alcoholics experience some form of denial, either minimizing their drinking or altogether denying adverse consequences. Furthermore, most (but not all), at some time or other, will try and quit or moderate their intake, occasionally with temporary success.

Lab: Lab abnormalities reflect complications, noted below. The combination of an elevated SGGT and MCV (reflecting, respectively, hepatic and bone marrow toxicity) is highly suggestive of alcoholism.

Crs: Episodic ("binge drinker") or chronic.

Episodic binges may last for days to weeks, and are separated by periods of abstinence of variable duration, from weeks to months.

Table 4.1-1. Complications of Alcoholism

Blackouts (see 4.2)
Alcohol withdrawal syndrome (see 4.3)
DTs (see 4.4)
Alcohol withdrawal seizures (see 4.5)
Wernicke's encephalopathy (see 4.6)
Korsakoff's syndrome (see 3.17)
Encephalopathic pellagra
Alcoholic dementia (see 3.14)
Alcoholic paranoia (see 5.8)
Alcoholic hallucinosis (see 5.9)
Alcohol-induced depression (see 6.8)
Gastritis
Hepatitis and cirrhosis
Hepatic encephalopathy
Acquired hepatocerebral degeneration
Bleeding esophageal varices
Pancreatitis
Head trauma (with, e.g., subdural hematoma)
Alcoholic cerebellar degeneration
Alcoholic polyneuropathy
Alcoholic myopathy
Central pontine myelinolysis
Marchiafava-Bignami disease
Alcoholic cardiomyopathy
Hypomagnesemia
Hypoglycemia
Megaloblastic anemia
Thrombocytopenia
Aspiration pneumonia

Chronic drinkers may become intoxicated daily or on a more or less regular basis (the "weekend drunk").

Spontaneous, full, and permanent remissions do occur, but are rare; for most alcoholics drinking continues until the pt is institutionalized, crippled, or dead.

Cmplc: See Table 4.1-1.

Suicidal ideation is almost ubiquitous; ~15% die by suicide.

Depressed, unemployed men without family or close friends who suffer from 1 of the general medical complications (e.g., cirrhosis) are at highest risk.

Fetal alcohol syndrome may occur in children born to alcoholic females who drink through pregnancy.

Etiol: Twin and adoption studies indicate a strong genetic component.

Ddx: Alcohol abuse distinguished by the absence of both tolerance and withdrawal.

Rx: Abstinence is the goal, and this must be clearly stated.

Hospitalization is often required, not only to treat complications but also to secure an enforced period of abstinence.

Concurrent conditions (e.g., major depression (see 6.1), bipolar disorder (see 6.6), schizophrenia (see 5.1), and panic disorder (see ch 7.1)) should be treated. Potentially addictive drugs (e.g., benzodiazepines) should not be prescribed to outpatients, and should be used only if absolutely necessary during hospitalization.

Give thiamine 100 mg im × 3 d then po thereafter (do not give glucose or food generally until 3 h after thiamine given, as this may precipitate Wernicke's encephalopathy); multivitamin 1 qd; assess for any complications (esp hypomagnesemia).

Measure CBC, electrolytes, liver enzymes, bilirubin, glucose, magnesium, ammonia, and if abdominal pain present, lipase and amylase.

Counsel pts to avoid all old "playgrounds" (e.g., bars, nightclubs) and "playmates" (e.g., drinking buddies).

AA should be recommended, and attendance at "outside" hospital meetings should begin during the inpatient stay. Pts should be encouraged to attend "90 meetings in 90 days," with the first of the 90 meetings being on the day of discharge.

Three medications may be helpful: disulfiram (Antabuse), naltrexone (ReVia), and acamprosate.

Disulfiram (Antabuse) may be useful for alcoholics committed to sobriety who continue to have "slips." Ethanol is metabolized first to acetaldehyde, then rapidly to acetic acid. Disulfiram (Antabuse) inhibits the conversion of acetaldehyde to acetic acid, leading to a rapid accumulation of acetaldehyde and a resultant "aldehyde reaction" characterized by the rapid onset of facial flushing, headache, vomiting, diaphoresis, dyspnea, palpitations, and chest pain—in some pts shock, myocardial infarction, or respiratory arrest may occur. SEs to disulfiram (Antabuse) include sedation, fatigue, headache, dizziness, tremor, restlessness, and impotence; a metallic taste and rash may also occur. Rarely, and generally only during the first few months of Rx, hepatitis (which may be fulminant) may occur and LFTs should be performed q 2 wk for 2 mo, and as indicated thereafter. Also, rarely, a sensory polyneuropathy and a dementia may occur. Treatment initiated at 500 mg qd for the first week, then 250 mg qd thereafter, with the dose generally taken in the morning, when the resolve to stay sober is generally strongest. The BAL *must* be 0 before disulfiram (Antabuse) is begun; furthermore, pts should be warned that the "acetaldehyde" reaction may still occur for up to 14 d after discontinuation of the disulfiram (Antabuse). Furthermore, the "acetaldehyde" reaction may occur not only with beverage alcohol but also with vinegars (as may be found in salad dressings), and alcohol-containing mouthwashes, cooking sauces, and even topical colognes, after-shave lotions, and perfumes.

Naltrexone (ReVia) 50 mg qd reduces the risk of a "slip": The mechanism is not clear—may reduce craving, may reduce reinforcing effect of alcohol taken during a "slip."

Acamprosate, not yet available in USA, reduces craving.

The overall place of these 3 medicines in the Rx of alcoholism is not yet clear.

4.2 BLACKOUTS

Am J Psychiatry 1969;126:191. Br J Psychiatry 1969;115:1033. J Stud Alcohol 1994;55:290.

Epidem: Seen in approximately one-third of alcoholics.

Sx: During moderate to severe intoxication, pts experience the abrupt onset of an amnestic episode (see 3.16) characterized primarily by anterograde amnesia, with relatively little retrograde amnesia. During the blackout, pts continue to act "in character," and often neither pts nor others recognize that anything is amiss. Pts may repeat the same joke after a few minutes, not remembering that they've already told it, and if tested formally, although digit span ability is intact and pts are able to recall events that happened until right before the onset of the blackout, they are unable to recall all 3 of 3 words after 5 min. Blackouts often remit suddenly, and pts may suddenly "come to," perhaps in the middle of a conversation, having no idea of what they were talking about, or how the conversation got started. The blackout itself, in retrospect, appears to the pt as an "island" of amnesia. Often, pts who continue drinking during the blackout will "pass out" before the blackout remits; upon waking the next morning, they may have no recall of how they got home. Such pts may anxiously inspect the car, to see if they had an accident on the way home.

Lab: NC.

Crs: Most blackouts last hours; occasionally they may last days (the "lost weekend"); recurrences are the rule.

Cmplc: Pts may be haunted by things said or done during the blackout.

Etiol: Alcohol-induced temporary dysfunction somewhere in the circuit of Papez is suspected.

Ddx: For a general discussion of the ddx of amnesia, see 3.16.

TGA is suggested by the pt's "out-of-character" repeated questioning during the episode; furthermore TGA tends to first appear in the 50s or 60s, in contrast to blackouts, which usually first occur early in the course of alcoholism.

Epileptic amnesia is suggested by the occurrence of complex partial or grand mal seizures at other times; in the alcoholic who also has alcohol-induced seizures, one may look to the absence or presence of intoxication during the episode to facilitate the dx.

Rx: Blacked-out pts should be observed until their ability to recall 3 of 3 words after 5 min is restored, thus indicating the resolution of the blackout. Abstinence is indicated to prevent future blackouts, and pts should be evaluated for alcoholism.

4.3 ALCOHOL WITHDRAWAL SYNDROME

Acta Psychiatr Scand 1981;64:254. Acta Psychiatr Scand 1984;69:398. Am J Psychiatry 1989;146:617.

Epidem: Seen in most alcoholics.

Sx: Sx appear as the BAL falls and then remains for several hours below the individual pt's "threshold" level for intoxication. Thus, when tolerance is minimal, withdrawal sx may not appear for 4–12 h after the last drink, whereas in those with high tolerance, sx may appear merely after the pt "cuts down."

Sx include anxiety, tremulousness, easy startability, diaphoresis, tachycardia, elevated BP, mydriasis, and hyperreflexia. Occasionally, there are brief, transient visual or auditory hallucinations. The tremor, when mild, is fine and may only be appreciated when the pt's hands are held out with the fingers parted; in severe cases, the tremor is coarse and obvious, at times involving not only the hands but also the tongue and eyelids. Although pts remain oriented, thinking becomes difficult and concentration poor. Insomnia may be severe.

Most alcoholics realize that a drink would "solve" the problem, and many will begin taking the "morning drink."

Lab: NC.

Crs: In most pts, sx peak in 1–2 d, then resolve gradually over the next 4–7 d. In a small minority, the withdrawal syndrome may be "protracted," with difficulty in thinking and concentration, and insomnia, persisting for up to a half year: Many alcoholics refer to this as the "fog."

In about 5% of pts with alcohol withdrawal syndrome, sx, rather than resolving, undergo a severe exacerbation, and the condition evolves into DTs (see 4.4); this is more likely in those with such conditions as pneumonia, hepatic failure, or gastrointestinal hemorrhage.

Cmplc: Work performance is impaired; concurrent conditions such as panic disorder, epilepsy, or cardiac disease may be aggravated.

Protracted withdrawal (the "fog") may impair the alcoholic's ability to participate in rehabilitative efforts, such as AA.

Etiol: Disturbances in GABAergic transmission are suspected.

Ddx: An almost identical syndrome may be seen after abrupt discontinuation of benzodiazepines or barbiturates.

Hypoglycemia is suggested by relief with food. Importantly, glucose preparations should *not* be given to alcoholics until after parenteral administration of thiamine, as a glucose load may precipitate Wernicke's encephalopathy.

Thyroid storm is suggested by proptosis and thyromegaly.

DTs are distinguished by the presence of delirium.

Rx: Mild sx may not require specific Rx.

See 4.1 for general Rx of alcoholism.

Moderate or severe sx may be treated with a benzodiazepine (e.g., lorazepam (Ativan)) or with carbamazepine (Tegretol).

Lorazepam (Ativan) given 2 mg po or 1 mg im q 2 h (using lower doses for the elderly or debilitated) until tremor is cleared; pts are then placed on a regularly scheduled dose approximately equivalent to the total required to abolish the tremor, with the total regular dose divided into 3 or 4 doses, and provision made for additional doses prn should tremor reappear. If prn doses are required, the regular dose is increased until tremor is controlled without need for prn doses. In most pts, sx are controlled within 48 h, and the total daily dose may then be tapered and discontinued over 3–5 days.

Carbamazepine (Tegretol) given in a total daily dose of 600–800 mg po (less in the elderly, debilitated, or those with significant hepatic failure), divided into 3 or 4 doses, with the dose adjusted over the next day or 2 in light of SEs and therapeutic effect. Carbamazepine (Tegretol) usually effective in less than 48 h, and may be used as single-agent Rx in mild to moderate cases; in severe cases, one may wish to use prn doses of lorazepam (Ativan) for the first day or 2, until the carbamazepine takes effect. Once carbamazepine (Tegretol) is effective, continue for ~7 d, then taper and discontinue over 2 d.

Although pts with mild to moderate withdrawal syndrome may be treated on an outpatient basis, severely affected pts require admission. Lorazepam (Ativan) should be prescribed to outpatients only with *great* caution.

4.4 DELIRIUM TREMENS (ALCOHOL WITHDRAWAL DELIRIUM)

Acta Psychiatr Scand 1961;36:443. Acta Psychiatr Scand 1965; 41(Suppl):1. J Gen Int Med 1989;4:432. Postgrad Med 1987;82:117.

Epidem: ~5% of pts with the alcohol withdrawal syndrome (see 4.3) will develop DTs.

Sx: Sx generally appear in the setting of the alcohol withdrawal syndrome, generally after 2 or 3 d; a h/o DTs generally predicts an earlier onset.

Concurrent with an exacerbation of the sx of the alcohol withdrawal syndrome, pts develop a delirium, with confusion, deficient short-term memory, and disorientation. The tremor of alcohol withdrawal often becomes very marked, and accounts for the name of this delirium (*delirium tremens* = "trembling delirium").

Typically, in the midst of the delirium, pts also develop hallucinations

Table 4.4-1. Differential Diagnosis of Delirium Tremens

Wernicke's encephalopathy (nystagmus, ataxia) (see 4.6)
Hepatic encephalopathy (asterixis; NH_3 >55 mcg/dL; caution: may be normal)
Subdural hematoma (focal signs)
Hypoglycemia (glucose <45 mg/dL)
Hypomagnesemia (myoclonus; Mg <1 mEq/L)
Meningitis (fever, stiff neck)
Encephalopathic pellagra (rigidity and dysarthria; urine *N*-methylniacinamide)
Postictal delirium
Respiratory failure (asterixis if hypercarbic; PaO_2 <55 mm Hg; PCO_2 >70)
Severe anemia

(visual > auditory) and delusions (most commonly of persecution). Pts may see insects, animals, or large scenes, and typically react to them appropriately, perhaps by stomping the floor to squash the "bugs." Auditory hallucinations are often of voices, which tend to be persecutory, telling pts that the medicine is poisoned or that they will be murdered.

As noted in 3.1, deliria may be either "noisy" or "quiet." Although in most pts, DTs are "noisy" and marked by agitation, occasionally there may be quiet DTs, with mild autonomic sx, and very little, if any, disruptiveness on the part of the pt.

Lab: Reflects common concurrent conditions, such as pneumonia, hepatic failure, gastrointestinal bleeding, etc.

Crs: 5%–15% die of arrhythmia, shock, or one of the complications of alcoholism (see 4.1). In those who survive, spontaneous remission occurs gradually in from several days up to 2–3 wk.

Cmplc: For general complications of delirium, see 3.1. Pts with DTs are often very uncooperative and may attempt to escape, or perhaps assault others.

Etiol: Prior episodes of alcohol withdrawal syndrome may "kindle" the limbic system.

Ddx: Of the many causes of delirium (see 3.1), those listed in Table 4.4-1 rank high on the ddx for alcoholism.

Rx: If not already in place, Rx as for the alcohol withdrawal syndrome (see 4.3) is rapidly instituted; psychotic sx may be treated with haloperidol (Haldol) 5 mg po or im (lower doses for the elderly, debilitated, or those with significant hepatic failure) qh until endpoint of satisfactory control, unacceptable SEs, or a maximum dose of 30 mg.

General Rx of delirium covered in 3.1.
General Rx of alcoholism covered in 4.1.

4.5 ALCOHOL WITHDRAWAL SEIZURES ("RUM FITS")

Epilepsia 1967;7:1. J R Soc Med 1987;9:571. NEJM 1976;294:757.

Epidem: Overall, ~1% of pts in the alcohol withdrawal syndrome (see 4.3) will have a grand mal seizure; among chronic alcoholics, the figure rises to ~10%.

Sx: From hours to 2 d after cessation of drinking, or in those tolerant to alcohol, a significant reduction in intake, a grand mal seizure occurs. In a minority, there may be a focal onset; the majority of these seizures, however, are generalized from the onset.

Lab: NC, except in pts with a focal onset, wherein MRI may reveal evidence of an old injury, e.g., a subdural hematoma.

Crs: Most pts have only 1–3 seizures; with repeated episodes, the likelihood of having seizures increases.

Cmplc: As for any grand mal seizure.

Etiol: Repeated episodes of alcohol withdrawal probably kindle the limbic system and related areas.

Ddx: Other alcohol-related disorders associated with seizures include hypoglycemia, hypomagnesemia, prior head trauma, Wernicke's encephalopathy, and Marchiafava-Bignami disease.

Pts with preexisting epilepsy are more likely to have seizures during withdrawal.

Rx: Isolated alcohol withdrawal seizures do not require treatment. Frequent seizures or status epilepticus may be treated with iv lorazepam (Ativan), 1–4 mg at a rate no faster than 2 mg/min, with concurrent administration of fosphenytoin (Cerebyx).

Alcoholics in the alcohol withdrawal syndrome who have a h/o alcohol withdrawal seizures should probably be treated with carbamazepine (Tegretol), as described in 4.3, in the hopes of preventing seizures.

4.6 WERNICKE'S ENCEPHALOPATHY

Ann Neurol 1987;22:595. J Neurol Neurosurg Psychiatry 1979;42:226.
J Neurol Neurosurg Psychiatry 1986;49:341. NEJM 1985;312:1035.

Epidem: Autopsy studies indicate that ~10% of all alcoholics have had Wernicke's encephalopathy and that in most it went undiagnosed in life.

Sx: Onset is subacute, over days.

The classic triad of delirium, nystagmus, and ataxia is in fact uncommon: Most pts present with delirium alone.

Grand mal seizures may accompany the delirium.

Lab: MRI may reveal increased signal intensity on T2-weighted scans in the mammillary bodies.

Crs: Mortality >50%; among those who survive, the majority will be left with Korsakoff's syndrome (see 3.17); residual nystagmus and ataxia may also be seen.

Cmplc: See 3.1.

Etiol: Thiamine deficiency leads to hemorrhagic necrosis in the mammillary bodies, dorsomedial nuclei of the thalamus, periaqueductal gray matter, and the cerebellum. Such severe thiamine deficiency is most commonly seen in alcoholics; it may also occur with prolonged vomiting (e.g., hyperemesis gravidarum, s/p gastrectomy) or hunger strikes. In pts with borderline adequate thiamine reserves, a glucose load may precipitate the encephalopathy.

Ddx: When the classic triad is present, the dx is fairly obvious. As most pts do not present with the classic triad, however, the dx often depends on a high index of suspicion. Thus, when delirium occurs in an alcoholic, as noted in Table 4.4-1, Wernicke's encephalopathy ought to be high on the ddx.

Rx: All alcoholics should be given thiamine 100 mg im × 3 d then po thereafter, and glucose loads should generally be withheld for 3 h after the thiamine is given. In pts in whom Wernicke's encephalopathy is strongly suspected, the initial dose of thiamine may be given iv, and then 100 mg im bid for the next 3 d, with oral administration thereafter. When Rx is timely, nystagmus may clear within hours, ataxia and delirium within days.

4.7 STIMULANT (AMPHETAMINE, METHAMPHETAMINE, DEXTROAMPHETAMINE)- AND COCAINE-RELATED DISORDERS

Am J Psychiatry 1991;48:495. Ann Int Med 1993;119:226. Arch Gen Psychiatry 1986;43:107. Biol Psychiatry 1970;2:95. J Clin Psychopharm 1995;15:63. NEJM 1988;318:1173.

Epidem: "Experimentation" with these substances is very common; prevalence of addiction in USA is uncertain, probably on order of several percent.

Sx: Addiction usually begins in the late teens or early 20s; the rate of progression from "social" use to addiction varies with the route of administration, from months with regular oral or intranasal use to within weeks or even days with iv or inhaled administration.

Mild intoxication characterized by euphoria, grandiosity, talkativeness, increased energy, and a generally increased level of activity; mydriasis, tremor, hyperreflexia, increased BP, and tachycardia (or occasionally, reflex bradycardia) are common.

Moderate intoxication may bring agitation, delusions of persecution and reference, and auditory or visual hallucinations; tactile hallucinations (classically with formication—"cocaine bugs") may also occur. Choreoathetosis and elevated temperature are seen in a minority.

Severe intoxication may cause delirium. Other sx may include seizures, arrhythmias, myocardial infarction, stroke, and respiratory arrest.

Withdrawal from stimulants or cocaine characterized by dysphoria, irritability, fatigue, and sleep change (generally insomnia), and may last from days to weeks.

After 2 yr or longer of repeated frequent intoxication, addicts may develop a psychosis during intoxication, which then persists for variable periods of time, and with frequent recurrences, may become chronic. Sx include delusions of persecution and reference and hallucinations, more commonly auditory than visual.

Lab: Serum or urine screens may reveal the parent compound or a metabolite.

Crs: Chronic course, with either frequent binges or daily use.

Cmplc: Chronic nasal insufflation may cause nasal septal necrosis.

Intravenous use with "dirty" needles risks AIDS or hepatitis, particularly hepatitis C.

Cerebral vasculitis and stroke may occur.

Etiol: Intoxication probably mediated by increased dopaminergic activity in the mesolimbic system.

Chronic psychosis may represent a "kindling" of the limbic system.

Ddx: Mania is distinguished by its persistence during periods of enforced abstinence.

Paranoid schizophrenia resembles the chronic psychosis, and if the addiction began early, may indeed be difficult to distinguish. The presence of mannerisms and similar bizarre features suggests schizophrenia.

Depression is distinguished from withdrawal by its persistence during enforced abstinence of several weeks or longer.

Rx: Mild intoxication generally requires only observation; moderate or severe intoxication may be treated with neuroleptics (e.g., chlorpromazine (Thorazine) 50–100 mg, or haloperidol (Haldol) 5–10 mg im qh until sx are controlled, unacceptable SEs occur, or a maximum dose of 1000 mg of chlorpromazine (Thorazine) or 60 mg of haloperidol (Haldol) is reached). Lower doses are used for the elderly, debilitated, or those with hepatic failure. Seizures may be treated with iv lorazepam (Ativan) (2–4 mg no faster than 2 mg/min), and arrhythmias with propranolol (Inderal).

Abstinence is the overall goal; some may do well with Cocaine Anonymous (CA) or Narcotics Anonymous (NA), and those with concurrent alcoholism may do well in AA.

4.8 CAFFEINE-RELATED DISORDERS

Arch Gen Psychiatry 1991;48:611. JAMA 1994;272:1043. NEJM 1992; 327:1109.

Epidem: Lifetime prevalence of caffeine intoxication in USA ~10%; prevalence of abuse uncertain.

Sx: >80% of Americans use caffeine (averaging ~200 mg/d): 1 cup coffee = 100 mg; 1 cup tea = ~50 mg; caffeinated soft drinks =

25–200 mg; chocolate bar = ~25 mg; various OTC and Rx medications. Caffeine is rapidly absorbed, with peak blood levels in 30–60 min and a half-life of ~5 h.

Intoxication, in nontolerant individuals, begins with acute consumption of 200–500 mg: anxiety, restlessness, apprehension, agitation; tremor, tachycardia; headache and insomnia. At doses of ~1000 mg, severe anxiety and agitation may occur, with muscle twitching and palpitations. Sx resolve over 6–12 h. Acute doses of >10 gm may cause seizures or respiratory failure.

Tolerance may appear after only ~2 wk of daily consumption of 500 mg or more.

Withdrawal may appear 12–24 h after the last dose: headache, poor concentration, fatigue, anxiety, irritability, and depressed mood, all clearing in 2–7 d.

Caffeine abuse is said to occur when pts recurrently take caffeine to the point of intoxication or continue their use despite the appearance of complications.

Lab: NC.

Crs: Uncertain.

Cmplc: Exacerbation of gastroesophageal reflux, peptic ulcer disease, and fibrocystic disease.

Etiol: Suggestive evidence that propensity to abuse caffeine is inherited.

Ddx: Panic attacks are distinguished by their acute onset and relative brevity (~15 min vs hours for caffeine intoxication). Although caffeine does not cause panic attacks in normal persons, it may exacerbate panic attacks in those with panic disorder.

Generalized anxiety disorder may be very difficult to distinguish and a trial of caffeine abstinence may be required.

Akathisia, as seen with neuroleptic Rx, is distinguished by the absence of tremor and tachycardia.

Hyperthyroidism is suggested by proptosis and confirmed by TFT.

Rx: Intoxication rarely requires treatment; diazepam (Valium) 5–10 mg po may be given for agitation.

Withdrawal does not require Rx.

Caffeine abusers are generally able to either moderate or discontinue use with education and minimal counseling.

4.9 CANNABIS-RELATED DISORDERS

Am J Psychiatry 1985;142:1325. Arch Gen Psychiatry 1970;23:204. Br J Psychiatry 1993;163:141.

Epidem: "Experimentation" is very common; addiction may be present in ~2.5% of those in their late teens or early 20s.

Sx: Cannabis dependence usually begins in the mid to late teens and is typically characterized by daily intoxication.

Mild intoxication characterized by euphoria, heightened awareness of sounds and colors, a sense that time is slowing down or disintegrating, illogical thinking, and often, a giggling hilarity; concentration and memory suffer. Conjunctival injection and a mild ataxia are not uncommon. In a minority, anxiety, which may be extreme, can appear. In most people, mild intoxication clears within 3–4 h. Occasionally, mild intoxication may be accompanied by fleeting delusions of persecution, and these may outlast the intoxication per se, clearing only after 1–3 d.

Severe intoxication may bring hallucinations (auditory or visual), which tend to clear with the intoxication, or a delirium, which may outlast the intoxication by 1–3 d.

Lab: Cannabinoid metabolites are present in the urine, and in heavy users may persist for a month. Importantly, low levels of metabolites may be seen in individuals exposed to large concentrations of "secondhand" smoke.

Crs: Long-term course of cannabis dependence not known.

Cmplc: Intoxicated pts may be unable to safely operate machinery, such as cars or airplanes, and this incapacity may extend for several hours after the euphoria has cleared.

Bronchitis may complicate chronic use.

There is controversy over whether or not chronic users may develop a personality change known as the "amotivational syndrome" with apathy, listlessness, and social withdrawal.

There is also controversy over whether chronic use can cause a chronic syndrome similar to paranoid schizophrenia.

Etiol: Cannabinoid receptors are present in the brain; their involvement in the development of addiction is not clear.

Ddx: Panic attacks are distinguished from the severe anxiety seen with some intoxications by the lack of other sx of intoxication that both precede and follow the anxiety.

Depression is distinguished from the amotivational syndrome by the presence of such sx as guilt and insomnia.

Rx: Mild intoxication generally requires only observation.

Anxiety, if severe, may be treated with a long-acting benzodiazepine (e.g., diazepam (Valium) 5–10 mg po).

Delusions and hallucinations may be treated with a neuroleptic (e.g., haloperidol (Haldol) 5–10 mg po).

Delirium may require admission; Rx proceeds as in 3.1.

Withdrawal sx and the amotivational syndrome generally require only abstinence.

Abstinence is the overall goal; hospitalization rarely required, except for pts with the amotivational syndrome who require a period of enforced abstinence to allow for the return of motivation. Denial and uncooperativeness are common. Some may benefit from AA; for those still living at home with parents, family counseling may be helpful.

4.10 HALLUCINOGEN-RELATED DISORDERS

Arch Gen Psychiatry 1972;27:437. Arch Gen Psychiatry 1993;40:884. Arch Gen Psychiatry 1994;51:98. Lancet 1992;340:384. Psychopharmacology 1995;119:247.

Epidem: Chronic abuse is rare; hallucinogens include lysergic acid diethylamide (LSD), psilocybin, dimethyltryptamine (DMT), mescaline, 2,5-dimethoxy-4-methylamphetamine (STP), dimethoxyamphetamine (DMA), methylenedioxyamphetamine (MDA), and 3,4-methylenedioxymethamphetamine (MDMA, or "Ecstasy").

Sx: Hallucinogen use typically begins in adolescence.

Intoxication is characterized by "altered" consciousness, a "cosmic" sense. Visual hallucinations (colors, geometric forms, scenes) are common; auditory ones less so. Mydriasis, fine tremor, and hyperreflexia are common, along with mild tachycardia and hypertension. In a minority, a "bad trip" may occur, with severe anxiety or delusions of persecution and reference. Intoxication generally clears within 6 h to a day, with the exception of DMT intoxication, which lasts only 2–6 h.

In contrast with other intoxicants, there is no craving for hallucinogens, and no withdrawal phenomena. Interestingly, though, tolerance can develop rapidly, over perhaps 3 or 4 days use; requiring several days of abstinence before intoxication is once again possible.

Lab: Gas chromatography is required to detect LSD in serum or urine.

Crs: It appears that hallucinogen use rarely persists beyond middle years.

Cmplc: "Flashbacks" are spontaneous, paroxysmal, transient recurrences of fragments of prior intoxications, often visual, that may occur with frequencies from several times daily to only weekly or monthly. With abstinence, the frequency generally wanes over several months; however, in some pts, they may persist for years or decades into abstinence.

Postintoxication mood changes (either depressive, or less commonly, manic) may occur in a minority, and tend to clear within a few days.

Postintoxication psychosis, which occurs in a small minority, consists of a prolongation of psychotic sx (hallucinations or delusions) past the intoxication, with, critically, a lack of insight. Intoxicated pts recognize that the psychotic sx are not "real," whereas pts in a postintoxication psychosis react as if they were real. Most postintoxication psychoses clear within days or weeks; exceptionally, they may persist chronically.

Recurrent intoxication with MDMA may damage serotoninergic neurons.

Etiol: Hallucinogens are mixed agonist-antagonists at postsynaptic serotonin receptors; those located in the dorsal raphe nucleus of the midbrain may be particularly important.

Ddx: Phencyclidine intoxication is distinguished by nystagmus.

Simple partial seizures are distinguished from flashbacks by the presence of other seizure types (complex partial, grand mal) at other times in the pt's life.

Depression or mania is distinguished from the postintoxication mood changes by the absence of a h/o immediately preceding intoxication and by their persistence beyond a few days.

Schizophrenia is distinguished from postintoxication psychosis by its subacute or gradual onset. Postintoxication psychoses are of sudden onset, emerging directly from an intoxication.

Rx: Intoxication generally requires only observation; "bad trips" may be managed with a long-acting benzodiazepine (e.g., diazepam (Valium) 2–10 mg po).

Postintoxication mood changes are managed with observation; suicidal ideation may necessitate hospitalization for a few days until the mood change resolves spontaneously.

Postintoxication psychosis, if prolonged, may be managed with neuroleptics, as described in 5.1.

Abstinence is the overall goal; specific treatments not as yet available.

4.11 INHALANT-RELATED DISORDERS

Am J Psychiatry 1987;144:903. Br J Psychiatry 1987;150:769. Neurology 1990;40:532.

Epidem: Experimentation occurs in ~10% of adolescents; a small minority go on to chronic use.

Sx: Inhalant use typically begins in early to mid teenage years, and is often done in groups.

Inhalation is accomplished by putting a small amount in the bottom of a paper or plastic bag, and then placing the bag across the nose and mouth, or by holding a soaked rag to cover the same area. Intoxicating aromatic hydrocarbons are found in glue ("airplane" or "model" glue), paint thinner, gasoline or kerosene, fingernail polish, etc. Intoxication occurs in minutes and is characterized by a dreamy euphoria, with drowsiness, dysarthria, ataxia, and nystagmus. Visual hallucinations may occur, as may confusion, and some users may become agitated or impulsive. In severe intoxication, ventricular arrhythmias, coma, and respiratory arrest may occur. In most pts, intoxication passes in a few hours.

Tolerance may develop, as may withdrawal, characterized by dysphoria, irritability, and tremulousness.

Lab: NC.

Crs: Most inhalant addicts use on a daily basis; the long-term course is not known.

Cmplc: School failure and truancy are common; some pts may suffocate on plastic bags.

Inhalant-induced dementia (see 3.15) may occur after years of use.

The common contaminant n-hexane may cause a motor peripheral polyneuropathy.

Etiol: Inhalants both increase neuronal membrane fluidity and interact with GABA receptors.

There is an association between inhalant dependence and antisocial personality disorder; however, the direction of causality is not clear.

Ddx: Alcohol or cannabis intoxication present in a similar fashion but is distinguished by the presence of conjunctival injection and the absence of an odor of solvents.

Rx: Uncomplicated intoxication requires only observation; benzodiazepines may increase sedation.

Abstinence is the overall goal, but few inhalant users stay in treatment.

4.12 NICOTINE-RELATED DISORDERS

Arch Gen Psychiatry 1991;48:52. JAMA 1993;269:1268. J Clin Psychopharm 1994;14:41. NEJM 1985;313:491.

Epidem: Lifetime prevalence of nicotine dependence ~30% in the USA.

Sx: Most nicotine-dependent pts obtain nicotine by smoking cigarettes; cigarette smoking usually begins in adolescence, and within from months to 3 yr dependence becomes established.

Inhaled nicotine is rapidly absorbed through the lungs and reaches the brain within seconds; nicotine has a half-life of ~2 h, and although none of its metabolites have substantial pharmacologic activity, one, cotinine, which has a half-life of ~20 h, may appear in drug screens.

Intoxication with nicotine is usually mild, esp with the first cigarette of the day; there is a mild sense of euphoria, associated with a decrease in any irritability, and a slightly enhanced ability to concentrate. Pulse and BP rise slightly, and peristaltic activity increases.

Tolerance may develop fairly rapidly; some smokers, initially only able to tolerate 2 or 3 smokes a day, eventually use up to 60 or more.

Withdrawal appears anywhere from 2 to 24 h after the last smoke and consists of a craving for a smoke, restlessness, irritability, difficulty concentrating, headache, and in some, insomnia. Sx peak in 1–2 d, and then gradually diminish over several weeks. Occasionally, withdrawal sx may persist for several months. Craving for a cigarette may occasionally recur over several years.

Cigarette use may range from 20 up to 100 or more qd; the denial

Table 4.12-1. Complications of Cigarette Smoking

Cancer	**Pregnancy Related**
Lung	Miscarriage
Larynx	Abruptio placentae
Mouth	Prematurity
Esophagus	Low birth weight
Bladder	
Pancreas	**Other**
	Gingivitis
Pulmonary	Esophageal reflux
	Peptic ulcer disease
Chronic bronchitis	
Emphysema	
Cardiovascular	
Coronary artery disease and myocardial infarction	
Stroke	
Peripheral vascular disease	
Raynaud's phenomenon	

SUBSTANCE-RELATED DISORDERS

seen in nicotine dependence is at times breathtaking. Postlaryngectomy pts may continue to smoke through the tracheostomy.

Lab: As noted, cotinine may appear in drug screens; other abnormalities reflect complications.

Crs: Generally chronic and lifelong.

Cmplc: These are listed in Table 4.12-1. Of all these, cancer (esp of the lung), COPD, and cardiac disease are the most important.

"Secondhand" exposure via passive inhalation by innocent bystanders increases the risk of cancer and pulmonary and cardiac complications.

Pipe smokers, if they inhale, incur the same risk that cigarette smokers do; if they abstain from inhaling, they remain at risk for gingivitis and oral cancer.

"Smokeless" tobacco, e.g., chewing tobacco, also incurs the risk of gingivitis and oral cancer.

Etiol: Adoption studies indicate a partial genetic liability to develop nicotine dependence, but it appears that nicotine is a very highly addictive substance. There are very few "social smokers"; most who begin smoking end up dependent.

Ddx: Nicotine abuse, that is to say, continued use despite consequences, without the appearance of tolerance or withdrawal, is unusual. Most quickly pass through this phase into dependence.

Rx: In a direct, nonjudgmental, yet forceful way, tell pts to stop smoking. For those in considerable denial, videotapes of, or visits with, pts with significant complications may be helpful.

For those who want to stop and are unable to do so, behaviorally oriented stop-smoking groups are helpful.

Bupropion (Wellbutrin, Zyban), used as described in 6.1, reduces the craving for nicotine.

Many pts also use a nicotine product to ease withdrawal. Nicotine transdermal patches (e.g., delivering 7, 14, or 21 mg over 24 h) are helpful, and for those who wish to individualize their dose, nicotine polacrilex gum (containing 2 or 4 mg) and the more rapidly effective nicotine nasal spray (containing 0.5 mg per metered spray) constitute alternatives. As a rough guide, 1 cigarette delivers ~1 mg of nicotine; thus, a "pack-a-day" smoker might require the 21-mg patch, 10 pieces of 2-mg gum, or 20 administrations of the nasal spray (1 administration = 1 metered spray to each nostril). Once pts have found a dose and product that prevent withdrawal and craving, then the dose may be reduced slowly. For those unable to successfully taper off the nicotine product, a case may be made for chronic use, as nicotine per se does little damage. It is the "tar" of the cigarette that contains carcinogens.

Weight gain is common after smoking cessation, and pts should be warned about this. If, however, it comes down to a choice between stopping smoking and gaining 10 lb, the weight gain is almost always the lesser of 2 evils.

4.13 OPIOID-RELATED DISORDERS

Acta Psychiatr Scand 1998;97:233. Arch Gen Psychiatry 1985;42:1063. Arch Gen Psychiatry 1993;50:577. J Clin Psychiatry 1984;45:42.

Epidem: USA lifetime prevalence ~0.5%; "epidemics" exist in some urban areas.

Sx: Opioid use typically begins in adolescence or early adult years.

Heroin is most commonly used; others include morphine, meperidine, hydromorphone, pentazocine, and fentanyl. Methadone, used in some treatment programs (see below), at times is diverted for use as an intoxicant.

Intoxication is generally by iv route, sc route is less common, some will "smoke" the opioid, and a few will ingest it. After iv use there is an intense euphoric "rush," which passes in a few minutes to be followed by a drowsy euphoria that may last for hours; some users may "nod off." Miosis, dysarthria, and constipation are common.

Intoxication with meperidine or pentazocine has distinctive features. Meperidine is metabolized to normeperidine, which may cause agitation, mydriasis, hyperreflexia, and seizures. Pentazocine may cause dysphoria, disturbed thoughts, and hallucinations.

Overdose with opioids causes stupor or coma; respiratory depression, pulmonary edema, and death may occur.

Tolerance develops to the effects of opioids *except* miosis, constipation, and respiratory depression.

Withdrawal begins with restlessness, yawning, lacrimation, rhinorrhea, dysphoria, and a craving for the drug. After several hours some pts fall into a restless sleep ("yen" sleep). Later all symptoms intensify and may be joined by waves of prominent gooseflesh (hence the phrase "going cold turkey"), nausea, vomiting, intestinal cramping, and diarrhea. Intense bone pain may also occur, often accompanied by spasmodic leg movements ("kicking the habit"). Temperature, pulse, and BP are all elevated, and mydriasis is present. Although opioid withdrawal per se is not lethal, copious vomiting and diarrhea may lead to hypovolemic shock. For most opioids, withdrawal sx begin within 6–12 h, peak in 2 or 3 d, and then gradually clear over 7–10 d. Meperidine and pentazocine have short half-lives, and the course of withdrawal is more rapid; methadone has a long half-life, with a correspondingly longer withdrawal syndrome.

Protracted withdrawal sx, including depression and insomnia, may persist for weeks to a half year.

Lab: With the exception of fentanyl, which requires specialized testing, urine or serum toxicology screens are generally positive.

Crs: Chronic: The majority of addicts end up incarcerated or dead, due to overdose or medical complications.

Cmplc: Shared needles spread AIDS and hepatitis; unsterilized needles may lead to bacteremia with endocarditis, meningitis, cerebral abscess, mycotic aneurysm, etc.

SUBSTANCE-RELATED DISORDERS

TB is becoming increasingly common among opioid addicts.

"Street" meperidine may be contaminated with 1-methyl-4-phenyl-1,2,3,6-tetrahydropyridine (MPTP), which may cause parkinsonism.

Etiol: Intoxication is mediated by endogenous opioid mu receptors.

Antisocial personality disorder may predispose to opioid dependence.

Ddx: Alcohol, inhalant, and cannabis intoxications are distinguished by the absence of the intense miosis seen with opioids (meperidine is an exception, as it may cause mydriasis, but is suggested by tremor and hyperreflexia).

Rx: Mild intoxication requires observation.

Severe intoxication, with stupor or coma, may be treated with naloxone (Narcan) 0.4–0.8 mg iv q 3–5 min until respirations are normal and pt approaches alertness; take care not to "overshoot" and precipitate withdrawal. Repeat doses required q 30–60 min until the opioid has "washed out."

Withdrawal is so extremely dysphoric that most addicts require admission to a locked unit to complete it. Some may elect to go "cold turkey"; most request some form of treatment, which may include methadone or clonidine (Catapres) and amitriptyline (Elavil). Methadone is available only in specialized facilities. Clonidine (Catapres), helpful for nausea and diarrhea, is given po 0.1–0.3 mg q 3 h until sx are relieved; most pts require 0.6–2.4 mg, which is then continued in divided doses for the duration of the withdrawal, after which it is tapered over 3–4 d and then discontinued. Amitriptyline (Elavil) 25–75 mg hs is helpful for insomnia. Adjunctive treatment includes prochlorperazine (Compazine) for nausea and diphenoxylate (Lomotil) for diarrhea.

Long-term Rx of the opioid addict is controversial: Some advocate "maintenance" Rx with methadone, while others stress abstinence from all opioids.

Methadone maintenance is followed by a reduction in criminal activity and the use of other opioids; most methadone pts, however, turn to other substances, such as alcohol, benzodiazepines, or cocaine.

Abstinence may be facilitated by referral to NA, or for those with concurrent alcohol abuse or dependence, AA. Some pts benefit from Rx with naltrexone (ReVia), a long-acting opioid antagonist, 50 mg qd: Blockade of receptors prevents the intensely reinforcing "rush," and thus reduces the risk of a "slip" turning into a sustained relapse.

4.14 PHENCYCLIDINE-RELATED DISORDERS

Am J Psychiatry 1977;134:1234. Am J Psychiatry 1978;135:1081. Am J Psychiatry 1987;144:1207.

Epidem: Several percent of adolescents "experiment"; prevalence of abuse uncertain.

Sx: Use begins in teenage years; drug taken orally or by smoking.

Mild intoxication is characterized by euphoria and a sense of detachment or dissociation, not only from environment but also from one's own body. Lethargy or agitation may occur, as may bizarre and unpredictable behavior; pts may complain of nausea or vertigo. Other sx include increased heart rate, elevated BP, miosis, nystagmus, dysarthria, ataxia, tremor, hyperreflexia, and myoclonus.

Moderate intoxication is characterized by delirium, often with delusions and hallucinations. Stuporous catatonia (see 3.19) may occur, along with dystonia and rigidity, which may be so extreme as to cause rhabdomyolysis, with possible renal failure. Occasionally, convulsions occur.

Severe intoxication is characterized by stupor or coma, with hyperreflexia and myoclonus; hyperthermia may occur and hypertension may be so severe as to cause hypertensive encephalopathy.

Intoxication may last for hours to days, depending on the dose; characteristically, sx wax and wane.

Postintoxication syndromes occur in a minority. Psychotic symptoms may persist for days to a week; manic sx, for days to a week; depressive sx, for days to several weeks; and delirium, for days to a week.

Tolerance and withdrawal do not appear to occur.

Lab: Urine toxicology is generally positive during intoxication.

Crs: Chronic use may follow a daily or binge pattern; most users eventually stop in their middle years.

Cmplc: Schizophrenia and related disorders are exacerbated by phencycli-

SUBSTANCE-RELATED DISORDERS

dine use; there is controversy over whether chronic phencyclidine use can cause a chronic psychosis.

Etiol: Phencyclidine has multiple pharmacologic effects: blockade of postsynaptic NMDA receptors; binding to sigma receptors; facilitation of dopamine release from presynaptic nerves; blockade of reuptake of dopamine, norepinephrine, and acetylcholine.

Ddx: Hallucinogen intoxication is distinguished by the *absence* of nystagmus, miosis, and ataxia.

Rx: Mild intoxication requires only observation in a quiet environment.

Moderate or severe intoxication requires admission. Both continuous gastric suction and acidification of the urine speed elimination of the drug: Acidification accomplished with 1 gm of either ascorbic acid or ammonium chloride po or iv q 6 h; furosemide (Lasix) is given, and serial U/As obtained to ensure acidification and to check for myoglobinuria. Antacids, H_2 blockers, and proton-pump inhibitors are contraindicated. Haloperidol 5 mg iv or lorazepam 2 mg iv, both q 1 h, may be given for agitation; restraints should be avoided, as they increase risk of rhabdomyolysis and renal failure. Dystonia and rigidity may be treated with lorazepam (Ativan), as above.

Postintoxication psychotic, manic, or delirious sx may be treated with a neuroleptic, such as haloperidol (Haldol) 5–10 mg/d; postintoxication depression requires observation (and generally resolves before any antidepressant could become effective).

Abstinence is the overall goal; as most phencyclidine users also abuse alcohol or cannabis, referral to AA or NA is appropriate.

4.15 SEDATIVE-, HYPNOTIC-, OR ANXIOLYTIC-RELATED DISORDERS

Acta Psychiatr Scand 1978;66(Suppl 270):1. Am J Psychiatry 1984;141: 1580. Am J Psychiatry 1989;146:536. J Clin Psychopharm 1990;10: 237.

Epidem: Dependence on sedatives, hypnotics, or anxiolytics has a lifetime prevalence in the USA of ~1%, and is often seen in combination with dependence on other substances, particularly alcohol and opioids.

Table 4.15-1. Sedatives, Hypnotics, and Anxiolytics

Short-acting Agents (Duration Generally <6 h)

Triazolam (Halcion)
Alprazolam (Xanax)
Paraldehyde (Paral)

Intermediate-acting Agents (Duration Generally 6–18 h)

Oxazepam (Serax)
Temazepam (Restoril)
Lorazepam (Ativan)
Chlordiazepoxide (Librium)
Meprobamate (Equanil, Miltown)
Chloral hydrate (Noctec)
Glutethimide (Doriden)
Ethchlorvynol (Placidyl)

Long-acting Agents (Duration Generally >24 h)

Quazepam (Doral)
Prazepam (Centrax)
Halazepam (Paxipam)
Flurazepam (Dalmane)
Clorazepate (Traxene)
Diazepam (Valium)
Amobarbital (Amytal)
Secobarbital (Seconal)
Pentobarbital (Nembutal)
Phenobarbital (Luminal)

Sx: Table 4.15-1 lists the various drugs in these groups.

Intoxication, when mild, is characterized by euphoria, some emotional lability, some decay in judgment, and often some disinhibition of sexual or aggressive urges. More severe intoxication is accompanied by slowed reaction times, lethargy, dysarthria, ataxia, and nystagmus. Blackouts, similar to alcoholic blackouts (see 4.2), may occur.

Tolerance develops gradually, but may become profound. Some pts may take 200 mg or more of diazepam daily, with little evidence of intoxication.

Withdrawal sx, with therapeutic doses of benzodiazepines, generally do not appear until after 4 mo of use; however, with high-dose use, esp of high-potency, short-half-life agents, sx may appear after only a few weeks. After abrupt discontinuation of the drug, withdrawal sx may appear in as little as 1 d with short-acting agents, 2–3 d for intermediate-acting agents, and 2–6 d for long-acting agents; in the case of some very-long-acting agents, such as diazepam or phenobarbital, a "self-tapering" process may occur, with blood levels falling so slowly that withdrawal sx either don't occur or are very mild. Withdrawal is characterized by anxiety, irritability, drug craving, and autonomic signs such as tremor, tachycardia, diaphoresis, and insomnia. Withdrawal sx tend to peak in 1–3 d for short- to intermediate-acting agents and then gradually resolve over 1–2 wk, whereas for long-acting agents the peak is generally at 5–7 d, with resolution taking 2–3 wk. In some pts, grand mal seizures may occur: These are more likely with barbiturates, and in contrast to alcohol withdrawal seizures ("rum fits"), these tend to be multiple, and status epilepticus may occur. In a minority of pts, generally those who have been dependent on sedative, hypnotics, or anxiolytics for years, and have experienced many episodes of withdrawal, a withdrawal delirium may supervene upon the withdrawal syndrome: While all the sx of the withdrawal syndrome worsen, delirium develops with confusion, disorientation, agitation, and often, hallucinations (visual > auditory) and delusions (typically of persecution).

Lab: Urine or serum toxicology screens are generally positive.

Crs: Chronic; even with treatment only a minority maintain abstinence.

Cmplc: Recurrent intoxication and withdrawal may disable pts; overdose, esp if combined with alcohol or opioids, may be lethal.

Etiol: A fhx of alcoholism increases the risk of sedative, hypnotic, or anxiolytic dependence.

Although some pts trace their dependence back to properly prescribed use of these agents, this is rare. The overwhelming majority of pts prescribed benzodiazepines do *not* become dependent on them. In most cases, these drugs are acquired illicitly.

Ddx: Abuse of sedatives, hypnotics, or anxiolytics is distinguished by the absence of tolerance and withdrawal.

Rx: Intoxicated or blacked-out pts may simply be observed. Should respiratory depression occur with benzodiazepines, flumazenil (Romazicon) may be given. For pts with tolerance, low doses should be used to avoid precipitating seizures (e.g., 0.1 mg iv q 3–5 min); otherwise one may give 0.2 mg iv, followed in 60 sec by 0.3 mg, then after another 60 sec, 0.5 mg, with the 0.5-mg dose repeated q 60 sec until the pt awakens or a total dose of 3–5 mg is given. A lack of response to 5 mg virtually rules out a benzodiazepine as the cause.

Withdrawal may be treated with the original agent, if known, with lorazepam (Ativan), or with carbamazepine (Tegretol). Lorazepam (Ativan) may be given in a dose of 2 mg po q 2 h, or im q 1 h, until the pt is calm or a maximum dose of ~12 mg is given. Once the pt is calm, a regular dose, approximately equal to the amount used in prn doses, is given on a tid or qid schedule, with provision of supplemental prn doses for the first few days. Once the pt is stable and no further prn doses are required, the dose may be tapered at ~10%/d. Carbamazepine (Tegretol) is given in a total daily dose of 400–800 mg, divided into a tid schedule. As the effect may not be seen for a day or so, it may be necessary to use lorazepam (Ativan) for that period of time, after which it may be rapidly tapered over 1–3 d. The carbamazepine (Tegretol) is then continued to cover the expected duration of the withdrawal syndrome, after which it may be tapered over a few days. Withdrawal from barbiturates may not respond to lorazepam (Ativan), or any other benzodiazepine, and the clinician may wish to give phenobarbital 60–90 mg po q 2 h until the pt is calm; a regular dose is then given, approximately equal to that required in prn doses, and may then be tapered at 5–10%/d.

Abstinence is the overall goal of Rx. Those with concurrent alcoholism or opioid dependence may be approached as described in 4.1 and 4.13. The optimum Rx of the minority that solely use sedatives, hypnotics, or anxiolytics is not as clear yet.

5. Schizophrenia and Other Psychoses

5.1 SCHIZOPHRENIA

Am J Psychiatry 1989;146:1267. Am J Psychiatry 1997;154:457. Am J
Psychiatry 1997;154(April Suppl):1. Arch Gen Psychiatry 1982;39:
784. Lancet 1995;346:678. NEJM 1992;327:604. NEJM 1994;330:
681.

Epidem: Lifetime prevalence ~1%.

Sx: Onset typically between late teens and early 30s, may be acute (over
weeks) or gradual (over a year or more), and may or may not be
preceded by a major stress, such as a death in the family.

Clinical features include hallucinations, delusions, loosening of associations, "negative" symptoms, mannerisms, and catatonia.

- *Hallucinations* may be auditory, visual, tactile, gustatory, or
olfactory. Auditory hallucinations generally consist of "voices"
that may command the pt to do things, comment on what the pt
is doing, or repeat the pt's thoughts out loud; the pt often talks
back to the voices. Visual hallucinations may be quite complex,
with scenes, people, or animals. Other types of hallucinations
less common: tactile (e.g., being pierced by needles), gustatory
(e.g., the taste of "poison"), olfactory (e.g., "poison gas").

- *Delusions* may be persecutory, grandiose, referential, or bizarre.
Importantly, with the exception of the paranoid subtype, the
delusions are generally not systematized, nor do they comprise
anything like a logically coherent system of belief. Persecuted pts
may be followed or stalked by the police, FBI, CIA, etc.; grandiose pts may declare their wealth or their confidential relationship
with high government officials. Pts with either persecutory or
grandiose delusions also typically have referential delusions,

wherein they believe that chance events in some way pertain or refer to them: The songs on the radio have special meaning; a passerby tips his hat, and the pt is convinced that his coronation is near. Bizarre delusions include Schneiderian First Rank symptoms: thought withdrawal, wherein thoughts are removed from the pt's mind; thought insertion, wherein alien thoughts are inserted into the pt's mind; thought broadcasting wherein the pt's thoughts are "picked up" and broadcast via television or radio, or perhaps "ESP"; and delusions of "influence" or "control" wherein pts believe that their thoughts, feelings, or actions are in some way directly controlled or influenced by some outside force or mechanical device.

- *Loosening of associations* is characterized by illogicalness, disconnectedness, and incoherence. In extreme cases, a "word salad" may appear where there are no connections between the pt's words and phrases.
- *Negative symptoms* include flattened affect (absence of emotion and facial expression), abulia (absence of urges, drives or motivation), or poverty of thought (absence of thoughts).
- *Mannerisms* consist of gestures, speech, or actions that have undergone bizarre transformation. Fingers may be splayed out and undulating; speech may be sing-song or dysmodulated; pts may walk with mincing or affected gaits.
- *Catatonia* is discussed in 3.19.

Subtypes of schizophrenia include paranoid, disorganized (hebephrenic), catatonic, simple, and a residual category, undifferentiated.

- *Paranoid schizophrenia:* predominance of delusions (often of persecution and reference) and hallucinations (typically auditory), with few other sx; pts often guarded and suspicious
- *Disorganized (hebephrenic) schizophrenia:* predominance of loosening of associations, mannerisms, and flattened, inappropriate, or bizarre affect
- *Catatonic schizophrenia:* predominance of catatonic sx (see 3.19), with the excited and stuporous forms often alternating in the same pt
- *Simple schizophrenia:* predominance of negative sx, often with few, if any, hallucinations or delusions

Lab: NC.

Crs: Chronic: After an initial decrement in overall functioning with the

Table 5.1-1. Differential Diagnosis of Schizophrenia

Schizophreniform disorder and brief psychotic disorder
Mania
Depression
Schizoaffective disorder
Delusional disorder
Secondary psychosis
Dementia and delirium
Personality disorders of the paranoid, borderline, schizotypal, and schizoid types

onset of the disease, subsequent course may be either essentially static or gradually waxing and waning.

Cmplc: Few pts are able to succeed in personal or business ventures. Suicide in ~10%.

Etiol: Genetic and intrauterine factors: Concordance rises from ~10% for first-degree relatives to ~50% for MZ twins, and adoption studies indicate a genetic rather than an environmental mechanism; intrauterine damage, perhaps due to a viral infection, may also be a factor.

MRI reveals ventricular dilatation and mild cortical atrophy, most prominent in the temporal lobes.

Neuropathologic studies reveal cortical neuronal disarray, esp in the temporal lobes, without gliosis or other evidence of inflammation.

Unifying theory states that there is a first-trimester infection with a neurotropic virus in a genetically susceptible fetus, leading to disordered neuronal migration with consequent neuronal disarray and cortical atrophy. Contrary to early theory, there is no evidence for any etiologic role of childhood trauma or faulty child rearing.

Ddx: See Table 5.1-1.

Schizophreniform disorder (see 5.2) and brief psychotic disorder (see 5.5), which are probably very rare, symptomatically are very similar to schizophrenia. Where they differ is in their course, with schizophreniform disorder lasting from 1 to 6 mo, and brief psychotic disorder, from 1 d to 1 mo.

Mania (as in bipolar disorder (see 6.6)) and depression (as in bipolar disorder or major depression (see 6.1)) may cause delusions and hallucinations; however, *critically,* here these psychotic sx occur only within the context of the episode of mania or depression. In the intervals between episodes, these pts are free of them.

Schizoaffective disorder, like schizophrenia, causes chronic psychotic sx; it is distinguished from schizophrenia, however, by the occurrence of sustained episodes of either mania or depression, during which the psychotic sx worsen.

Delusional disorder is distinguished by the general absence of all sx except delusions; furthermore, in contrast with schizophrenia, the delusions seen in delusional disorder are highly systematized and often appear plausible.

Secondary psychoses are discussed in 5.10.

Dementia and delirium may be characterized by delusions and hallucinations, but are distinguished from schizophrenia by the presence of significant intellectual deficits. At times, during exacerbation, pts with schizophrenia may also experience confusion and be unable to calculate or do abstractions. Here, however, in the natural course of events, these sx eventually clear, leaving the pt only with the typical clinical picture described above.

Paranoid personality disorder (see 14.1) is distinguished by the general absence of hallucinations, delusions, loosening of associations, etc. Borderline personality disorder (see 14.5) may, under great stress, produce hallucinations or delusions; however, these are transient, in contrast to the enduring nature of sx in schizophrenia; schizotypal (see 14.3) and schizoid (see 14.2) personality disorders are distinguished from simple schizophrenia by their stability over time, without any initial decrement in functioning.

Rx: Almost all pts require a neuroleptic; see Figure 5.1-1.

Select a neuroleptic from those listed in Table 5.1-2. Neuroleptics are divided into 2 overall groups: "typical" (or "classical") and "atypical." By and large, atypical neuroleptics are therapeutically superior to the typical neuroleptics, and of the 3 atypical neuroleptics, 2 of them, risperidone (Risperdal) and olanzapine (Zyprexa), overall have fewer SEs than any of the typical neuroleptics. Clozapine (Clozaril), the other atypical neuroleptic, although clearly therapeutically superior to any other neuroleptic in the world, has so many SEs (including agranulocytosis) that it is held in reserve for treatment-resistant cases. The place of quetiapine (Seroquel) relative to risperidone, olanzapine, and clozapine is not clear: It may or may not have atypical characteristics, and further study is needed. In general, if the pt can afford either risperidone (Risperdal) or olanzapine (Zyprexa), then 1 of these should be chosen first: Of the 2, olanzapine (Zyprexa) is probably marginally supe-

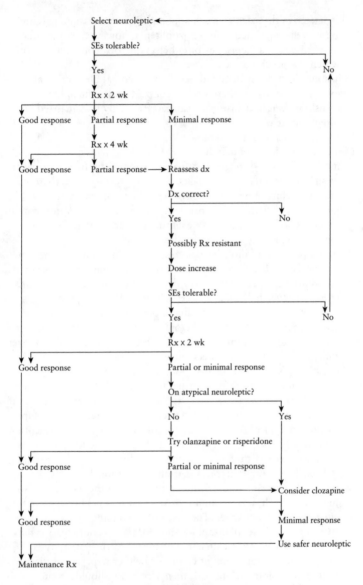

Figure 5.1-1. Algorithm for neuroleptic treatment.

Table 5.1-2. Neuroleptics

	Sedation	Orthostatic Hypotension	Anticholinergic	Extrapyramidal SEs	Average Dose (Range) in mg
Typical					
Low Potency					
Chlorpromazine (Thorazine)	+++	+++	+++	+	100–300 (50–1500)
Thioridazine (Mellaril)	+++	+++	+++	+	100–300 (50–800)
Mesoridazine (Serentil)	+++	+++	+++	+	100–300 (50–800)
High Potency					
Trifluoperazine (Stelazine)	+	+	+	+++	5–15 (2.5–40)
Perphenazine (Trilafon)	+	+	+	+++	8–16 (2–48)
Thiothixene (Navane)	+	+	+	+++	5–15 (2–40)
Pimozide (Orap)	+	+	+	+++	4–8 (2–15)
Fluphenazine (Prolixin)	+	+	+	+++	5–15 (2.5–40)
Haloperidol (Haldol)	+	+	+	+++	5–15 (2–40)
Medium Potency					
Loxapine (Loxitane)	++	++	++	++	50–100 (25–300)
Molindone (Moban)	++	++	++	++	50–100 (25–300)
Atypical					
Risperidone (Risperdal)	+–	++	+–	+–	4–8 (3–12)
Olanzapine (Zyprexa)	+–	+–	+–	+–	7.5–12.5 (5–15)
Clozapine (Clozaril)	+++	+++	++	+– –	300–450 (150–900)
Quetiapine (Seroquel) *(possibly atypical)*	+	++	+	+–	300–350 (200–750)

+++ = severe; ++ = moderate; + = mild; +– = minimal; +– – = negligible.

SCHIZOPHRENIA AND OTHER PSYCHOSES

rior to risperidone, in terms of SEs and therapeutic efficacy. If circumstances dictate using a typical neuroleptic, the choice is based, for the most part, on SE profile: "Low-potency" agents tend to cause sedation, hypotension, and anticholinergic effects (dry mouth, blurry vision, urinary hesitancy or retention, constipation), but have a low potential for extrapyramidal SEs (see below); conversely, "high-potency" agents, although having little tendency to cause sedation, hypotension, or anticholinergic effects, are much more likely to cause extrapyramidal SEs. The "medium-potency" agents fall between these extremes. Further data regarding the neuroleptics are provided in 16.1.

Extrapyramidal SEs include parkinsonism, dystonia, and akathisia, discussed, respectively, in 15.1, 15.2, and 15.4.

In some cases, choosing among the typical neuroleptics is straightforward: Cardiovascular pts (who would poorly tolerate a fall in BP) or pts with benign prostatic hypertrophy (who are prone to develop urinary retention) should generally not be given a low-potency agent; conversely, pts, say, in traction who would not tolerate a dystonia or an akathisia should probably not be started on a high-potency agent. All other things being equal, if a typical neuroleptic is indicated, choose a high-potency agent, and of the high-potency agents, either fluphenazine (Prolixin) or haloperidol (Haldol) should be selected, as both of these are available in long-acting "depot" preparations (see below).

Initial dosage should be somewhere in the "average" range, with lower doses for the elderly, debilitated, or those with significant hepatic failure. Low-potency typical neuroleptics should be titrated up in approximately one-third to one-half total dose increments q 2–3 d. High-potency typical neuroleptics and risperidone (Risperdal) and olanzapine (Zyprexa), in general, do not require titration.

SEs such as sedation, hypotension, and anticholinergic effects lessen with time or dose reduction; extrapyramidal SEs are often treatable, as described in 15.1 for parkinsonism, 15.2 for dystonia, and 15.4 for akathisia.

SEs, to a minimal degree, are present in almost all pts, and tolerability varies from pt to pt; intolerable SEs call for selecting a different neuroleptic, based on the SE profiles in Table 5.1-2.

Rx initially should last ~2 wk in order to assess effectiveness. In case of a minimal response, the dx should be reassessed; in case of a partial response, an additional 4 wk is allowed to assess full effect; and if the response is still only partial, then the dx should be reassessed.

Diagnosis should be suspected if there is only a minimal or no response at this point, as discussed in ddx, above.

Possible treatment resistance calls for a significant dose increase; if SEs tolerable, then give a 2-wk trial; if intolerable, then select a different neuroleptic based on the SE profile in Table 5.1-2, and repeat the algorithm. If the pt is not already on olanzapine (Zyprexa) or risperidone (Risperdal), then 1 of these should be tried; if the response to 1 of these is only partial, then clozapine (Clozaril) should be considered.

Clozapine consideration takes into account the risk of agranulocytosis. If the clinical condition justifies this risk, then clozapine (Clozaril) should be tried, and if a good response follows, continued. Clozapine is begun at 25–50 mg/d, and the dose is increased in 25–50-mg increments daily until unacceptable SEs occur or a total dose of ~400 mg is reached; during the initial titration the total daily dose is divided into a tid schedule; once a dose of ~400 mg is reached, the daily dose is divided into a bid schedule. Preliminary data suggest that steady-state clozapine levels >350 ng/mL are more likely to be therapeutic. Some patients may require up to 900 mg daily to achieve a response. Although it may take 6 mo to see a full response, most pts show significant benefit after ~6 wk; a lack of significant benefit at this point should prompt discontinuation of the drug rather than continuation of the risk of agranulocytosis. WBC count is obtained before Rx, then weekly for the first 6 mo, and biweekly thereafter. Should clozapine be stopped, WBC counts should be continued for 4 wk. Once a response has been achieved, the dose may often be gradually reduced, often to ~300 mg, without loss of effectiveness.

Maintenance treatment is indicated in almost all pts. As a chronic disease, schizophrenia generally requires chronic Rx with dosages generally "titrated" to the severity of any remaining sx. Dose adjustments generally are made no more frequently than q 3–4 mo.

Depot preparations of either fluphenazine (Prolixin) or haloperidol (Haldol) are long-acting decanoate preparations, given im, and greatly facilitate compliance. Fluphenazine decanoate (Prolixin Decanoate) is given at 12.5–50 mg (average 25 mg) q 14 d; haloperidol decanoate (Haldol Decanoate) at 150–250 mg (average 200 mg) q 28 d. Pts not previously exposed to the short-acting oral preparations should be started on these first, before giving a decanoate, to ensure safety and tolerability.

Tardive dyskinesia (discussed further in 15.7) is a late-appearing (typically after years of treatment) SE of neuroleptics, which, in contrast to the extrapyramidal SEs discussed above, does not promptly clear with cessation of Rx. Indeed, although in some pts, sx of tardive dyskinesia may gradually resolve several months after discontinuation of the neuroleptic, in the majority, sx are chronic. Generally, tardive dyskinesia presents with choreiform movements; tardive akathisia or dystonia occur in a minority.

Psychosocial measures complement neuroleptic treatment, and may include case management and half-way houses.

5.2 SCHIZOPHRENIFORM DISORDER

Am J Psychiatry 1994;151:815. Arch Gen Psychiatry 1967;16:693. Arch Gen Psychiatry 1986;43:324. Br J Psychiatry 1990;157:351.

Epidem: Probably rare, perhaps very rare.

Sx: Onset from the late teens to the early 30s, typically acute following a major stress, in a pt with an essentially normal premorbid personality.

Sx are similar to those seen in schizophrenia, and may include delusions, hallucinations, and loosening of associations. In most pts, these are accompanied by confusion or perplexity, depressive sx, or agitation. "Negative" sx, such as flattening of affect, abulia, and poverty of thought, are conspicuously absent.

Lab: NC.

Crs: In the natural course of events, sx persist for at least a month, and remit *spontaneously* and *fully* within 6 mo.

Cmplc: These are similar to those seen in schizophrenia.

Etiol: Uncertain, but a similarity with schizophrenia is suspected.

Ddx: Schizophrenia is distinguished by its chronic, *non*remitting course, with pts remaining ill at least for 6 mo, typically for their entire lives. The ddx between schizophrenia and schizophreniform disorder *cannot* be made with certainty unless the pt is observed to undergo a spontaneous complete remission within 6 mo; thus, in evaluating a pt who is currently psychotic but has been ill for less than 6 mo, or a pt who has been treated before 6 mo has passed and has fully remitted *with treatment,* the dx of schizophreniform must be considered provisional only. Furthermore, in considering the dx of schizophreniform disorder, you must be certain that there has been a *full* and *complete* remission of sx. Many pts with schizophrenia experience partial, but far-reaching, spontaneous remissions that leave them, to casual inspection, well. Close inspection, however, will reveal residual sx, such as mannerisms, quietly bizarre thoughts, etc. If these strict ddx considerations are applied, the dx of schizophreniform disorder is very rarely, if ever, warranted.

Brief reactive psychosis is distinguished by its extreme brevity, with sx remitting spontaneously in <1 mo.

Manic episode, as may be seen in bipolar disorder, is distinguished by the presence of hypomanic sx *preceding* the appearance of psychotic sx. As stage I mania can be very brief, lasting sometimes only a day or less, not only the pt but also collateral sources must be *carefully* interviewed regarding this point.

Secondary psychoses are discussed in 5.10; particular attention should be paid to the possibility of drug intoxication with hallucinogens, phencyclidine, or stimulants.

Rx: This is similar to that described for schizophrenia. In pts in whom sx remit entirely with treatment, it is appropriate, after a matter of months, to gradually taper the neuroleptic, watching for any signs of relapse. If the dx is correct, then Rx will not be required beyond 6 mo of the onset of the illness; if sx persist beyond that point, then the dx must be revised.

5.3 SCHIZOAFFECTIVE DISORDER

Arch Gen Psychiatry 1974;31:632. Can J Psychiatry 1992;37:335. J Nerv Ment Dis 1982;170:646.

Epidem: Uncertain; probably substantially less prevalent that schizophrenia.

Sx: Onset similar to that for schizophrenia.

Disorder characterized by *chronic, unremitting* psychotic symptoms, similar to those seen in schizophrenia, in the course of which appear discrete episodes, each lasting >2 wk, of mood disturbance, either depressive or manic (for a description of a depressive episode, see 6.1; for a manic episode, see 6.6). Importantly, although the psychotic sx undergo an exacerbation during the episode of mood disturbance, and then partially resolve after the mood episode clears, the psychotic sx do *not* clear completely, but *persist* in between the episodes of mood disturbance. The episodes of mood disturbance themselves occur at various times, generally with long intervals between them.

In pts in whom only depressive episodes occur, the dx is schizoaffective disorder, depressed type; in pts who have at least 1 manic episode, the dx is schizoaffective disorder, bipolar type.

Lab: NC.

Crs: Chronic.

Cmplc: Similar to those for schizophrenia (see 5.1) and during episodes of mood disturbance, to those described for depression (see 6.1) and for mania (see 6.6). During depressive episodes, pts with schizoaffective disorder are at high risk for suicide.

Etiol: Familial; not clear if schizoaffective disorder is a disease sui generis and "runs true," or whether it represents an inheritance of 2 separate illnesses (i.e., schizophrenia plus either major depression or bipolar disorder), which then present as an "amalgamation" in the individual pt.

Ddx: Schizophrenia is distinguished by the *absence* of sustained episodes of mood disturbance. Pts with schizophrenia not uncommonly experience depression, and at times may experience certain manic sx, but in schizophrenia these mood sx are generally not severe, and more importantly, are not sustained, lasting perhaps hours or days at the most.

Major depression and bipolar disorder are characterized by discrete, sustained, episodes of mood disturbance, which at times may be accompanied by psychotic sx. Critically, however, these psychotic sx occur only in the "context" of the mood disturbance and do *not* persist in the intervals between them.

Rx: Neuroleptics are given on a chronic basis, using the procedure as outlined in 5.1

Schizoaffective disorder, depressed type, when a depressive episode occurs, often requires Rx with an antidepressant, as discussed in 6.1. Importantly, unlike major depression, the depression seen in schizoaffective disorder does not respond to psychotherapy.

Whether or not chronic Rx with an antidepressant is required depends on the frequency and severity of the depressive episodes, as discussed in 6.1.

Schizoaffective disorder, bipolar type, requires treatment with a mood stabilizer, as discussed in 6.6.

Psychosocial measures are as noted for schizophrenia in 5.1.

5.4 DELUSIONAL DISORDER

Am J Psychiatry 1989;146:1261. Arch Gen Psychiatry 1980;37:699. Br J Psychiatry 1982;141:344. J Clin Psychiatry 1996;57(Suppl 3):32.

Epidem: Lifetime prevalence ~0.05%.

Sx: Onset gradual, in middle years.

Characterized by *systematized, encapsulated* delusions, which, rather than being bizarre, retain a certain *plausibility*. Hallucinations may or may not be present; if present they are mild and play a very minor role in the overall clinical picture.

- *Systematization* is evident in the orderly development of a logically coherent set of beliefs which stem from 1, or at the most, a few delusional premises.
- *Encapsulation* is evident in that outside the area covered by the delusional system, the pt's behavior is typically normal.
- *Plausibility* of the pt's delusional system may mislead the diagnostician; e.g., the belief that one's coworkers are colluding in an attempt to have someone fired is, on the face of it, believable. Bizarre delusions (e.g., that a computer has been implanted in the pt's brain) are conspicuously absent.

Delusional disorder is divided into several subtypes, based on the predominant delusional theme: persecutory, grandiose, erotomanic, jealous, and somatic. In all subtypes, pts also typically have delusions of reference, wherein they misinterpret actual events in a way that reinforces the primary delusion (e.g., the delusion that coworkers were conspiring to fire a pt might be reinforced by the misinterpretation that a group of workers on a coffee break were, in fact, actively plotting).

- The persecutory subtype is characterized by delusions of conspiracy or persecution, often involving the FBI, CIA, judiciary, etc.

- The grandiose subtype is characterized by delusions of grandeur, high descent, or wealth. Pts may believe themselves to be confidantes of presidents, descendants of kings, or possessors of huge, but secret, fortunes.
- The erotomanic subtype is characterized by a delusion to the effect that the pt is secretly loved by someone else, usually someone of high public station, such as a politician or film star. Such pts are convinced that the other person for some reason is constrained from a show of love, and may follow, or even stalk the other person.
- The jealous subtype is characterized by a delusion on the pt's part that the significant other, whether lover or spouse, has been unfaithful. All manner of trivial phenomena are taken as "proof," and the significant other may be punished or placed under "house arrest."
- Somatic subtype is characterized by a belief that something is wrong with a body part. In the "olfactory reference syndrome," pts are convinced that they have loathsome body odor; in "parasitosis," pts are convinced that they are infested with vermin or bugs of some sort, and may excoriate themselves.

Lab: NC.

Crs: Chronic, waxing and waning.

Cmplc: Related to the primary delusion: Persecuted pts may take flight to escape their persecutors, sometimes to other states or countries; erotomanic pts may kidnap their "secret" lovers; jealous pts may murder their significant others. Importantly, as noted above, outside the area of delusional concern, these pts typically behave normally and thus incur no complications. The jealous pt, outside the home, may be a model employee, and helpful to neighbors.

Etiol: Uncertain; delusional disorder is not related to schizophrenia.

Ddx: Schizophrenia is distinguished by the unsystematized and implausible nature of its delusions. Even in paranoid schizophrenia, the most "organized" of the subtypes, the various delusions are often contradictory, and often include bizarre beliefs (e.g., computer chips controlling thoughts). Furthermore, in schizophrenia, other sx, such as hallucinations and loosening of associations, play a major role.

Depression, as in major depression (see 6.1) when severe, may include delusions, often of persecution. In contrast to delusional disorder, however, the depressed pt typically feels the persecution is justified, perhaps as punishment for multiple sins; furthermore, once the depressive episode clears, either spontaneously or by virtue of Rx, the delusion of persecution clears also.

Mania, as seen in bipolar disorder (see 6.6), is often characterized by delusions of grandeur when the pt is euphoric, and by delusions of persecution when the pt is irritable; here, however, as in depression, the delusions clear when the episode of mood disturbance does.

Intoxication with cocaine, amphetamines, or cannabis may be accompanied by delusions of persecution, which, in some pts, may persist beyond the intoxication per se. The inception of the delusions during intoxication suggests the correct dx.

Alcoholic paranoia (see 5.8) is suggested by the severity of the preceding, long-established alcoholism.

Dementia (see 3.2) may be accompanied by delusions, generally of persecution; here the coexistence of a global intellectual deficit suggests the correct dx.

Secondary psychoses are discussed in 5.10.

Paranoid personality disorder (see 14.1) is distinguished by, at most, transient delusions, in contrast to the chronic presence of delusions in delusional disorder.

Rx: Neither agree nor disagree with pt, but adopt an attitude of studied neutrality and make suggestions with tact and diplomacy.

Consider a neuroleptic, but offer it, not for "delusions," but for a more neutral, though still appropriate, indication, such as "nerves," or perhaps for sleep if the pt complains of insomnia. If the pt agrees to a trial of a neuroleptic, select 1 using the algorithm presented in Figure 5.1-1. Olanzapine (Zyprexa) 10 mg hs is probably the best choice. If the pt is not compliant, but willing to consider a decanoate preparation, then try a low dose of haloperidol decanoate (Haldol Decanoate) (e.g., 50–100 mg q 28 d), increasing the dose very gradually, always being careful to avoid SEs, as these pts often tolerate SEs poorly.

Hospitalization, on an involuntary basis if necessary, is indicated when violence threatens.

5.5 BRIEF PSYCHOTIC DISORDER

Acta Psychiatr Scand 1988;78:627. J Nerv Ment Dis 1982;170:657.
    J Nerv Ment Dis 1988;176:72. J Nerv Ment Dis 1988;176:82.

Epidem: Uncertain; probably very rare.

Sx: Onset from the late 20s to the early 30s, typically acute following a major stress, in a pt with an essentially normal premorbid personality.

Sx are similar to those seen in schizophrenia, and may include delusions, hallucinations, and loosening of associations. In most pts, these are accompanied by profound confusion and emotional turmoil. "Negative" sx, such as flattening of affect, abulia, and poverty of thought, are conspicuously absent.

Lab: NC.

Crs: In the natural course of events, sx persist for at least a day, and remit *spontaneously* and *fully* within 1 mo.

Cmplc: These are similar to those seen in schizophrenia.

Etiol: Uncertain.

Ddx: Schizophreniform disorder is distinguished by its course, with sx persisting longer than 1 mo. The ddx between schizophreniform disorder and brief psychotic disorder *cannot* be made with certainty unless the pt is observed to undergo a spontaneous complete remission within 1 mo; thus, in evaluating a pt who is currently psychotic but has been ill for <1 mo, or a pt who has been treated before 1 mo has passed and has fully remitted *with treatment,* the dx of brief psychotic disorder must be considered provisional only. Furthermore, in considering the dx of brief psychotic disorder, you must be certain that there has been a *full* and *complete* remission of sx. If these strict ddx considerations are applied, the dx of brief psychotic disorder is very rarely, if ever, warranted.

Manic episode, as may be seen in bipolar disorder, is distinguished by the presence of hypomanic sx *preceding* the appearance of psychotic sx. As stage I mania can be very brief, lasting sometimes only a day or less, not only the pt but also collateral sources must be *carefully* interviewed regarding this point.

Postpartum psychosis is distinguished by its appearance early in the puerperium. Some authors consider postpartum psychosis to be a "brief psychotic disorder," but given its etiologic relationship to the puerperium and the neuroendocrine events accompanying it, this seems inappropriate.

Secondary psychoses are discussed in 5.10; particular attention should be paid to the possibility of drug intoxication with hallucinogens, phencyclidine, or stimulants.

Rx: This is similar to that described for schizophrenia. In pts in whom sx remit entirely with treatment, it is appropriate, after a matter of time, to gradually taper the neuroleptic, watching for any signs of relapse. If the dx is correct, then Rx will not be required beyond 1 mo of the onset of the illness; if sx persist beyond that point, then the dx must be revised.

5.6 POSTPARTUM PSYCHOSIS ("PUERPERAL PSYCHOSIS")

Acta Psychiatr Scand 1985;71:451. Arch Gen Psychiatry 1981;38:829. Br J Psychiatry 1983;142:618. J Clin Psychiatry 1985;46:182.

Epidem: 1/1000 primiparous females affected.

Sx: Onset typically acute, even explosive, 3–14 d postpartum.
Confusion, labile mood, agitation, accompanied by hallucinations (auditory > visual) and delusions. Delusions often center on the newborn, who is often considered either divine or demonic.

Lab: NC.

Crs: Spontaneous remission within weeks to several months.
30%–40% risk of relapse during subsequent postpartum periods.

Cmplc: Formation of mother-infant bond disturbed.
Infanticide in ~4%.

Etiol: No conclusive correlation with changing hormonal levels; although this psychosis is clearly related to CNS changes in the postpartum period, it is not clear how.

Ddx: Schizophrenia, schizoaffective disorder, and delusional disorder may all undergo an exacerbation in the postpartum period; they are distinguished by their existence prior to delivery.
Bipolar disorder, in some females, may become "entrained" to the postpartum period, but is distinguished by the occurrence of mood episodes at other times in the pt's life.

Rx: Hospitalization is imperative.

SCHIZOPHRENIA AND OTHER PSYCHOSES

Neuroleptics are very useful, and may be chosen according to the algorithm in Figure 5.1-1.

Mood stabilizers (e.g., divalproex (Depakote), as discussed in 6.6) are useful when agitation and lability are prominent.

Pharmacologic Rx should continue for at least 3 mo, and then tapered gradually, watching closely for any evidence of relapse.

ECT effective, and should be considered in emergency situations.

As pt improves, and while still hospitalized, she may be gradually reintroduced to the infant under the 1:1 supervision of an experienced nurse.

In long-term f/u, should pt desire to have another child, preventive Rx may be considered immediately postpartum, before onset can occur.

5.7 SHARED PSYCHOTIC DISORDER (FOLIE À DEUX)

Am J Psychiatry 1987;144:658. Can J Psychiatry 1995;40:389. Comp Psychiatry 1993;43:120.

Epidem: Rare.

Sx: Onset gradual, typically after living for many years under the influence of a person with an illness such as paranoid schizophrenia or delusional disorder.

Typically the pt has lived an isolated existence, more or less cut off from society, with a dominating individual who openly expresses a delusion, often of persecution, sometimes of grandeur. The pt is generally submissive, impressionable, and dependent, and over time comes to adopt what the dominant person says as true; indeed, given enough time, the pt may come to vigorously defend the delusional beliefs of the dominant partner.

Although in most cases only 1 person has come under the sway of the dominant individual (hence folie à deux), in some cases there may be 3 (à trois) people involved, or even an entire family (folie à famille).

Lab: NC.

Crs: Chronic until the pt is separated from the dominant individual and placed in the company of normal people. Subsequent to such a separation, most pts gradually lose conviction, and finally drop the belief expressed by the dominant one.

Cmplc: Pts, expressing clearly false beliefs, and guided by them, may be further hampered in any efforts to break away from the dominant partner.

Etiol: The adoption of the false belief by the pt appears to be a placating move; it may not be proper to speak of the pt's false belief as a delusion, for it is not autonomous, but rather fades upon separation from the dominant person.

Ddx: The dx is suspected upon interviewing relatives and finding a relative who expresses the same belief, but much more vigorously and confidently. The dx is confirmed when the pt improves upon separation from the dominant one or upon successful Rx of the dominant one.

Rx: Separation or successful treatment of the dominant one.

5.8 ALCOHOLIC PARANOIA (ALCOHOL-INDUCED PSYCHOTIC DISORDER WITH DELUSIONS)

Acta Psychiatr Scand 1961;36(Suppl):7. Br J Psychiatry 1995;167:668. Kraepelin E, Clinical psychiatry, Scholars Facsimiles and Reprints, Delmar, New York, 1981.

Epidem: Uncertain, may be far from rare.

Sx: Onset is gradual, even insidious, after many years of chronic, severe alcoholism.

Pts develop delusions, of either persecution or jealousy, accompanied by delusions of reference; occasionally, bizarre delusions, such as Schneiderian First Rank symptoms, may occur.

Persecutory delusions are often accompanied by guardedness and irritability. Pts may keep the blinds drawn, or carry weapons when they venture outside. Many suspect that others, perhaps the police, or employers, are leagued together, and see "evidence" for this in the police cars that cruise the street, or the "unjustified" reprimands at work.

Jealous delusions typically leave pts angry, even enraged, at their sexual partners for being unfaithful, and pts see "evidence" of this infidelity, even in trivial things: "wrong number" telephone hang ups, the partner arriving home a few minutes late, an unusual smell on the sheets. Some pts become abusive toward their partners, and some may hold them captive to ensure their fidelity.

Auditory hallucinations may occur, but play a minor role. Footsteps may be heard on the roof; there may be some "talking" going on in the heating vents.

Lab: NC.

Crs: With continued drinking, sx gradually worsen, but eventually plateau. With abstinence, sx fade very slowly, over months to a year or more, and eventually either resolve completely or reach a baseline level, which then persists.

Cmplc: Irritability and assault may bring legal consequences.

Alcoholic paranoia, especially with prominent delusions of persecution, makes participation in rehabilitative efforts, like AA, difficult if not impossible.

Etiol: Uncertain; may be related to "kindling" of the limbic system by repeated episodes of alcohol withdrawal.

Ddx: The dx is often missed. After establishing some rapport with an alcoholic, it is *critical,* in a calm, matter-of-fact way, to ask pts how "paranoid" they became.

Paranoid schizophrenia and delusional disorder (persecutory or jealous type) are distinguished by, in most pts, the absence of alcoholism. However, alcoholism may coexist with either of these 2 disorders in the same pt, and in such cases, the timing of the onset of the psychosis relative to the onset of the alcoholism is critical: Should psychotic sx appear early in the course of the alcoholism, then a dx of alcoholic paranoia is very unlikely. When psychotic sx appear after a decade or more of chronic alcoholism, then making a ddx becomes very difficult. The presence of loosening of associations or mannerisms strongly suggests paranoid schizophrenia, as such sx are not seen in alcoholic paranoia; in their absence, however, it may be impossible to make a reliable ddx.

Paranoid personality disorder is distinguished by its early onset, long before the alcoholism could become sufficiently chronic to cause alcoholic paranoia.

Alcohol hallucinosis is distinguished by its relatively acute onset, often during DTs or the alcohol withdrawal syndrome and by the prominence of auditory hallucinations.

Rx: Abstinence is essential.

Neuroleptics, such as haloperidol (Haldol), risperidone (Risperdal), or olanzapine (Zyprexa), used as described in 5.1, may relieve sx sufficiently to allow pts to participate in rehabilitative efforts. In the expectation that the disorder will gradually remit, efforts should be made to gradually taper the dose, and hopefully to discontinue the medication entirely.

5.9 ALCOHOL HALLUCINOSIS (ALCOHOL-INDUCED PSYCHOTIC DISORDER WITH HALLUCINATIONS)

Acta Psychiatr Scand 1990;81:255. Br J Psychiatry 1971;119:549. Can J Psychiatry 1980;25:57.

Epidem: Uncertain.

Sx: Onset typically after many years of chronic alcoholism punctuated by numerous episodes of the alcohol withdrawal syndrome, or more especially, DTs; in most pts the onset itself occurs during withdrawal or DTs.

Auditory hallucinations, often of 2 or more voices (which at times speak with each other), are typical and are often critical or persecutory. Pts have no "insight" into the pathologic nature of the voices, and may strain to "overhear" them, or try and find out where they are coming from. Delusions of persecution, jealousy, and reference may also occur, but these play only a minor role.

Querulousness and irritability are common.

Lab: NC.

Crs: With continued drinking, sx worsen to a certain plateau, then remain chronic. If pts become abstinent soon after the onset, then sx gradually fade over 3–6 mo. With resumption of drinking, however, sx eventually reappear, and importantly, if pts then become abstinent, the sx take longer to resolve, and in some, may never resolve completely.

Cmplc: Absorbed in their hallucinatory experience, pts are often unable to participate in rehabilitative efforts.

Etiol: Strongly suspected that alcohol hallucinosis results from repeated "kindling" of the limbic system by repeated and frequent episodes of alcohol withdrawal or DTs.

SCHIZOPHRENIA AND OTHER PSYCHOSES

Ddx: DTs are distinguished by the prominent autonomic sx, and by the fact that all sx spontaneously resolve after several weeks.

Paranoid schizophrenia is distinguished as suggested for alcoholic paranoia in 5.8.

Rx: As for alcoholic paranoia, in 5.8.

5.10 SECONDARY PSYCHOSIS (PSYCHOTIC DISORDERS SECONDARY TO GENERAL MEDICAL CONDITIONS, AND SUBSTANCE-INDUCED PSYCHOTIC DISORDERS)

Acta Psychiatr Scand 1977;56:421. Arch Neurol 1987;44:289. Br J Psychiatry 1985;146:184. Epilepsia 1991;32:225. Epilepsia 1996;37:551. J Neurol Neurosurg Psychiatry 1997;63:434.

Epidem: Uncertain; certainly commonly seen in hospital or ER practice.
Sx: Onset determined by underlying cause (see below), and ranges from paroxysmal (ictal psychosis) to gradual (e.g., a slowly growing frontal meningioma).

Hallucinations and delusions, in various combinations, are seen.
Lab: Determined by the underlying etiology (see below).
Crs: Determined by the underlying etiology.
Cmplc: Depending on the content of the hallucinations and delusions, and the pt's reactions to them, complications may range from minimal to, in some cases wherein pts act on the psychotic sx, disabling.
Etiol: See Table 5.10-1.

  I. *Medication-induced* psychosis is suggested by the temporal relationship between starting or increasing the dose of a drug and the onset of the psychosis.
 II. *Intoxicants* are suggested by evidence of present or recent intoxication; in the case of alcohol-induced psychoses, there is a long h/o chronic alcoholism.
III. *Epilepsy-related* psychoses are suggested by the h/o seizures. Ictal psychoses are a kind of complex partial seizure and are suggested by their paroxysmal onset; postictal psychoses are separated from the seizure proper by a "lucid interval," lasting $1/2$–6 d; the psychosis of forced normalization makes its

Table 5.10-1. Etiology of Secondary Psychosis

I. Medication Induced

Dopaminergic agents (levodopa-carbidopa (Sinemet), bromocriptine (Parlodel), pergolide (Permax), pramipexole (Mirapex), ropinirole (Requip))
Sympathomimetics
Corticosteroids (e.g., prednisone)
Anabolic steroids
Others (e.g., disulfiram (Antabuse))

II. Intoxicants

Stimulants (amphetamines, cocaine; see 4.7)
Cannabis (see 4.9)
Hallucinogens (see 4.10)
Phencyclidine (see 4.14)
Chronic alcoholism (alcoholic paranoia and alcohol hallucinosis)

III. Epilepsy Related

Ictal psychosis
Postictal psychosis
Psychosis of forced normalization
Interictal psychosis

IV. Choreiform Disorders

Huntington's disease (see 3.11)
Sydenham's chorea (laboratory evidence of rheumatic fever (ASO, ESR) may or may not be present)

V. Endocrinologic Disorders

Cushing's syndrome (in endogenous Cushing's syndrome, violaceous abdominal striae, "buffalo hump"; serum cortisol and ACTH, 24-h urine for free cortisol)
Hypothyroidism ("myxedema madness": cold sensitivity, deepening of voice, hair loss, facial puffiness; thyroid profile with TSH)
Hyperthyroidism (tachycardia, proptosis, tremor, generalized hyperreflexia; thyroid profile with TSH)

VI. Miscellaneous

Associated, often, with focal findings on neurologic exam: tumors, infarction, or MS, esp when any of these involve the frontal or temporal lobes
Wilson's disease (tremor, dystonia, dysarthria; serum copper and ceruloplasmin levels)
Metachromatic leukodystrophy (peripheral polyneuropathy; leukocyte arylsulfate A level)
Systemic lupus erythematosus (arthralgia, rashes, pleurisy, cytopenias, constitutional sx; ANA)
B_{12} deficiency (macrocytosis; B_{12} level, and in doubtful cases, serum methylmalonic acid and homocysteine levels)
Encephalitis (often accompanied by fever and seizures; MRI, LP)

Table 5.10-2. Laboratory Screen for Secondary Psychosis

Urine and serum toxicology
B_{12} level
Thyroid profile with TSH
Serum cortisol and ACTH with 24-h urine for free cortisol
ANA
MRI
Further testing if index of suspicion high:
  EEG
  Genetic testing for Huntington's disease
  Copper and ceruloplasmin levels for Wilson's disease
  Leukocyte arylsulfatase A level for metachromatic leukodystrophy
  LP for encephalitis

appearance when anticonvulsants have not only stopped seizures but also "normalized" the EEG; and the interictal psychosis is suspected when, after years of uncontrolled seizures, pts gradually develop a psychosis which, symptomatically, resembles that seen in schizophrenia.

IV. *Choreiform* disorders are suggested by the concurrence of psychosis and chorea. Huntington's disease is the most common cause

V. *Endocrinologic* disorders are suggested by their specific clinical features, noted in Table 5.10-1.

VI. *Miscellaneous* causes are suggested by clinical features noted in Table 5.10-1; a meticulous hx, general PE, and neurologic examination are required.

Should a secondary psychosis be suspected, but the clinical findings be nondiagnostic, a laboratory "screen," as in Table 5.10-2, may be appropriate.

Ddx: Dementia and delirium are distinguished by the presence of cognitive deficits.

Primary psychoses (i.e., schizophrenia and schizoaffective disorder) are distinguished by the absence of the associated items from hx and exam noted in pts with secondary psychosis.

Rx: Rx the underlying cause, if possible.

Symptomatic Rx, if necessary, is similar to that described for schizophrenia (see 5.1).

6. Mood Disorders

6.1 MAJOR DEPRESSION (UNIPOLAR DEPRESSION)

Am J Psychiatry 1976;133:905. Am J Psychiatry 1986;143:18. Arch Gen Psychiatry 1971;24:215. J Clin Psychiatry 1998;59(Suppl 16):13. NEJM 1986;314:1329.

Epidem: Lifetime prevalence ~10%; male-female ratio 1:2.

Sx: Major depression is characterized by episodes of depression separated by more or less sx-free intervals; the first episode of depression typically appears in the mid-20s, with a wide range, from childhood to old age.

Depressive episodes last anywhere from 2 wk up to several years, averaging about 6–12 mo. During the episode, pts experience a persistent sense of depression or anhedonia. Pts may describe their mood as depressed, sad, blue, or irritable; *anhedonia* indicates an inability to take pleasure in formerly pleasurable activities, often coupled with a pervasive lack of interest. In addition, pts typically experience other sx, such as anergia, difficulty with concentration, changes in appetite and weight, sleep changes, and psychomotor change. *Anergia* refers to a loss of energy, often accompanied by a definite sense of fatigue. Difficulty with concentration may appear when pts attempt to follow a conversation or read, and find themselves unable to "take in" the material. Appetite and weight are often lost; however, at times these may increase. Sleep is often lost, and insomnia may be initial (trouble falling asleep), middle (awakening in the middle of the night and having trouble getting back to sleep), or terminal (awakening early and being unable to get back to sleep); in a minority, pts may become hypersomnic and experience an increased need for sleep, sometimes sleeping 12 or 16 h a day. Psychomotor change generally tends toward agita-

MOOD DISORDERS

tion; however, at times there may be psychomotor retardation, with thought and behavior being generally slowed down.

Psychotic sx, in some pts, may occur within the context of the depressive episode, and may consist of either delusions or hallucinations. Typically, these psychotic sx are "mood congruent" in that they "make sense" in the light of the pt's mood (e.g., guilt-ridden pts might well believe that they had committed unpardonable sins and hear voices telling them they'd been condemned). Bizarre delusions (e.g., a computer chip controlling the pt's thoughts) do not occur. Occasionally, the depressive episode will evolve into a catatonic stupor (see 3.19).

Lab: Dexamethasone suppression test (DST) may show a positive result; however, false-negative results do occur, and the test is not recommended for dx purposes.

Crs: Major depression is characterized by the occurrence of 1 or more depressive episodes during the pt's lifetime; in between episodes most pts are free of depressive sx; in a minority residual, mild sx may "cloud" the interval.

The duration of the depressive episodes and of the intervals between them, although demonstrating wide *inter*patient variability, tend to show significant *intra*patient stability. Thus, in some pts, it may be possible, based on a sufficiently long past hx, to predict with considerable accuracy when the next episode will occur, and how long it will last.

Cmplc: Occupational performance and the ability to sustain personal relations are impaired, and some pts may give up on treatment efforts.

"Self-medication" with alcohol or anxiolytics may lead to substance dependence.

Suicide attempts are common, and completed suicide seen in ~10%.

Etiol: Familial pattern: Prevalence in first-degree relatives is higher than general population, concordance is ~30% for DZ and ~50% for MZ twins.

Disturbance in biogenic amine functioning; e.g., CSF levels of 5-HIAA (a metabolite of serotonin) are low, and platelets (models for CNS neurons) have a decreased number of serotonin uptake sites.

Disturbance in neuroendocrine functioning; e.g., CSF levels of corticotropin-releasing factor (CRF) are high and the DST, as noted above, typically shows nonsuppression of cortisol.

Ddx: "Normal" depression, such as grief or bereavement, may follow closely upon a loss or misfortune, and is proportional, with regard to both severity and duration, to the severity of the precipitant. By contrast, depressive episodes are generally "autonomous" from the environment. Some episodes lack precipitants entirely ("out of the blue"); other episodes may follow upon precipitants but their severity or duration is out of proportion to the severity of the precipitant (e.g., a severe depression after being turned down for a dinner invitation, or any duration of depression >12 mo, regardless of the precipitant).

Bipolar disorder (see 6.6) characterized by episodes of depression and episodes of mania, and a h/o a manic episode rules out the dx of major depression. Since in bipolar disorder, the first episode of the illness is often a depressive episode, the question arises, when evaluating pts who are experiencing a depressive episode for the first time, as to whether the depressive episode is caused by major depression (in which case these pts will experience only depressive episodes for the remainder of their lives) or by bipolar disorder (in which case these pts will, at some point in the future, have a manic episode). Long-term f/u is the *only* way to reliably resolve the ddx. In the natural course of events, pts with bipolar disorder whose first episode of illness is a depressive one will eventually have a manic one either within 10 yr from the end of the initial depressive episode or within the first 5 subsequent episodes of illness, whichever comes first. Thus, if, after a depressive episode, either 10 yr pass or 5 subsequent depressive episodes occur, then the odds that this pt has major depression and not bipolar disorder are >90%.

Dysthymia (see 6.2) is distinguished by a chronic course characterized by low-level sx.

Premenstrual syndrome (see 6.5) is characterized by very brief episodes of depression that are "entrained" to the menstrual cycle, occurring during the luteal phase.

Postpartum depression is characterized by depressive episodes occurring *solely* within the puerperium.

Secondary depression (e.g., as seen in Cushing's syndrome) is discussed in 6.8.

Generalized anxiety disorder (see 7.7), if severe, may resemble a psychomotorically agitated depressive episode; however, in generalized anxiety disorder anhedonia and middle or terminal insomnia are generally absent.

Alcoholism may cause depressive sx; however, these clear spontaneously after 3–4 wk of abstinence.

Stimulant withdrawal may be accompanied by depressive sx but these clear spontaneously, generally within the first week of abstinence.

Rx: Rx proceeds in 3 phases: (1) acute, to effect recovery from the current episode; (2) continuation, to sustain the recovery until, in the natural course of events, the depressive episode in question undergoes spontaneous remission; and (3) maintenance (or prophylactic), to prevent future episodes.

Cognitive behavior therapy is effective for acute and continuation treatment of depressive episodes of mild to moderate intensity, but has not been shown effective for severe depressive episodes; there is suggestive evidence that it may also be effective as maintenance treatment in some pts with major depression wherein the episodes, again, are generally of mild to moderate intensity. Antidepressants are effective for all 3 phases of treatment, and are effective not only for depressive episodes of mild to moderate severity but also for severe episodes.

Acute-phase antidepressant treatment is outlined in the algorithm presented in Figure 6.1-1.

Life-threatening depression (e.g., high risk of suicide, emaciation) should prompt consideration of ECT. ECT, discussed in 16.2, is the *most* effective and most rapidly effective treatment for depression, and in experienced hands, is quite safe.

Select an antidepressant from those listed in Table 6.1-1. By and large, all antidepressants are equally effective from a therapeutic point of view; where they differ is in (1) their potential SEs; (2) lethality in overdose; and (3) drug-drug interactions. In selecting an antidepressant, consider any h/o antidepressant Rx: A good response in the past predicts a good one now, and vice versa. Notable SEs are listed in Table 6.1-1; in addition to these, all the antidepressants, with the exception of nefazodone (Serzone), mirtazapine (Remeron), and bupropion (Wellbutrin), may cause sexual dysfunction (e.g., impotence, delayed ejaculation, decreased vaginal lubrication, delayed orgasm, decreased libido). Lethality in overdose is a major concern: Of the antidepressants listed in Table 6.1-1, the SSRIs (with the exception of fluvoxamine (Luvox)) are safe in overdose, and it appears that venlafaxine (Effexor),

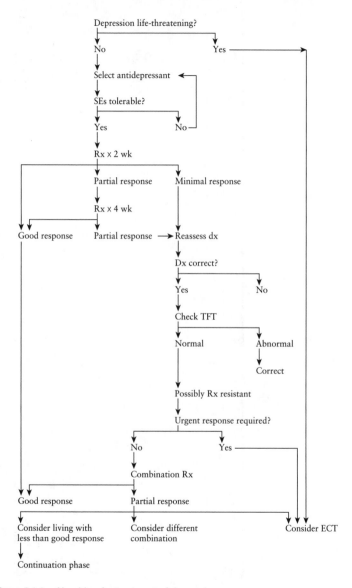

Figure 6.1-1. Algorithm for treatment of depression.

Table 6.1-1. Antidepressants								
	1	2	3	4	5	6	7	8
SSRI								
Citalopram (Celexa)	–	–	–	–	+–	+–	–	20–40
Sertraline (Zoloft)	–	–	–	–	+–	+	–	50–150 (25–200)
Fluoxetine (Prozac)	–	–	–	–	+–	+	–	20 (10–80)
Paroxetine (Paxil)	–	–	–	–	+–	+	–	20–40 (10–60)
Fluvoxamine (Luvox)	–	–	–	–	+–	+	–	100–200 (50–300)
Heterocyclic								
Tricyclic								
Secondary Amine								
Nortriptyline (Pamelor)	+	+	+–	+	–	–	+–	50–100
Desipramine (Norpramin)	++	++	+–	+–	+–	–	+–	150–200 (100–300)
Protriptyline (Vivactil)	++	+++	+	+	+–	–	+–	20–40 (10–60)
Tertiary Amine								
Amitriptyline (Elavil)	+++	+++	+++	+++	–	–	+–	150–200 (100–300)
Imipramine (Tofranil)	+++	++	++	++	–	–	+–	150–200 (100–300)
Trimipramine (Surmontil)	+++	+++	++	+++	–	–	+–	150–200 (100–300)

	1	2	3	4	5	6	7	8
Clomipramine (Anafranil)	+++	+++	++	+++	−	−	+	150–200 (100–250)
Doxepin (Sinequan)	+++	++	++	+++	−	−	+−	150–200 (100–300)
Tetracyclic								
Maprotiline (Ludiomil)	+++	+	+−	+	−	−	+	150 (100–225)
Amoxapine (Asendin)	++	++	++	++	−	−	+	150–300 (100–600)
MAOI								
Phenelzine (Nardil)	+++	+	+	+++	−	−	−	60–75 (45–90)
Tranylcypromine (Parnate)	++	−	−	−	+	−	−	30–40 (20–60)
Others								
Mirtazapine (Remeron)	++	+	++	++	−	−	−	30–45
Nefazodone (Serzone)	++	+	−	++	−	+−	+−	300–400 (200–600)
Bupropion (Wellbutrin, Zyban)	+	−	−	−	++	+	+	300–450
Venlafaxine (Effexor)	+−	+−	−	−	+	+	+	150–225 (100–375)
Trazodone (Desyrel)	+++	−	−	+++	−	−	−	400–500 (300–600)

1 = orthostatic hypotension; 2 = dry mouth, blurry vision, constipation; 3 = weight gain; 4 = sedation; 5 = agitation and restlessness; 6 = nausea, vomiting, diarrhea; 7 = lowered seizure threshold; 8 = average dose (range), in mg. +++ = severe; ++ = moderate; + = mild; +− = minimal; +−− = negligible; −− = absent.

MOOD DISORDERS

nefazodone (Serzone), and mirtazapine (Remeron) may also be safe; the heterocyclic and MAOI antidepressants are all much more dangerous. Drug-drug interactions and other aspects of the antidepressants are discussed in 16.1. All things considered, reasonable first choices include the following: from the SSRIs, citalopram (Celexa); from the heterocyclic agents, nortriptyline (Pamelor); and from the "other" group, mirtazapine (Remeron). In general, MAOIs, given their potential for producing a hypertensive crisis, should not be used as "first-line" agents.

Once an antidepressant is chosen, it must be used at an adequate dose for an adequate duration. Average doses are listed in Table 6.1-1; lower doses are indicated for the elderly, frail, or those with hepatic failure. With the exception of citalopram (Celexa), sertraline (Zoloft), fluoxetine (Prozac), and paroxetine (Paxil) (all of which may generally be started out at the average dose), the antidepressant dose should be "titrated" up in increments of from one-fourth to one-third the total average dose q 3–4 d in order to reduce the impact of SEs. Correlations between blood levels and therapeutic response have been made for the heterocyclic agents, but not other agents. All the heterocyclic agents, with the exception of nortriptyline (Pamelor), have only a "minimum" level, below which a response is not expected; nortriptyline (Pamelor) alone has a true therapeutic "window" such that a response is not only unlikely if the level is below a minimum but also unlikely should the level be above a maximum.

SEs must be closely assessed, and if not tolerable it is reasonable to select another antidepressant that is unlikely to cause that SE.

Treat for an adequate duration. Although 6 wk or longer may be required for a full response, an initial response is generally seen within 2 wk. If the response is at least partial, then continue Rx for ~4 wk further; if the response is good, Rx is then continued, whereas if the response is still only partial (or if it were minimal after the initial 2-wk trial), then the accuracy of the dx should be reassessed.

Thyroid function should be assessed at this point, because hypothyroidism, even if minimal, may blunt the response to an antidepressant. If adequate thyroid function is ensured and the pt still has not responded, then the pt may be considered possibly treatment resistant.

Treatment resistance is first approached by asking if an urgent response is required (e.g., ongoing suicidal ideation, threatened job loss or divorce). If not, then another trial with a single antidepressant may be considered, either by substantially increasing the dose of the present antidepressant (with the exception of nortriptyline (Pamelor), wherein the level must not rise above the therapeutic maximum), or by switching to a different one from a different class; if, however, the situation is urgent, then either proceed to ECT or consider combination antidepressant Rx.

Combination treatments include (1) lithium (Eskalith, Lithobid) (discussed in 6.6 and 16.1) plus either a heterocyclic or an SSRI; (2) triiodothyronine (T_3), 50 mcg qd plus a heterocyclic or an SSRI; (3) MAOI plus a tricyclic (although effective, this is a potentially dangerous combination, and should be left to a specialist). The combination of a tricyclic (with the exception of clomipramine (Anafranil)) and an SSRI (with the exception of fluvoxamine (Luvox)), although not yet confirmed in double-blind studies, is becoming popular; however, the potential for drug-drug interactions is high. Should the combination provide a good response, it is continued; if not, one may opt for ECT, another combination, or perhaps for living with a less than good response.

The above approach to the acute-phase antidepressant Rx of depression is a rough guide only, and good clinical judgment must prevail. Some clinicians routinely check thyroid function at the outset, esp for the severely ill, and some, again for the severely ill, will move to high-dose single-drug treatment immediately.

Continuation-phase antidepressant treatment involves ongoing antidepressant Rx until the underlying depressive episode has had time to run its course. In some pts given single-agent Rx, if SEs are a problem, it may be possible to reduce the dose, and in case of combination Rx, it may be possible to lower the dose or dispense entirely with the augmenting agent. After the depressive episode has had time to run its course, the decision must be made as to whether to discontinue Rx or enter a maintenance phase. Pts with frequent or severe episodes should be encouraged to consider maintenance Rx. If the decision is to discontinue antidepressant Rx, then you should wait until the pt has been sx free for at least 6 consecutive mo, after which the dose may be tapered by one-third to one-half the full continuation dose q 3–4 mo until either discontinued or until sx resurface, at which point the dose should be

raised to the last effective one and further time allowed for the episode to run its course.

Maintenance-phase antidepressant Rx generally consists of the same
Rx as was effective during the continuation phase.

6.2 DYSTHYMIA

Acta Psychiatr Scand 1994;89(Suppl 383):19. Br J Psychiatry 1995;166:
174. Psychiatr Clin 1996;19:121.

Epidem: Lifetime prevalence ~6%.

Sx: Onset gradual, typically in teenage years (type I), or less commonly,
early adult years (type II).

Most of the time, pts experience a depressed or sorrowful mood,
accompanied by low self-esteem, difficulty with concentration or
decision making, pessimism, and fatigue; insomnia and poor appetite may also occur. Sx typically are low level, "smoldering," and
not disabling. Most pts "bear up" under them and succeed in plod-
ding through a joyless life.

Lab: NC.

Crs: Chronic, waxing and waning over many years or decades.

Cmplc: Pts often fail to achieve what they are otherwise capable of; with
onset in early teens, the effect may be crippling as pts fail to complete school or establish mutually satisfying relationships.

Etiol: Dysthymia probably represents a very mild but extremely long-
duration depressive episode of the type seen in major depression.

Ddx: By convention, the appearance of a full depressive episode within
the first 2 yr of chronic depressive sx rules out a dx of dysthymia
in favor of major depression; in pts in whom the chronic mild
depressive sx have persisted for at least 2 yr before a full episode
occurs, convention dictates diagnosing both dysthymia and major
depression.

The appearance of hypomanic or manic sx rules out dysthymia and
suggests either cyclothymia or bipolar disorder.

Normal human unhappiness can be chronic in situations where
repeated misfortunes occur, but most individuals "bounce back"
between misfortunes. In doubtful case, a dx by Rx response may
be appropriate.

Rx: Cognitive behavioral therapy is helpful.

Antidepressants may be used as described in 6.1; given the chronicity of dysthymia, chronic maintenance-phase Rx is generally indicated.

6.3 POSTPARTUM DEPRESSION (MAJOR DEPRESSION WITH POSTPARTUM ONSET)

Br J Psychiatry 1984;144:35. Br J Psychiatry 1988;152:799. Br J Psychiatry 1995;166:191.

Epidem: Uncertain; some studies suggest an incidence as high as 10%–15%.

Sx: Onset is gradual, between 3 wk and 4–5 mo postpartum.

Sx are very similar to those seen in a depressive episode of a major depression, as described in 6.1; anxiety, crying spells, and fatigue tend to be prominent. Occasionally, pts may experience a particularly disturbing obsession: an urge ("horrific temptation") to kill the infant.

Lab: NC.

Crs: In most pts there is a gradual spontaneous remission within months to a year. In a small minority, however, the depression is chronic, lasting for years or even longer. Of those pts who do recover, the chances of another episode after a subsequent pregnancy are as high as 50%.

Cmplc: The pt's ability to care for her child may be severely compromised, and relations with family members become strained. Suicide may occur, and very rarely, infanticide.

Etiol: Uncertain: Some authors believe that postpartum depression represents a major depression that has become "entrained" to the puerperium, with depressive episodes occurring only during those times; others suggest that postpartum depression is a disease sui generis, related, in some as yet unknown way, to the neuroendocrine changes occurring during the puerperium.

Ddx: Postpartum blues are distinguished by an onset within several days.

Postpartum psychosis is distinguished by lability, agitation, and psychotic sx, such as auditory hallucinations.

Major depression is distinguished by the occurrence of depressive episodes outside of the puerperium.

MOOD DISORDERS

Sheehan's syndrome is distinguished by diminished lactation, a failure of menses to resume, and loss of pubic and axillary hair.

Rx: Pharmacologic treatment is essentially the same as that described for major depression (see 6.1) in the acute and continuation phases. Given that most agents are excreted in the breast milk, consideration should be given to bottle feeding. If hospitalization is required, the infant should be cared for by others until the pt has recovered to the point where she can begin to enjoy some success in her attempts at child care. If infanticidal urges were ever present, all mother-infant visits must be supervised until the risk is past. In psychotherapy, pts should be helped to see that it is the illness, and not their character, that has interfered with child care.

Should pts become pregnant again, consideration may be given to instituting preventive treatment in the next puerperium.

6.4 POSTPARTUM BLUES

Arch Gen Psychiatry 1968;18:16. Arch Gen Psychiatry 1991;48:801. Br J Psychiatry 1973;122:431.

Epidem: Seen in >50% of postpartum women.

Sx: Onset acute, usually within the first few days postpartum.

Mood is depressed, anxious, or fearful; occasionally an unstable and brittle euphoria may be admixed. The most striking feature of the postpartum blues is the lability of mood and affect: Uncontrollable crying may occur "at the drop of a hat" or for no reason, and may clear just as suddenly; some women, although unable to stop the tears cascading down their cheeks, may yet insist that they are happy. Minor degrees of fatigue, difficulty with concentration, and insomnia may occur.

Lab: NC.

Crs: Sx remit spontaneously and fully within 2 wk.

Cmplc: Women may doubt their ability to care for the infant, and family members may be upset at the "irrationality" of the sx.

Etiol: Beyond saying that there is a connection with the neuroendocrine events of the puerperium, little is known.

Some authors, citing the high prevalence of the postpartum blues, doubt that it represents a disorder at all, but should be considered normal. The striking symptomatology, however, which is at odds with the pt's functioning outside the puerperium, suggests that it is a disorder, and most women who go through it find it to be one also.

Ddx: Postpartum depression is of later onset, generally >3 wk postpartum.

Postpartum psychosis may have an onset within 3 d postpartum, and may present with striking lability. The subsequent appearance of psychotic sx clearly differentiates it from postpartum blues.

Rx: Reassurance is indicated, and family members may be counseled to provide extra help until the "blues" pass. Antidepressants are not indicated, as the "blues" resolve before they could become effective. Benzodiazepines are occasionally prescribed if insomnia is severe; however, they are excreted in the breast milk and must be used with caution. Lorazepam (Ativan) 2 mg is a reasonable choice.

6.5 PREMENSTRUAL SYNDROME (PREMENSTRUAL DYSPHORIC DISORDER, LATE-LUTEAL-PHASE DISORDER)

Am J Psychiatry 1990;147:1634. Arch Gen Psychiatry 1993;50:467. J Clin Psychiatry 1997;58(Suppl 14):54. NEJM 1995;322:1529.

Epidem: >5% menstruating females.

Sx: Onset anytime after menarche, but usually in late teens or early 20s. Anywhere from 3 to 10 d before menstruation begins, pts experience significant dysphoria (depression, anxiety, lability, or irritability) coupled with other sx, such as fatigue, difficulty in concentration, anhedonia, sleep change (insomnia or hypersomnia), and appetite change (loss or more commonly, increase, often for sweets, particularly chocolates). Concurrently, pts also generally have headache, bloating, breast swelling or tenderness, nausea, or constipation.

Critically, sx resolve spontaneously within 3 d of the onset of menses, and pts then remain free of sx until at least past the halfway point of their cycle.

Lab: NC.

Crs: Over the years or decades, the premenstrual episodes typically gradually become longer and more severe.

Episodes cease after menopause.

MOOD DISORDERS

Cmplc: Work and personal life suffer during the episode; some pts may isolate themselves and stay isolated until the episode passes.

Etiol: Familial.

Hysterectomy does *not* relieve sx, indicating that the episodes themselves are not a psychological reaction to menstruation.

Speculated that an "entrainment" has occurred in the hypothalamus (or related structures) between the processes that regulate the menstrual cycle and those that regulate mood.

Ddx: Dysthymia and depressive episodes (e.g., as in major depression) may undergo an exacerbation premenstrually, but are distinguished from the premenstrual syndrome by the fact that they do not clear within days after menses begins.

Dysmenorrhea (painful menses) begins with menses and not before it.

Rx: Fluoxetine (Prozac) 20 mg qd taken continuously is effective. Alprazolam (Xanax) 1–4 mg qd taken at the start of the luteal phase and continued into the first few days of menses is also effective.

6.6 BIPOLAR DISORDER (MANIC-DEPRESSIVE ILLNESS, CIRCULAR TYPE)

Acta Psychiatr Scand 1998;97:387. Arch Gen Psychiatry 1970;22:262. Arch Gen Psychiatry 1973;28:1641. J Clin Psychiatry 1998;59(Suppl 6):13. J Clin Psychiatry 1998;59(Suppl 6):74. Psychiatr Clin 1996; 19(2):215.

Epidem: Lifetime prevalence ~1.2%; equally common in males and females.

Sx: Over pt's lifetime there are 1 or more manic episodes, and in almost all pts, also 1 or more depressive episodes; critically, in between episodes, pts are generally euthymic and free of sx.

The first episode usually has an onset in the late teens or early 20s, and in a little more than half of pts, the first episode is a depressive one. Over 90% of pts will have their first episode of illness by the time they reach 50.

Manic episodes may appear gradually, over days or weeks, or acutely, over hours to a few days; most episodes last from weeks to several months. Manic episodes are divided into 3 stages: stage I, or hypomania; stage II, or acute mania; and stage III, or delirious mania (many authors lump stages II and III and refer to the combination as psychotic mania). Stage I, hypomania, is characterized by a heightened mood (either predominantly euphoric or irritable), grandiosity, pressured speech, flight of ideas, heightened distractibility, hyperactivity, increased energy, and a decreased need for sleep. In stage II, acute mania, all the sx seen in hypomania are intensified and are joined by delusions, either of grandeur or of persecution. In stage III, delirious mania, a further intensification of sx occurs, and hallucinations (often auditory), incoherence, and bizarre behavior (including catatonia) may appear. In all manic episodes, stage I sx are seen; in the majority of pts, there is an evolution to stage II, but only in a minority of pts does the evolution proceed to the height of mania, stage III. Once the individual episode has reached its peak, there is a more or less orderly devolution of sx, back to stage II, then stage I, and finally euthymia.

Depressive episodes typically appear gradually, over several weeks or longer. The pt with fully developed bipolar disorder experiences depressed (or irritable) mood, poor concentration and memory, anhedonia, fatigue, appetite change (loss or more often, increase), psychomotor change (agitation or more commonly, retardation), and sleep change (insomnia or more commonly, hypersomnia). Delusions, often of guilt and well-deserved punishment, are not uncommon and may be joined by hallucinations, often of voices that condemn or persecute the pt. Most of the depressive episodes seen in bipolar disorder last about 6 mo and resolve gradually.

Mixed manic episodes are seen in a minority of pts and consist of an admixture of both manic and depressive sx. Elated pts may suddenly sink into despair; depressed pts may energetically proclaim themselves as the greatest of all sinners.

Lab: NC.

Crs: The *sequence* of episodes varies from pt to pt; it is rare to find a pt who experiences regularly alternating depressive episodes and manic episodes. Most pts experience a preponderance of 1 type of episode over another.

The *interval* between episodes also varies widely from pt to pt: from as little as weeks to a decade or more. Although in most pts the intervals are sx free and pts remain euthymic, a minority may have mild, residual sx that persist in between full-fledged episodes. In general, the "coloring" of the interval, whether depressive or manic, is consistent with the preponderance of episodes; thus,

MOOD DISORDERS

Table 6.6-1. Precipitants of Manic Episodes

Drugs

Antidepressants
Stimulants (e.g., cocaine, amphetamines)
Sympathomimetics (e.g., pseudoephedrine)
Theophylline
Dopaminergic agents (e.g., levodopa-carbidopa (Sinemet), bromocriptine (Parlodel))
Corticosteroids

Drug Withdrawal

Alcohol withdrawal
Benzodiazepine withdrawal
After discontinuation of chronic Rx with clonidine

Other

Light therapy
Sleep deprivation

---

when the majority of episodes in any given pt are depressive, the interval, if not sx free, will most likely be "colored" by mild depressive sx.

The *number* of episodes during the pt's lifetime depends on the duration of the episodes and of the intervals between them, and ranges from as few as 1 or 2 per lifetime to 4 or more per year ("rapid cycling").

Manic episodes, at times, may be triggered by various precipitants (see Table 6.6-1), and it is critical that pts avoid these.

Cmplc: Manic pts often engage in spending sprees and impulsive sexual relations, and often come into conflict with others, including officers of the law; suicide is seen in ~10%.

For complications of depressive episodes, see 6.1.

Etiol: Adoption and twin studies indicate a strong genetic component, and in some pedigrees linkage has been established to a locus on chromosome 18. Disturbances in functioning of biogenic amines, particularly serotonin, are strongly suspected.

Ddx: Major depression is distinguished by the fact that these pts never, during their lives, have a manic episode; thus, a h/o a manic episode in a pt currently depressed rules out a dx of major depression. Difficulty occurs when a pt has had only 1 or a few depressive episodes, but never a manic one, and the question arises as to whether the pt has major depression and will never have a manic episode, or bipolar disorder, wherein a manic one will eventually appear at some point in the future. This ddx is discussed in 6.1.

Cyclothymia (see 6.7) is distinguished by the "subsyndromal" nature of the sx, which remain mild and never approach the severity of stage I.

Schizoaffective disorder, bipolar type (see 5.3) is characterized by manic episodes and depressive episodes but is distinguished by the fact that in the euthymic intervals between the episodes, the pts *remain* psychotic. In contrast, in bipolar disorder, although pts may be psychotic during the episodes, the intervals between episodes are *never* characterized by psychotic sx.

Postpartum psychosis (see 5.6) is distinguished by the restriction of sx to the postpartum period; by contrast, in bipolar disorder, episodes occur at other times in the pt's life.

Secondary depression and secondary mania are discussed in 6.8 and 6.9.

Rx: *Mania and mixed mania* treated with divalproex (Depakote), lithium (Eskalith, Lithobid), or carbamazepine (Tegretol): see Table 6.6-2 (lamotrigine (Lamictal) and gabapentin (Neurontin) are currently under investigation). Lower doses are used in the elderly or debilitated, and dosage adjustments are made on the basis of SEs, blood levels, and clinical response. For divalproex (Depakote) and carbamazepine (Tegretol), lower doses are indicated with significant hepatic failure, and for lithium (Eskalith, Lithobid), with renal failure.

Divalproex (Depakote) is the most rapidly effective, generally best tolerated, and easiest to use. Load at ~20 mg/kg, and continue the loading dose (divided into bid schedule) beginning the next day: response usually seen in 2–4 d.

Lithium (Eskalith, Lithobid) begun at a total daily dose of 900–1800 mg/d (divided into tid or qid schedule), with higher doses generally required for younger, heavier, and more severely manic pts. Response usually seen in 7–10 d. Lower doses required for those with renal failure, or those taking diuretics, NSAIDs (except sulindac), some ACE inhibitors, and metronidazole, all of which increase lithium levels. Theophylline may decrease lithium levels. The combination of lithium (Eskalith, Lithobid) and fluvoxamine (Luvox) may cause seizures. Once the pt is stable, a time-release

MOOD DISORDERS

Table 6.6-2. Mood Stabilizers

	Divalproex (Depakote)	Lithium Carbonate (Eskalith, Lithobid)	Carbamazepine (Tegretol)
Time to peak	3–8 h	1–2 h	4–8 h
Protein binding	93%	0	75%
Metabolism	Liver; active metabolite	Excreted unchanged in urine	Liver[a]; active metabolite
Half-life	14 h	18–24 h	25–65 h initially; with autoinduction, 12–17 h
Therapeutic range	50–100 mcg/mL	0.6–1.2 mEq/L	4–12 mcg/mL
Notable SEs	Nausea	Nausea	Sedation
	Vomiting	Vomiting	Ataxia
	Sedation	Diarrhea	Dizziness
	Weight gain	Weight gain	Constipation
	Hair loss	Hair loss	Dry mouth
	Hepatitis	Fine tremor	Blurry vision
	Thrombocytopenia	Incoordination	Rash
	Hyperammonemia	Hypothyroidism[b]	SIADH with hyponatremia
		Nephrogenic diabetes insipidus (polyuria and polydipsia)	Agranulocytosis
		Worsening of acne or psoriasis	Aplastic anemia

[a] Carbamazepine induces its own metabolizing enzymes over ~21 d, and with this autoinduction, the half-life falls dramatically and dose increases are generally required to maintain a therapeutic level.

[b] In a substantial minority, lithium induces a primary hypothyroidism, with a fall in thyroxine and a rise in TSH. In most cases, the changes are minor and clear spontaneously; in a minority they progress. The development of hypothyroidism, in addition to bringing the risk of myxedema, also blunts the response to mood stabilizers and to antidepressants, and one of the first signs of developing hypothyroidism in a pt on lithium may be the appearance of a depressive episode. Thyroid profile with TSH should be checked at least q 6 mo in pts on lithium, and exogenous thyroxine is given if sx develop. The risk of clinically significant hypothyroidism is higher in pts with antimicrosomal or antithyroglobulin antibodies, and it is prudent to check for these early on.

preparation is used and the entire daily dose is given hs. Although more difficult to use than divalproex (Depakote), lithium (Eskalith, Lithobid) is a very valuable drug, and every psychiatrist should master its use.

Carbamazepine (Tegretol) begun in a total daily dose of 300–800 mg, divided into a tid or qid schedule. Response usually seen in 7–10 d. With autoinduction (see Table 6.6-2), dose increases to 600–1200 mg usually required; once stable, a time-release preparation may be used, allowing for a bid schedule. Carbamazepine (Tegretol) is difficult to use, and is probably a third-choice agent.

Stage I mania at times may be treated with a mood stabilizer alone; however, in stages II and III, adjunctive treatment is generally required until the mood stabilizer has taken effect. Rapid control may be obtained with adjunctive use of lorazepam (Ativan) 2 mg, haloperidol (Haldol) 5 mg, or chlorpromazine (Thorazine) 50–100 mg, each given q 1–2 h im until the pt is calm, unacceptable SEs occur, or a maximum dose (12 mg lorazepam (Ativan), 60 mg haloperidol (Haldol), 1000 mg chlorpromazine (Thorazine)) is reached. The adjunctive agent is then continued at a total daily dose approximately equivalent to that required in the initial prn doses (divided into a tid or qid schedule), with provision for extra prn doses should breakthrough sx be troublesome. Once the mood stabilizer has become effective, the adjunctive Rx may be tapered and discontinued over a day or 2.

Once the mania has been controlled by a mood stabilizer, Rx must be continued, at a minimum, until the manic episode, in the natural course of events, has had time to run its course. Preventive Rx is then considered (see below).

Depression is treated *first* with 1 of the mood stabilizers (if not already in place), for 2 reasons: (1) Some depressive episodes of bipolar disorder will respond to a mood stabilizer alone; and (2) treatment of a depressed bipolar pt who is not "covered" with a mood stabilizer runs a high risk of precipitating a manic episode. If the depression does not respond to a mood stabilizer alone, then an antidepressant may be added, using the method outlined in 6.1. Once the depression has fully cleared, it is important to taper and discontinue the antidepressant as soon as clinically feasible. Mood stabilizers, although reducing the risk of an antidepressant-precipitated mania, do not eliminate that risk.

MOOD DISORDERS

Preventive treatment with a mood stabilizer should be strongly recommended in any of these situations: episodes (either manic or
depressive) occurring q 2 yr, or more frequently; a h/o episodes of
such severity that a recurrence would be catastrophic; or manic
episodes of such acute onset that there would not be time to insti-
tute effective Rx on an outpatient basis.

6.7 CYCLOTHYMIA (CYCLOTHYMIC DISORDER)

Am J Psychiatry 1977;134:1227. Arch Gen Psychiatry 1983;40:801.
J Nerv Ment Dis 1993;181:485.

Epidem: Lifetime prevalence ~0.4%–1.0%; equally common in males
and females.

Sx: Onset insidious, typically in teenage years.

Pts chronically experience periods of very mild hypomanic sx alternating in irregular sequence with periods of very mild depressive sx;
the periods may last from days to weeks, and between them there
may or may not be euthymic intervals, which never last more than
a month.

Manic periods are characterized by enthusiasm or irritability; pts are
energetic, talkative, and active, and typically seek out other people
and undertake numerous projects.

Depressive periods characterized by depression or irritability;
fatigue and apathy are common and pts tend to be quiet and
withdrawn.

Lab: NC.

Crs: Chronic, perhaps lifelong.

Cmplc: During manic periods, gifted individuals, rather than complications, may experience considerable success in life; those with only
average gifts, however, are prone to ill-considered and rash ventures that often end up in failure. During depressive periods, most
pts fail to live up to their potential. The constant "mood swings"
generally impair personal relationships.

Etiol: Probably a forme fruste of bipolar disorder (see 6.6).

Ddx: Bipolar disorder is distinguished by a full manic or a full
depressive episode. In about one-third of pts with apparent cyclothymia, a full episode eventually appears, and in such pts, the

cyclothymia represents, in fact, a long prodrome to the full bipolar disorder.

Schizoaffective disorder, bipolar type, is distinguished by the presence of psychotic sx, which are never seen in cyclothymia.

Stimulant intoxication, alternating with withdrawal, may closely resemble cyclothymia, and all pts considered for this dx should be screened for drug use.

Borderline personality disorder is distinguished by the reactivity of the pt's mood swings to environmental events. This reactivity is in contrast to the mood swings in cyclothymia, which are autonomous and occur regardless of environmental changes.

Secondary mania is discussed in 6.9.

Rx: Divalproex (Depakote), lithium (Eskalith, Lithobid), or carbamazepine (Tegretol), as described in 6.6, should be used chronically.

6.8 SECONDARY DEPRESSION (MOOD DISORDER DUE TO A GENERAL MEDICAL CONDITION WITH DEPRESSIVE FEATURES)

Arch Gen Psychiatry 1988;45:247. Arch Neurol 1986;43:766. Br J Psychiatry 1983;142:16. J Nerv Ment Dis 1985;173:118. Lancet 1984;1: 297.

Epidem: Probably common.
Sx: Essentially the same as those seen in a depressive episode (see 6.1).
Lab: Reflects etiology.
Crs: Determined by underlying etiology.
Cmplc: Similar to those described in 6.1; importantly, such pts may give up on Rx of the underlying condition that is causing the depression.
Etiol: See Table 6.8-1.
Ddx: Major depression and bipolar disorder are distinguished by their episodic courses, and by the absence of associated features noted in Table 6.8-1.

Dysthymia is suggested by early onset and lack of associated features.

Postpartum depression and premenstrual syndrome are distinguished by their connection with delivery and menstruation, respectively.

Rx: Etiologic condition treated, if possible.

Table 6.8-1. Etiologies of Secondary Depression

I. Focal CNS Lesions

Strokes (esp of left frontal cortex or left caudate)
Tumors (esp of anterior corpus callosum)
Traumatic brain injury
Subdural hematoma

II. Dementing Diseases

Alzheimer's disease (see 3.3)
Parkinson's disease (see 3.9)
Huntington's disease (see 3.11)
Wilson's disease (tremor, dysarthria; MRI, copper and ceruloplasmin levels)

III. Endocrinologic Conditions

Cushing's syndrome (cushingoid habitus, violaceous abdominal striae, hypertension; serum cortisol and ACTH levels, 24-h urine for free cortisol)
Hypothyroidism (hair loss, voice change, cold sensitivity; thyroid profile)
Hyperthyroidism ("apathetic" variant in elderly with atrial fibrillation being a common clue; thyroid profile)
Adrenocortical insufficiency (nausea, vomiting, dizziness, hypotension; in primary adrenal failure, hyperkalemia; serum cortisol and ACTH levels, 24-h urine for free cortisol)
Hyperparathyroidism (nausea, vomiting, colic; decreased Q-Tc interval, hypercalcemia)
Hypoparathyroidism (tetany, seizures; increased Q-Tc interval, hypocalcemia)

IV. Infectious Diseases

AIDS (HIV)
Neurosyphilis (FTA, LP)
Lyme disease (h/o erythema chronicum migrans, arthritis; anti-*Borrelia* antibodies)
Infectious mononucleosis (malaise, fatigue, headache, pharyngitis, cervical adenopathy; "monospot" test)

V. Epilepsy

Interictal depression (h/o chronic, recurrent grand mal or complex partial seizures)
Ictal depression (paroxysmal onset, brief duration; EEG)

VI. Vitamin Deficiency

B_{12} deficiency (macrocytosis; B_{12} level, serum methylmalonic acid and homocysteine levels)
Pellagra (dermatitis, diarrhea; 24-h urine for *N*-methylniacinamide)

VII. Medications

Reserpine
Alpha-methyldopa

Table 6.8-1. (*Continued*)

VII. Medications (*cont.*)

Propranolol
Oral contraceptives
Metoclopramide
Ranitidine
Nifedipine
Pimozide
Clonidine
After abrupt discontinuation of chronic Rx with a drug with strong anticholinergic
    effects ("cholinergic rebound," with dysphoria, nausea, insomnia, seen, e.g., after
    discontinuation of benztropine or heterocyclic antidepressants)

VIII. Associated with Drugs of Abuse

Alcoholism (see 4.1)
Stimulant withdrawal (see 4.7)
Opioid withdrawal (see 4.11)

IX. Miscellaneous

MS (usually with evidence, clinical or MRI, of numerous cerebral plaques)
Pancreatic cancer (weight loss and abdominal pain; abdominal CT, ERP)
Systemic lupus erythematosus (arthritis, rashes, pleurisy, constitutional sx; ANA)
Paraneoplastic limbic encephalitis (seizures; MRI, serum antineuronal antibodies)
Lead encephalopathy (abdominal pain, constipation or diarrhea, anemia; blood lead
    level, erythrocyte protoporphyrin level)
Obstructive sleep apnea (sleep attacks, heavy snoring; polysomnography)

Antidepressant Rx, as outlined in 6.1, useful if etiologic condition
    not readily treatable; citalopram (Celexa) is a good choice. With
    conditions that might lower the seizure threshold, antidepressants
    that may do the same (see Table 6.1-1) should be avoided. Nor-
    triptyline (Pamelor) is effective for poststroke depression.
In case of oral contraceptive–induced secondary depression, pyridox-
    ine 50 mg/d is effective and may allow for continued Rx with the
    contraceptive.

MOOD DISORDERS

6.9 SECONDARY MANIA (MOOD DISORDER SECONDARY TO A GENERAL MEDICAL CONDITION WITH MANIC FEATURES)

Am J Psychiatry 1984;141:1084. Ann Neurol 1990;27:652. Arch Gen Psychiatry 1978;35:1333. JAMA 1979;241:1011.

Epidem: Much less common than secondary depression (with the exception of mania secondary to exogenous corticosteroids, which is not at all uncommon).

Sx: Essentially the same as those seen in a manic episode (see 6.6).

Lab: Reflects etiology.

Crs: Determined by underlying etiology.

Cmplc: Similar to those described in 6.6; in addition, medical care may be greatly disrupted.

Etiol: See Table 6.9-1.

Ddx: The overwhelming majority of cases of manic sx are caused by bipolar disorder, cyclothymia, or schizoaffective disorder, bipolar type. Secondary mania should be suspected in the presence of some of the associated features and conditions listed in Table 6.9-1.

Rx: Treat the underlying etiology, if possible.

With the exception of corticosteroid-induced mania, which responds quite well to lithium (Eskalith, Lithobid), either divalproex (Depakote) or carbamazepine (Tegretol) is preferred for secondary mania, as discussed in 6.6. In pts in whom secondary mania is anticipated (e.g., in a pt with a h/o prednisone-induced mania who requires another course of steroid Rx), preventive Rx is appropriate.

Table 6.9-1. Etiologies of Secondary Mania

I. Drug Induced

Corticosteroids (e.g., prednisone)
Anabolic steroids
Stimulants (cocaine, amphetamines)
Levodopa-carbidopa (Sinemet)
Zidovudine (Retrovir)
Procyclidine
Withdrawal from either reserpine or baclofen (Lioresal)

II. Focal Lesions (e.g., infarctions, tumors), esp affecting the right hemisphere (MRI)

Frontal or temporal lobe cortex or subcortical white matter
Caudate nucleus
Thalamus
Hypothalamus
Mesencephalon

III. Closed Head Injury (MRI)

IV. MS (MRI)

V. AIDS (HIV)

VI. Epilepsy

Postictal
Ictal (simple or complex partial; EEG)

VII. Endocrinologic Conditions

Hyperthyroidism (tremor, proptosis; thyroid profile)
Cushing's syndrome (cushingoid habitus, violaceous abdominal striae, hypertension; serum cortisol and ACTH levels, 24-h urine for free cortisol; note, with endogenous hypercortisolemia, depression is much more likely than is mania)

VIII. Dementing Diseases

Huntington's disease (see 3.11)
Adrenoleukodystrophy (cortical hemianopia or blindness; very-long-chain fatty acid level)
Metachromatic leukodystrophy (motor polyneuropathy; leukocyte arylsulfatase A level)

IX. Miscellaneous

Neurosyphilis (FTA, LP)
Systemic lupus erythematosus (arthritis, rash, pleurisy, constitutional sx; ANA)
Sydenham's chorea
Chorea gravidarum

MOOD DISORDERS

7. Anxiety Disorders

7.1 PANIC DISORDER

Am J Psychiatry 1991;148:361. Am J Psychiatry 1994;151:413. Am J
Psychiatry 1998;155(May Suppl):1. Comp Psychiatry 1994;35:349.
J Clin Psychiatry 1998;59(Suppl 8):47.

Epidem: Lifetime prevalence ~1%–2%; at least twice as common in
females than males.

Sx: First attack typically in late teens or early 20s; onset ranges from
childhood to middle age.

Panic attacks erupt suddenly, often without any precipitants at all,
and sx mount in intensity and number over perhaps a minute or
so: extreme anxiety (sense of "impending doom"), tremor, palpitations, diaphoresis, dyspnea, dizziness, and acral paresthesias. Chest
pain may appear, and may radiate to the left side of the neck. Sx
persist for 5–15 min, rarely for as long as an hour, and then sub-
side over several minutes, often leaving pts "shaken," drained, and
apprehensive for several hours afterward. Most are terrified during
the attack, and fear dying or "going crazy."

Rare variant of "panic attack without panic" wherein the attacks are
identical in all respects to typical attacks with the remarkable
exception that there is little or no sense of panic or anxiety.

Nocturnal panic attacks occur in most pts, and arise out of NREM
sleep; in a small minority, panic attacks occur only at night.

Lab: NC.

Crs: Frequency of attacks varies from daily to monthly; some pts have
an "episodic" course wherein long stretches of frequent attacks
are separated by long intervals of no attacks.

Cmplc: Most common complication is agoraphobia (see 7.2), wherein
the growing anticipatory anxiety over having another attack
makes pts even more reluctant to leave the safety of home.

Abuse or dependence on alcohol or sedative-hypnotics is not uncommon; during withdrawal from these, pts typically experience an increased frequency of attacks, thereby setting a vicious cycle in motion.

Etiol: Panic disorder is strongly familial.

Panicogens are agents that, though innocuous in normal persons, reliably precipitate attacks in pts: lactate infusion; inhalation of 5% CO_2; cholecystokinin; isoproterenol; and the benzodiazepine antagonist flumazenil (Romazicon).

PET reveals asymmetric metabolism in the parahippocampal gyri.

Current theory focuses on the locus ceruleus and the temporal lobes. The locus ceruleus is the source of noradrenergic innervation to most of the brain, and paroxysmal activity here could lead to a panic attack; simple partial seizures arising from foci in the temporal lobes are at times almost identical to panic attacks. Speculatively, paroxysmal activity in the locus ceruleus could, via stimulation of the temporal lobes or their parahippocampal gyri, cause the attacks; panicogens could be exerting their effects via an action on sensitized cells in any of these structures.

Mitral valve prolapse is strongly associated with panic disorder; this association, however, is probably not causal, but reflects some common denominator between them.

Ddx: Anxiety attacks, similar to panic attacks, may be seen with specific phobia (see 7.3), social phobia (see 7.4), posttraumatic stress disorder (see 7.6), and obsessive-compulsive disorder (see 7.5). Critically, however, in all these disorders the anxiety attacks do not occur spontaneously, but only in the presence of specific precipitants. By contrast, in panic disorder, the attacks, for the most part, come "out of the blue." The simple phobic has attacks only on exposure to the phobic objects (e.g., snakes); the social phobic, only in certain social situations (e.g., public speaking); the posttraumatic pt, only on exposure to events reminiscent of the original trauma (e.g., war movies in combat veterans); and the obsessive-compulsive pt, only to certain objects or situations (e.g., a "contaminated object" in a compulsive hand washer).

Secondary causes of panic attacks are discussed in 7.8.

Rx: See Table 7.1-1 for agents that may prevent attacks.

Antidepressants are first choice: of the SSRIs, sertraline (Zoloft); of the tricyclics, nortriptyline (Pamelor). The antidepressant should be started in a very low dose (e.g., 12.5–25 mg sertraline (Zoloft)

Table 7.1-1. Agents Effective for Preventing Panic Attacks

Antidepressants	Benzodiazepines
SSRIs	Alprazolam (Xanax)
Fluoxetine (Prozac)	Clonazepam (Klonopin)
Paroxetine (Paxil)	
Sertraline (Zoloft)	**Anticonvulsants**
Fluvoxamine (Luvox)	Divalproex (Depakote)
Citalopram (Celexa)	
Tricyclics	
Nortriptyline (Pamelor)	
Desipramine (Norpramin)	
Imipramine (Tofranil)	
Clomipramine (Anafranil)	
MAOIs	
Phenelzine (Nardil)	

or 10 mg nortriptyline (Pamelor)) and increased in similar increments very slowly (e.g., q 1 wk). Although most (but not all) pts require a "full" dose (see 6.1), rapid titration to this dose often provokes a "flurry" of attacks. Full prevention may not occur for 4–6 wk.

Benzodiazepines are viable alternatives. Dose is rapidly titrated up (over 3–7 d) to 2–6 mg for alprazolam (Xanax) and 2–4 mg for clonazepam (Klonopin), both given on a tid divided schedule. Given the short half-life of alprazolam (Xanax), pts are at risk for withdrawal-induced attacks should they miss doses, and therefore clonazepam (Klonopin), with a longer half-life, may be preferable. In either case, if Rx is continued >6 wk, pts are at high risk for withdrawal, and the dose must be tapered *very* slowly, over perhaps 10 wk.

Divalproex (Depakote) is used as described in 6.6.

Pharmacologic Rx should be chronic, given the chronicity of the disorder.

Cognitive behavior therapy also appears effective in preventing attacks; in some pts a combination of this and pharmacotherapy gives the best results.

7.2 AGORAPHOBIA (INCLUDING AGORAPHOBIA WITHOUT HISTORY OF PANIC ATTACKS AND PANIC DISORDER WITH AGORAPHOBIA)

Am J Psychiatry 1993;150:1496. Am J Psychiatry 1995;152:1438. Arch Gen Psychiatry 1986;43:1029.

Epidem: Lifetime prevalence as high as 1%–2%; twice as common in females as males.

Sx: Onset typically in the 20s or early 30s. Pts gradually come to fear and more or less completely avoid situations or places wherein either help is not immediately available or escape is difficult. Examples include bridges, tunnels, escalators, or even riding in the back seat of a 2-door car; in severe cases, pts become housebound, unable to step foot outside the front door without paralyzing anxiety. Importantly, the presence of a friend or companion may serve as a kind of "portable" security, allowing pts to go places they could not if they were alone.

Lab: NC.

Crs: Chronic, often waxing and waning.

Cmplc: Jobs dependent on travel may be lost; housebound pts may be totally disabled. Demoralization and alcohol or sedative-hypnotic abuse or dependence may occur.

Etiol: In the vast majority, agoraphobia evolves as a complication of panic disorder (see 7.1). In a small minority there is no h/o panic attacks, and the source of the pt's dread remains unknown.

Ddx: Social phobia is distinguished by the source of the pt's avoidance of situations, namely, a fear of humiliation or embarrassment; by contrast in agoraphobia, the fear is of having a panic attack.

Major depression may cause depressive episodes wherein pts fail to leave their houses: here, however, the "housebound" status reflects not a fear of what may happen outside the house (as in agoraphobia) but rather a lack of interest in anything outside the house.

Schizophrenia may produce delusions of persecution that keep pts in the house for fear of the surveillance that awaits them outside.

Severe disfigurements and embarrassing sx (e.g., incontinence, tremor) may make some pts avoid public view.

Rx: Panic disorder, if present, *must* be successfully treated first. Subsequently, graded, hierarchically ordered, and progressively longer forays away from home and safety are established.

ANXIETY DISORDERS

7.3 SPECIFIC PHOBIA (SIMPLE PHOBIA)

Am J Psychiatry 1988;145:1207. Br J Psychiatry 1998;173:212. Comp Psychiatry 1969;10:151.

Epidem: Lifetime prevalence ~11%; almost twice as common in females as males, with the exception of the blood-injury type of specific phobia, wherein the ratio is almost equal.

Sx: Specific phobic objects may consist of animals (e.g., snakes, insects, dogs), situations (e.g., heights, closed spaces), or blood or injury. Typically, upon approach or contact with the phobic object, pts experience severe anxiety, often accompanied by tremor, tachycardia, and diaphoresis. Some will attempt to flee, while others attempt to endure. Blood-injury phobia is unique in that after this initial "sympathetic" reaction, there follows immediately a "parasympathetic" reaction with bradycardia, hypotension, dizziness, and at times, syncope.

Onset of animal and blood-injury phobias typically in childhood; other specific phobias may appear first in childhood or during early adult years.

Lab: NC.

Crs: Early-onset animal phobias tend to remit by adult years; adult-onset phobias tend to persist indefinitely.

Cmplc: When the phobic object is easily avoided, complications are minimal; in other situations (e.g., a coal miner who develops a fear of closed spaces), the phobia may be disabling.

Etiol: Specific phobias (esp blood-injury phobia) are familial and "run true." "Nature" and "nurture" components are not clear: In some cases, parents, by modeling, may "teach" children to be afraid of, say, dogs; in some instances, e.g., fear of snakes, there may be good Darwinian reasons for the phobia.

Ddx: Social phobics, rather than having a fear of specific things, have a fear of doing things in public that they otherwise can do without difficulty in private; e.g., the pt with a fear of public speaking may be unable to deliver a speech to an audience yet be able to do it flawlessly in an empty auditorium.

Panic disorder is distinguished by the presence of spontaneously occurring attacks.

Rx: Repeated contact with the phobic object is required. In some pts, only supportive counseling is required; in others systematic desensitization or "modeling" by a therapist may help. Medications, e.g., benzodiazepines, are inferior to behavioral approaches.

7.4 SOCIAL PHOBIA

Am J Med 1982;72:88. J Clin Psychiatry 1995;56(Suppl 5):5. J Clin Psychiatry 1997;58(Suppl 14):32. J Clin Psychiatry 1998;59(Suppl 17): 54.

Epidem: Lifetime prevalence ~3%; in general population, female > male; in clinic samples, male > female.

Sx: Onset typically in mid teenage years.

Two types:
- *Circumscribed* social phobia, characterized by anxiety over engaging in specific activities in public for fear of embarrassment or humiliation: public speaking, eating in public, urinating in public restrooms. Critically, if the pt is alone, the activity may be approached and accomplished without anxiety.
- *Generalized* social phobia, characterized by a fear of acting foolishly or being embarrassed in most social situations (e.g., dating, school activities, casual social engagements) and despite a desire for social contact, a consequent avoidance of being with others in social situations.

Some pts may be able to endure the phobic situation while others, if forced to stay, may experience an anxiety attack with severe anxiety, tremulousness, diaphoresis, and palpitations, which does not resolve until the pt is out of the situation.

Lab: NC.

Crs: Chronic.

Cmplc: Circumscribed social phobia has complications only when avoidance of the phobic situation interferes with the pt's life (e.g., a public speaking phobia in a politician).

Generalized social phobia may leave pts isolated and housebound. Demoralization and alcohol or sedative-hypnotic abuse or dependence may follow.

Etiol: Familial; in some pts preceded by childhood shyness and inhibition.

Ddx: Facilitated by considering each of the 2 types of social phobias individually.

Circumscribed Social Phobia: Specific phobia is distinguished by pts' anxiety regardless of whether they are in public or in private.

Normal performance anxiety is distinguished by being readily overcome with a few "dress rehearsals."

Generalized Social Phobia: Agoraphobia is distinguished by the motive of the pt's withdrawal. The agoraphobic pt fears leaving the safety of home and risking a panic attack; the generalized social phobic fears, not leaving home per se, but encountering a social situation.

Body dysmorphic disorder is distinguished by the source of potential embarrassment: imaginary disfigurements in body dysmorphic disorder vs various faux pas in generalized social phobia.

Schizotypal and schizoid personality disorders may be characterized by social isolation, and such pts may feel awkward in public. In distinction with generalized social phobia, however, these pts have little interest in social contact.

Avoidant personality disorder is difficult to distinguish, but is suggested by an earlier onset (childhood) and by the presence of a well-elaborated self-image centered around the conviction of social ineptness. In generalized social phobia, pts often have trouble elaborating an explanation for their reluctance to appear in public.

Normal social embarrassment may be experienced by pts with disfiguring or embarrassing signs (e.g., facial rashes, tremor).

Normal shyness in new situations is distinguished by its evaporation with familiarity.

Rx: Circumscribed social phobia, in some instances (e.g., fear of speaking, writing, or eating in public), esp when tremor is prominent, may be treated with propranolol (Inderal) 20–60 mg taken ~2 h before the anticipated public exposure. Phenelzine (Nardil) 60 mg or fluoxetine (Prozac) 20 mg may help some pts.

Generalized social phobia often responds to phenelzine (Nardil) 60 mg and may respond to fluoxetine (Prozac) 20 mg; alprazolam (Xanax) ~4 mg or clonazepam (Klonopin) ~2–3 mg may also be effective, but after ~6 wk of chronic Rx, the pt is exposed to the risk of withdrawal sx. Cognitive behavioral therapy may be as effective as phenelzine (Nardil); other psychotherapies (social skills training, progressive relaxation, and gradual exposure) may also be effective.

7.5 OBSESSIVE-COMPULSIVE DISORDER

Am J Psychiatry 1986;143:1527. Arch Gen Psychiatry 1994;51:302. Br J Psychiatry 1975;127:342. Br J Psychiatry 1998;173(Suppl 35):64. J Clin Psychiatry 1997;58(Suppl 12):18.

Epidem: Lifetime prevalence 2%–3%; equally common in males and females.

Sx: Onset typically in late teens or early 20s; range from childhood to late 30s.

Most pts have both obsessions and compulsions; ~15%–25% have obsessions only; ~5% have only compulsions.

Obsessions are unwanted, intrusive, recurrent thoughts, impulses, or images that although at times are neutral in content, generally concern sexual or violent themes: A young mother was plagued with the image of her baby lying dead on the street; a preacher was beset with recurrent urges, which he never acted on, to utter obscenities from the pulpit. Efforts to stop obsessions are generally futile, and some pts may avoid situations that pertain to the obsessions (e.g., the mother might never go near the street with her baby; the preacher may stop ascending to the pulpit).

Compulsions are overwhelming and irresistible urges to engage in activities that pts recognize as senseless, purposeless, and without pleasure. One pt, for fear the gas had not been turned off, repeatedly went back into the house to check on it; another, for fear of having been contaminated, engaged in repeated hand washing to the point of causing a dermatitis. Some pts have difficulty articulating the fear motivating their compulsive behavior; thus, "touchers" are compelled to touch things a certain number of times, and "arrangers" are compelled to order things perfectly and "just so," often striving for an impossible symmetry. Although most compulsions consist of publicly observable behavior, in a minority the compulsion may be a private event, e.g., repeatedly and silently thinking the same prayer.

Although most pts retain "insight" into the senselessness of their behavior and offer at least some resistance before giving in, in a minority insight is lost, and such pts come to see their compulsions as reasonable. Thus, a "washer" finally came to believe that in fact, there *was* invisible contamination on the hands; subsequently, rather than resisting the urge to wash, the washer went at the task with a great sense of purpose. Such pts are said to have "psychotic" obsessive-compulsive disorder.

Lab: NC.

Crs: In most pts, chronic with waxing and waning intensity; in a minority, there may be an episodic course.

Cmplc: The content of obsessions, as in the examples given, may lead pts to restrict their lives; the time spent in compulsions may cut into other, more productive activities, and in the case of "washers" may lead to serious dermatologic complications.

Etiol: Familial, with some evidence for the existence of a common diathesis for obsessive-compulsive disorder and Tourette's syndrome; in an as yet unknown number of pts, obsessive-compulsive disorder is a sequela to Sydenham's chorea.

PET suggests involvement of the head of the caudate and the orbitofrontal cortex.

Serotoninergic functioning is disturbed. Only drugs with serotoninergic activity are effective, and metachlorophenylpiperazine (mCPP), a mixed agonist-antagonist at postsynaptic serotonin receptors, if given orally, exacerbates sx.

Ddx: See Table 7.5-1.

Depressive episodes may be accompanied by obsessions or compulsions; however, these clear as the episode does.

Sydenham's chorea is suggested by the chorea; however, in a majority of pts, the obsessions or compulsions precede the chorea.

Table 7.5-1. Differential Diagnosis for Obsessions or Compulsions

Depressive episode of major depression or bipolar disorder
Sydenham's chorea
Focal lesions (basal ganglia or right parietal lobe)
Postencephalitic
Simple partial seizure
Medications (e.g., clozapine (Clozaril))

Focal lesions of the basal ganglia may be suggested by the presence of AIMs along with the obsessions or compulsions.

Encephalitis lethargica often produces obsessions or compulsions, which are often associated with oculogyric crises.

Simple partal seizures are suggested by the presence of other seizure types, e.g., grand mal or complex partial.

Rx: Behavior therapy (exposure and response prevention) is effective for compulsions, but has little effect on obsessions.

SSRIs or clomipramine (Anafranil) are effective for both compulsions and obsessions. Although some pts may respond to doses similar to those used for depression (see 6.1), many pts require higher doses: fluoxetine (Prozac) 80 mg, sertraline (Zoloft) 200 mg, paroxetine (Paxil) 60 mg, fluvoxamine (Luvox) 300 mg, clomipramine (Anafranil) 250 mg. Most pts tolerate an SSRI better than clomipramine (Anafranil).

When single-agent Rx is not fully effective, search for a h/o tics, as such pts will improve with the addition of a neuroleptic (e.g., haloperidol (Haldol) 5 mg, risperidone (Risperdal) 6 mg, olanzapine (Zyprexa) 10 mg). Importantly, neuroleptics are *not* helpful in pts lacking a h/o tics.

Combination of behavior therapy and medication is often superior to either alone.

7.6 POSTTRAUMATIC STRESS DISORDER

Arch Gen Psychiatry 1980;37:85. J Clin Psychiatry 1997;58(Suppl 9):29. Psychiatr Clin 1994;17:409.

Epidem: Estimates of lifetime prevalence range from 1% to 14%; conservative estimates around 2%–3%.

Sx: Onset may be immediate, within days or weeks of the inciting trauma, or delayed, with months or years passing until sx appear.

In 1 fashion or another, pts repeatedly reexperience the original trauma, perhaps in nightmares or vivid, intrusive memories; some pts may experience "flashbacks" of almost hallucinatory quality wherein they virtually reexperience the original trauma. Pts also become "numb" to the world around them; interest in former activities is lost and pts may complain of feeling dead or lifeless inside, and often appear listless or detached.

Typically, pts are chronically apprehensive, anxious, and easily startled, as if forever on guard. Events reminiscent of the original trauma are avoided; unavoidable exposure may provoke severe anxiety, to the point of an anxiety attack, with tremor, diaphoresis, palpitations, etc.

Additional sx include irritability, lability, poor concentration, and insomnia, which may be severe.

Lab: NC.

Crs: Approximately half of pts gradually recover within 3 mo; in the other half, sx wax and wane chronically. Immediate onsets are more likely to end in recovery, while delayed onsets often predict chronicity.

Cmplc: Preoccupation with the trauma, and a detachment from current life often lead to failure in personal and business endeavors.

Etiol: Extreme trauma (e.g., torture) is more likely to be followed by PTSD than milder traumas (e.g., divorce). Individual factors that determine why some individuals develop the illness while others, exposed to the same trauma, do not are unknown.

In contrast to depression, PTSD is associated with hypersuppression of cortisol on the DST.

Ddx: Depression following a traumatic event resembles PTSD in that pts may be anxious and irritable, with poor concentration and insomnia; in depression, however, although pts may at times ruminate on past misfortunes, one does not see the virtual reexperiencing typical of PTSD.

Generalized anxiety disorder with its persistent anxiety, easy startability, and poor concentration resembles PTSD but is distinguished from PTSD by the lack of a precipitating trauma.

Malingering and factitious illness may be difficult to detect, and whenever suspected should prompt a review of original records related to the purported trauma, e.g., hospital or armed service records.

Rx: Cognitive behavioral therapy is helpful. Amitriptyline (Elavil), imipramine (Tofranil), phenelzine (Nardil), and fluoxetine (Prozac) are all useful, and are used as in the treatment of depression (see 6.1), with the exception of fluoxetine (Prozac), for which doses of 80 mg are often required.

Concurrent substance abuse or dependence must be treated first.

7.7 GENERALIZED ANXIETY DISORDER

Acta Psychiatr Scand 1997;95:444. Acta Psychiatr Scand 1998;98(Suppl 393):102. Arch Gen Psychiatry 1993;50:884. J Clin Psychopharm 1995;15:12.

Epidem: Lifetime prevalence 1%–2%; female-male ratio 1:2.

Sx: Onset in late teens or early 20s.

Chronic "free-floating" anxiety, excessive worrying, persistent apprehensiveness that something untoward will occur; typically accompanied by tremulousness, heightened muscle tension, difficulty with concentration, easy fatigability, and broken sleep.

Lab: NC.

Crs: Chronic waxing and waning.

Cmplc: In severe cases, pts may be "paralyzed" by the anxiety and unable to function in most situations.

Etiol: Disturbances of GABAergic or serotoninergic function are suspected.

Ddx: Dysthymia or a depressive episode of either major depression or bipolar disorder is distinguished by guilt, crying spells, persistent fatigue (rather than easy fatigability), and anhedonia; furthermore, in depressive episodes, there are generally sx-free intervals, phenomena not seen in generalized anxiety disorder.

Phobias (specific or social) are distinguished by the presence of anxiety only in proximity to the phobic object or event.

Panic disorder may be accompanied by considerable anticipatory anxiety; however, it is distinguished by the h/o discrete attacks of panic.

PTSD may entail considerable "free-floating" anxiety but is distinguished by the h/o a severe inciting trauma.

Alcohol or sedative-hypnotic withdrawal may be characterized by prominent anxiety but is distinguished by the h/o recurrent intoxication.

Secondary anxiety is discussed in 7.8.

Rx: Cognitive therapy, combined with progressive relaxation, is often effective.

Antidepressants (e.g., nortriptyline (Pamelor) or paroxetine (Paxil), as described in 6.1), buspirone (BuSpar) 30–60 mg/d (in 3 divided doses), hydroxyzine (Vistaril) (as described in 16.1), and benzodiazepines (e.g., chlordiazepoxide (Librium), diazepam (Valium), lorazepam (Ativan), alprazolam (Xanax), all as described in 16.1) are effective (antidepressants and buspirone (BuSpar) take weeks to become effective, whereas hydroxyzine (Vistaril) and benzodiazepines are effective almost immediately; benzodiazepines, unlike all the others, are subject to abuse).

7.8 SECONDARY ANXIETY (ANXIETY DISORDER DUE TO A GENERAL MEDICAL CONDITION)

Acta Neurol Scand 1993;87:14. Am J Psychiatry 1983;140:342. J Clin Psychiatry 1983;44:31. J Nerv Ment Dis 1993;181:100.

Epidem: Probably common.

Sx: Secondary anxiety may present in 1 of 2 ways:
- *Discrete attacks* of secondary anxiety resemble panic attacks (see 7.1). Over a relatively short period of time pts develop anxiety, tremulousness, tachycardia, diaphoresis, etc. Secondary anxiety attacks may last from minutes to hours.
- *Chronic* secondary anxiety may present either insidiously or semi-acutely, depending on the etiology. Pts experience waxing and waning sx of anxiety, restlessness, and easy startability, with or without autonomic sx, such as tremor and tachycardia. These sx persist for variable periods of time, depending on the etiology, from days to weeks or longer.

Lab: Reflects the etiology.

Crs: Determined by the etiology.

Cmplc: Similar to those described for panic disorder (see 7.1) or generalized anxiety disorder (see 7.7).

Etiol: See Table 7.8-1. Most of the etiologies are fairly straightforward; some deserve comment.

Supraventricular tachycardia is suggested by hyperacute onset and offset, and by relief with a Valsalva maneuver.

Angina, myocardial infarction, or pulmonary embolus is suggested by presence of risk factors, e.g., for pulmonary embolus, immobilization, and thrombophlebitis.

Hypoglycemia is suspected in pts on insulin or oral hypoglycemic agents; in untreated pts, postprandial onset is suggestive. In any

Table 7.8-1. Etiologies of Secondary Anxiety

Secondary Anxiety Attacks

Drugs
   Stimulants (cocaine, amphetamines)
   Sympathomimetics
   Caffeine
   Hallucinogens (e.g., LSD)
   Phencyclidine
   Cannabis
Cardiopulmonary conditions
   Supraventricular tachycardia
   Angina or myocardial infarction
   Pulmonary embolus
   Asthmatic attack
   Hyperventilation
Pheochromocytoma
Hypoglycemia
Parkinson's disease
Simple partial seizure

Secondary Chronic Anxiety

Drug withdrawal
   Alcohol
   Benzodiazepines
   Nicotine
   Clonidine (Catapres)
Drugs
   Sympathomimetics
   Theophylline
   Caffeine
   Yohimbine (Yocon)
   Various antidepressants (SSRIs, tricyclics, MAOIs, bupropion (Wellbutrin, Zyban))
Cardiopulmonary conditions
   COPD
   CHF
Endocrinologic conditions
   Hyperthyroidism
   Hypoparathyroidism (with hypocalcemia)
Stroke (right frontal cortex)
Traumatic brain injury

case, "Whipple's triad" must be demonstrated: appropriate sx, documented hypoglycemia, and relief with sugar.

Parkinson's disease pts are liable to attacks of anxiety during "off" periods.

Simple partial seizures are suspected in pts with other seizure types, e.g., complex partial or grand mal.

Ddx: Panic disorder (in contrast to secondary anxiety attacks) and generalized anxiety disorder (in contrast to chronic secondary anxiety disorder) are essentially dx of exclusion; however, the ddx task here is not difficult, as most of the causes of secondary anxiety are readily assessed.

Rx: Secondary anxiety attacks rarely require Rx per se, except for treating the underlying cause.

Secondary chronic anxiety may, in addition to attending to the underlying cause, require symptomatic Rx, e.g., diazepam (Valium) 5–10 mg/d or chlordiazepoxide (Librium) 25–50 mg/d.

8. Somatoform and Related Disorders

8.1 SOMATIZATION DISORDER (BRIQUET'S SYNDROME)

Am J Psychiatry 1986;143:873. Arch Gen Psychiatry 1984;41:334. NEJM 1962;266:421. NEJM 1986;314:1407.

Epidem: Lifetime prevalence ~1%; male-female ratio 1:9.

Sx: Onset typically in teenage years, with full clinical picture evident by early 20s.

Full syndrome characterized by multiple sx, suggesting disease in multiple systems, all of which are medically unexplained. Hx often presented in a dramatic but vague and imprecise manner; physicians often comment that ROS is "diffusely positive." PE typically normal or reveals only minor changes inadequate to explain the pt's complaints.

Sx occur in each of the 4 groups presented in Table 8.1-1.

A negative workup, rather than reassuring pts, often leaves them resentful. "Doctor shopping," with demands for ever-more invasive dx maneuvers, is common.

Lab: Dx tests appropriate to the pt's complaints generally negative.

Crs: Chronic, with stress-induced exacerbations.

Cmplc: Excessive sick days may cost jobs; tyrannical demands for sympathy may alienate friends and family; unwarranted invasive procedures may bring their own complications.

Etiol: Adoption studies suggest that the same genotype produces antisocial personality disorder in males and somatization disorder in females.

Table 8.1-1. Symptoms of Somatization Disorder

Conversion Symptoms	Sexual Dysfunction
Ataxia	Decreased libido
Weakness or paralysis	Impotence
Dysphagia or globus	Ejaculatory delay
Aphonia	Irregular menses
Urinary retention	Heavy menstrual bleeding
Anesthesia	Prolonged and frequent vomiting during pregnancy
Blurry vision	
Diplopia	**Pain**
Blindness	
Deafness	Headache
Pseudoseizures	Abdominal pain (often vague or poorly localized)
Amnesia	Backache
Dizzy spells	Arthralgia
Syncope	Chest pain
	Rectal pain
	Painful menses
Gastrointestinal Symptoms	Dyspareunia
	Dysuria
Nausea	
Bloating	
Vomiting	
Diarrhea	
Constipation	
Multiple food intolerance	

Ddx: Conversion disorder (see 8.2) is a monosymptomatic disorder, in contrast to the polysymptomatic nature of somatization disorder; furthermore, sx in conversion disorder are suggestive only of neurologic disease, in contrast to the multiple organ systems implicated in somatization disorder.

Hypochondriasis (see 8.4) is distinguished by the focus of the pt's concern. In hypochondriasis the pt is principally concerned with what the particular sx means, i.e., that there might be some as yet undiagnosed serious disease; in contrast, in somatization disorder, the focus is more on the sx themselves, and on the suffering caused by them.

Pain disorder (see 8.3) is distinguished by its monosymptomatic nature, limited essentially to the complaint of pain.

Depressive episodes, as seen in major depression or bipolar disorder, esp in the elderly, may present with multiple unfounded complaints. Here, however, one also sees an episodic course and promi-

nent vegetative sx of depression (weight loss, insomnia, psychomotor change, etc.).

Malingering and factitious illness are distinguished by the purposeful
nature of the pt's complaints.

Multisystem disease, such as systemic lupus erythematosus or sarcoid-
osis, may present with a picture similar to somatization disorder,
esp after pts have been referred from 1 doctor to another, without
a dx being made. Thus, the dx of somatization disorder cannot be
made until a thorough dx evaluation has been unrewarding.

Complications of invasive diagnostic procedures may add to the pt's
complaints.

Rx: Pts should be seen by 1 primary care physician on a scheduled
basis, and a conservative approach to dx and Rx is appropriate.
For the first year, monthly visits are appropriate; in subsequent
years the frequency of visits is titrated to the pt's condition. At the
end of each office visit, it is critical to make a scheduled f/u
appointment; open-ended return dates tend to generate anxiety
and increase the pt's sx.

When the structured primary care approach fails, some pts may benefit from highly focused, time-limited "Briquet's groups."

8.2 CONVERSION DISORDER

Am J Psychiatry 1963;119:960. Br J Psychiatry 1996;169:282. J Neurol
Neurosurg Psychiatry 1995;58:750. NEJM 1981;305:745.

Epidem: Uncertain; probably uncommon.

Sx: Onset typically in adolescence or early adult years, typically after a
major life stress.

Typically, pts develop sx that resemble, to a greater or lesser degree,
those that do occur secondary to diseases of the nervous system,
such as anesthesia or paralysis. Critically, however, conversion sx,
in 1 way or another, "violate" the "laws" of anatomy and physiology. Thus, a pt with conversion anesthesia of the arm may report
that the boundary between normal sensation and anesthesia precisely encircles the elbow joint; such a boundary, clearly, cannot
occur with lesions of the central or peripheral nervous system, and
it is in this sense that the pt's sx "violate" the anatomic "law."

Importantly, although conversion sx do not arise secondary to lesions of the nervous system, they are not under the voluntary control of the pt and they may cause suffering or disability. Some pts with conversion paralysis may develop contractures.

Common conversion sx are noted in the appropriate part of Table 8.1-1. Some of the "violations" are noted below.

In conversion ataxia, despite the pt's (often wildly) unsteady gait, examination in bed reveals normal finger-to-nose and heel-to-knee-to-shin test results, along with an absence of truncal ataxia.

In conversion paralysis, e.g., conversion hemiplegia, the "paralyzed" foot is often dragged, rather than circumducted, and the DTRs are symmetric. Result on Hoover's test may also be positive: Place the hands, palms up, under the pt's heels and ask the pt to lift the "paralyzed" leg off the bed; for a positive result, one will fail to feel the normal auxiliary downward pressure from the normal leg.

Conversion aphonia is suggested when during auscultation of the lungs, the pt is asked to cough and does so successfully.

Conversion monocular blindness is betrayed by the bilaterally intact light reflex.

Conversion deafness, if bilateral, is indicated by the intact blink reflex to a sudden, unexpected loud noise.

Conversion seizures ("pseudoseizures") of the grand mal type are distinguished by gradual onset, nonrhythmic motor activity, and in general, an absence of tongue biting or incontinence. If the physician is present, the pt's face may be suddenly touched by an ice cube, or an attempt may be made to elicit the corneal reflex. Pts in a pseudoseizure typically withdraw from such maneuvers in contrast to pts with actual seizures, where typically there is no response. Prolactin or neuron-specific enolase levels, measured 15–30 min postictally, are often elevated with actual seizures, and typically normal with pseudoseizures.

Lab: NC.

Crs: Chronic or self-remitting: Acute onset, precipitating factors, and an absence of other psychopathology predict spontaneous remission; however, of those who do experience remission, within a year, approximately one-fourth will develop another conversion sx, not necessarily identical to the preceding one.

Cmplc: Pts may feel disabled from work, and lose jobs. With conversion paralysis, contractures or disuse atrophy may occur.

Etiol: Conscious intent or purpose is absent. The conversion sx appears to represent, symbolically, what the pt is unable to say or do.

Ddx: A failure to determine a cause for any given sx does not, by itself, indicate a dx of conversion, for many diseases, e.g., MS and systemic lupus erythematosus, are elusive and subtle. To make the dx one *must* demonstrate that the sx in question "violates" one of the laws of anatomy or physiology. Also bear in mind that the same pt may have both bona fide sx and conversion sx (e.g., both epileptic seizures and pseudoseizures).

Somatization disorder is distinguished by a multitude of sx spanning several organ systems, in contrast to conversion disorder, where there is typically only 1 sx, restricted to the central or peripheral nervous system. Although conversion sx may appear in somatization disorder, they are always accompanied by a multitude of other sx.

Pain disorder and its distinction from conversion disorder are discussed in 8.3.

Malingering and factitious illness are distinguished by the presence of intentionality and purpose.

Rx: Present the truth to the pt constructively: Rather than "there's nothing wrong," consider saying, "Neither my exam nor the tests I've ordered have revealed any damage to your brain or nerves," and then offer firm reassurance that such sx usually clear up on their own. In some cases, a short course of physical therapy will get pts with conversion paralysis or ataxia "moving" again.

8.3 PAIN DISORDER

J Affect Disord 1989;16:21. Pain 1990;40:3. Psychosomatics 1993;34: 494.

Epidem: Uncertain, but probably uncommon.

Sx: These pts are typically in chronic pain, and typically do not bear up well with it. In some pts, a lesion (that might reasonably be expected to be painful) is present, but the pt's complaints appear disproportionately severe relative to what an experienced physician might expect from pts with this sort of lesion. In other pts, despite a thorough diagnostic evaluation, no lesion can be found.

Often, there are significant depressive sx: Pts appear beaten down and are often bitter or irritable; their attention is focused on the pain and their need for relief, and there is very little interest in anything else. Fatigue is common, and pts rarely have restful nights. Others may view these pts as demanding and difficult (if not impossible) to please.

Typical complaints center on low-back pain, arthralgia, headache, and abdominal or pelvic pain.

At times, these pts are said to have "functional" pain, or if a lesion is present but the complaints seem magnified and exaggerated, to have significant "functional overlay."

Lab: If a lesion is present, appropriate findings noted (e.g., disk narrowing); otherwise NC.

Crs: Typically chronic, with sx persisting for 6 mo or longer.

Cmplc: Family members and friends (and indeed, often medical personnel) are often put off; jobs may be lost due to missed work; pts may suffer iatrogenic injury due to unnecessary dx procedures; some may become dependent on opioids.

Etiol: Predicting how much pain pts "should" be in for any given lesion is very difficult. Some pts with extensive myocardial infarction will have none (a "silent" myocardial infarction), and some pts whose lesions have been removed will have an intense amount (i.e., "phantom" pain after amputations). Furthermore, the pain that pts experience with any given lesion may vary dramatically, depending on their situation; e.g., some soldiers, sustaining horrific wounds in the heat of battle, may have no pain for hours, and only eventually begin to experience pain after being evacuated. Thus, although it is natural (and appropriate) to extrapolate from the lesion to an estimate of how much pain a pt "should" be in, exceptions to this extrapolatory rule obviously exist.

In addition, it is also difficult to infer the degree of pain pts are in from observation of their facial expression, tone of voice, posture, etc. On the one hand, some individuals tend toward "stoicism," and rather than complaining, may withdraw from company and downplay their suffering. On the other hand, dramatic or emotional individuals who are in pain may be dismissed on the assumption that their complaints reflect more their general tendency to exaggerate than anything else. Most physicians (if they're honest) can recall thinking "functional" and sending the pt home, only to have the pt show up later in the ER with "objective" evidence of disease (e.g., Q waves on the EKG, a mass on the MRI).

It is currently unclear why pts with little or nothing in the way of a lesion end up in severe, chronic pain, the expression of which comes to dominate their lives and the lives of those around them. In the past, such pts have been characterized as being "pain prone"; however, this is at best a descriptive phrase and says little about mechanism.

Ddx: Somatization disorder is distinguished by a multiplicity of complaints in addition to pain.

Hypochondriasis is distinguished by the focus of the pt's complaints, which is not so much the pain and its attendant suffering, but on the fear that the pain signifies some serious and as yet undiagnosed disease.

Conversion disorder generally involves a disturbance in function (e.g., blindness, paralysis) rather than pain. Theoretically, a case could be made for saying that pain disorder without a lesion represents a rare variety of conversion disorder. Clinically, however, treatment of the pain would be the same.

Malingering and factitious disorder are suggested by the presence of a purpose behind the pt's complaints, such as winning a lawsuit, avoiding military service or work, or simply being a pt in the hospital.

Schizophrenia may cause pain, which is relieved with neuroleptics. The dx is suggested by the presence of other sx, such as delusions or hallucinations.

Depressive episodes, of either a major depression or bipolar disorder, may present with complaints of pain, and this is particularly true in the elderly, where one speaks of a "masked" depression. The dx is suggested by the presence of marked vegetative sx before the complaints of pain appear.

In all pts, it is imperative to conduct a thorough search for any lesion, and to treat that lesion if possible. Furthermore, if the search is unrevealing, it is appropriate to periodically reevaluate the pt for any new evidence of a lesion.

Rx: When a lesion is present, it is appropriate to conservatively employ the pain relief measures generally offered most pts with such lesions, including physical therapy and analgesics (beginning, if appropriate, with acetaminophen, and progressing successively from NSAIDs (e.g., ibuprofen) to propoxyphene, codeine, or oxycodone, and finally agents such as morphine). In most pts it is appropriate to administer medications on a scheduled basis, with provision for prn doses, with the regular dose being adjusted relative to how much is used in prn doses, to the point where pts are generally able to function, free of undue SEs, and able to go without prn doses. Other measures, such as TENS units, nerve blocks, etc., are used on an individualized basis.

All pts should be given a trial of a TCA. These drugs are effective for chronic pain *regardless* of whether pts are depressed or not. Importantly, the SSRIs are not effective in this regard. Although amitriptyline (Elavil) is commonly used, SEs (sedation, dizziness, etc.) are often limiting, and a better choice is nortriptyline (Pamelor). Antidepressants are used in the same fashion as described in 6.1, and require the same amount of time to see a response. When success is only partial, the addition of fluphenazine (Prolixin) 1–2 mg po daily may be effective. An alternative to antidepressants is carbamazepine (Tegretol), but the evidence here is far less substantial than for tricyclics.

Psychotherapy using a cognitive behavioral approach, hypnosis, and progressive relaxation may be helpful. Placebos may be very helpful. Although there is controversy regarding the ethics of using placebos, they should probably be considered before using any approach that carries a risk, such as surgery.

Clinical progress is generally slow, and successful treatment requires tact and patience. As pts improve, it is appropriate to introduce the notion that the goal is not "cure" or complete pain relief, but rather a reduction in pain and a reentry into normal life.

8.4 HYPOCHONDRIASIS

Arch Int Med 1981;141:723. Br J Psychiatry 1996;169:189. Br J Psychiatry 1998;173:212. J Clin Psychopharm 1993;13:438. NEJM 1981; 304:1394.

Epidem: In general medical population, prevalence ~5%–10%; prevalence in general population uncertain.

Sx: Onset typically in 20s or 30s.

Hypochondriacal pts, despite appropriate reassurance from the physician, are persistently worried that they have some serious, as yet undiagnosed, disease. Minor sx or signs are viewed with alarm: The cough of a cold indicates lung cancer; simple constipation, colon cancer; diffuse aches and pains, AIDS.

"Doctor shopping" is common; pts, often already resentful over what they consider to be poor medical attention in the past, often arrive with excruciatingly detailed lists of signs, sx, and the results of prior investigations. Although some pts may be reassured after a careful exam, such reassurance is typically only temporary, and doubts quickly arise.

Lab: NC.

Crs: Chronic.

Cmplc: Invalidism may occur, and pts may submit to unwarranted invasive dx procedures.

Etiol: In some pts, prior experience, either personal or vicarious, with serious illness may be followed by hypochondriasis; in most pts, however, the cause is unknown.

Ddx: Conversion disorder and somatization disorder are distinguished by the focus of concern. The pt with conversion disorder or somatization disorder is most concerned with the suffering or disability "caused" by their sx, whereas the pt with hypochondriasis is more concerned with the import of the sx, namely, that there is some serious underlying disease (indeed, the hypochondriacal sx itself may cause no pain or disability at all).

Pain disorder is distinguished by the focus of the pt's concerns about the pain. In pain disorder it is on the suffering inherent in the pain, whereas in hypochondriasis it is not so much on the pain per se, as it is on what the pain might indicate, namely, the presence of a serious disease.

Body dysmorphic disorder also is distinguished by focus of concern. Pts with body dysmorphic disorder are concerned about the disfiguring aspect of their sx, and not with the possibility of some serious, underlying disease.

Depressive episodes, as seen in major depression or bipolar disorder, are often accompanied by unfounded concerns regarding disease; here, however, one sees the vegetative sx of depression (weight loss, insomnia, psychomotor change), which are absent in hypochondriasis.

Transient hypochondriacal concerns are common (e.g., "doctor's diseases" among medical students), but clear within 6 mo.

Undiagnosed medical illness must always be considered. Occult cancers, systemic lupus erythematosus, and similar diseases may elude the best of diagnosticians, leaving resentful pts who then begin "doctor shopping." Each complaint must be carefully assessed before being considered hypochondriacal.

Rx: Scheduled visits with a conservative primary care physician may reduce doctor shopping and avoid iatrogenic disease; cognitive behavioral therapy is effective in reducing hypochondriacal concerns. Preliminary results suggest that fluoxetine (Prozac) may reduce hypochondriacal concerns. Group psychotherapy may also be helpful.

8.5 BODY DYSMORPHIC DISORDER (DYSMORPHOPHOBIA)

Am J Psychiatry 1991;148:1138. Am J Psychiatry 1993;150:302. Am J Psychiatry 1995;152:1207. J Clin Psychiatry 1993;54:389.

Epidem: Prevalence in general population unknown; in cosmetic surgery clinics, ~2%; equally common in males and females.

Sx: Onset typically in mid to late teens.

Pts are concerned that in some way or other, they are disfigured, deformed, or ugly despite the fact that there are no abnormalities, or if some are present, that they are minor and unlikely to attract attention.

The face or head is often the focus of concern. The nose is too long, or is disfigured; hair is misplaced; the eyes are too close together. Concern may settle on other body parts. The breasts are too large (or too small) or asymmetric; the hips are too wide.

Reassurance from physicians has little effect, and pts often seek out cosmetic surgery.

Ideas of reference are common, and pts often are concerned that others are staring at them or talking about them. Some pts may spend hours checking their appearance in the mirror; conversely, some will avoid any reflecting surface for fear of seeing their deformity. Some may avoid contact with others, to the point of only going out at night.

In a minority of pts, the concern may become delusional. There is no longer any doubt, and medical reassurance has absolutely no effect.

Lab: NC.

Crs: Chronic, with the level of concern waxing and waning over time; the focus of concern may change over time, and pts often have concerns about multiple body parts. Delusions, should they occur, generally fade over time, leaving a more typical clinical picture.

Cmplc: Some pts become housebound. Plastic surgery may have complications, and pts are rarely satisfied with the results, no matter how good. Suicide attempts may occur.

Etiol: A relationship with obsessive-compulsive disorder is suspected.

Ddx: Transsexual pts may despise their primary or secondary sexual characteristics, not because they are disfiguring in some way or other, but simply because they aren't consistent with their gender identity.

Anorexia nervosa is accompanied by a concern over being fat; here, however, the goal of the pt is not to become normal in appearance but to become thin.

Narcissistic personality disorder may be accompanied by requests for cosmetic surgery. However, here the goal is not to look normal, but to become perfect; furthermore, the desire for perfection covers not only bodily appearance, but also dress, jewelry, family, and friends.

Normal concerns about appearance (as commonly seen in teenagers) are transient and respond to reassurance.

Rx: Fluoxetine (Prozac) or clomipramine (Anafranil), used as described in 7.5 on obsessive-compulsive disorder, are generally effective. Neuroleptics, including pimozide (Orap), are not.

8.6 MALINGERING AND FACTITIOUS ILLNESS

Acta Psychiatr Scand 1988;77:497. Am J Psychiatry 1982;139:1480. Ann Int Med 1979;90:230. Br J Psychiatry 1983;143:8. J For Sci 1982;27:401. Med J Aust 1970;2:349.

In both malingering and factitious illness, pts voluntarily, deliberately, and purposefully feign illness in order to achieve some more or less readily discernible goal. In malingering, the goal is often obvious: to escape legal consequences, obtain narcotics, secure disability payments, or escape the draft. In factitious illness the goal is simply to be a pt in the hospital.

Malingerers may feign headache, low-back pain, chest pain, or voices; occasionally malingerers may stage accidents, or if suffering from an actual disease, may elaborate and inflate their complaints out of proportion to what is typical for the actual disease in question.

In factitious illness, pts typically present at the ER with dramatic and more or less convincing complaints that earn them admission. Once admitted, these pts are typically irritable and often demand 1 test after another, proceeding even to invasive procedures. Occasionally, one may see factitious illness "by proxy" wherein a parent intentionally produces illness in a child such that the child is admitted. Children have been injected with feces, given insulin or warfarin, or been subjected to trauma. Pts with factitious illness may make a "career" out of going from 1 hospital to another, and here one speaks of "hospital hoboes" or "Munchausen's syndrome."

Malingering may be suspected when a possible "goal" becomes apparent; indeed, some malingerers may bring their claims forms with them. Factitious illness may be harder to spot: Often it is the accumulation of negative and ever-more invasive tests that first raises suspicion. Some malingerers or factitial pts may be quite sophisticated, to the point of biting their tongues, the better to feign a grand mal seizure.

Malingering and factitious illness are distinguished from conversion disorder, hypochondriasis, and somatization disorder primarily by the purposeful and deliberate nature of the sx.

Once malingering or factitious illness has been confirmed, it is appropriate to tell the pt in a nonjudgmental, yet firm way that there is nothing wrong. Allowing such pts to "save face" by giving them an unsupported dx may be easier for the physician but is a disservice to the pt, for it only reinforces lying and makes feigning in the future more likely. Most pts, when apprised of the facts, react with some anger; some will escalate their complaints whereas others will beat a hasty retreat. Such pts should not be admitted to psychiatric wards, as it does little or no good, and may do harm by exposing the pt to other illnesses that may be feigned in the future.

9. Dissociative Disorders

9.1 DISSOCIATIVE AMNESIA

Am J Psychiatry 1939;96:711. Am J Psychiatry 1962;119:57. Arch
  Neurol Psychiatry 1935;34:587. BMJ 1973;4:593.

Epidem: Probably rare.
Sx: Onset typically in late teens or early 20s.
  By convention, dissociative amnesia is classified as follows:
  - *Localized* dissociative amnesia, characterized by an inability to
    recall events of a circumscribed period of time, events usually
    highly emotionally charged. Memory for events preceding and
    following the circumscribed period is intact.
  - *Systematized* dissociative amnesia, characterized by an inability
    to recall multiple events scattered in the past, all of which share
    some common emotional denominator. Thus, the periods of
    amnesia may be systematized around episodes of abandonment,
    lost love, or angry confrontation. Events falling outside of these
    periods are recalled.
  - *Generalized* dissociative amnesia, characterized by an inability to
    recall anything from the past at all.

Lab: NC.
Crs: Most pts eventually experience a spontaneous resolution of the
  amnesia and can recall the events in question.
Cmplc: An inability to recall the past restricts the ability to learn from
  experience.
Etiol: The name of the disorder reflects the current speculation that disso-
  ciation is causal here; earlier theories emphasized repression or the
  easy hypnotizability of these pts.
Ddx: The localized type of dissociative amnesia is distinguished from
  TGA by the later age at onset of TGA, from epileptic amnesia by

the presence of other epileptic phenomena and the brevity of the
episode, and from blackouts by the evidence of intoxication.

Both the systematized and generalized types are unique, and are not
mimicked by any of the other amnesias discussed in 3.16.

Rx: Psychotherapy may facilitate recall of relevant emotional events; hypnosis and amobarbital "interviews" have also been used.

9.2 DISSOCIATIVE FUGUE

Am J Psychiatry 1982;139:552. J Clin Psychiatry 1979;40:381. S Med J
1988;81:568.

Epidem: Rare.

Sx: Onset generally in late teens or early 20s.

Fugue typically precipitated by some highly emotionally charged
event; the onset of the fugue itself is generally abrupt, with pts simply leaving off whatever they were doing and traveling. During
their travels, pts have no recall of their former lives; furthermore,
and critically, when their travels cease, they adopt a new name
accompanied by a new identity. In most cases this new identity is
simple and unassuming. Pts may rent an apartment, get a non-
descript job, and lead an uneventful life. Furthermore, while in the
new identity pts have no recall of their prior identity. Fugue may
last anywhere from hours to years. When the fugue ends, pts
"come to" in their original identity and experience some surprise
at finding themselves where they are and seeing evidence of events
that transpired during the fugue, events of which they have no
recall.

Lab: NC.

Crs: Inadequate information.

Cmplc: Personal, financial, and occupational affairs, left untended, deteri-
orate.

Etiol: Current speculation invokes dissociation as the mechanism underlying fugue.

Ddx: There is only 1 other disorder in which pts adopt a new identity
and new name: multiple personality disorder (or as it has recently
been renamed, dissociative identity disorder). Multiple personality
disorder is distinguished by the fact that there are usually multiple

different personalities (in contrast to just 1 in fugue) and by the fact that at least 1 of the alternative personalities is quite familiar with the original one.

Rx: Psychotherapy, hypnosis, and amobarbital interviews have been advocated.

9.3 DISSOCIATIVE IDENTITY DISORDER (MULTIPLE PERSONALITY DISORDER)

Br J Psychiatry 1988;153:593. Br J Psychiatry 1992;160:327. Br J Psychiatry 1994;164:600.

Epidem: Controversial: Some believe it is common; others hold that it is rare and that most, if not all, cases are iatrogenic.

Sx: Onset typically in adolescence or early adult years.

The "primary" personality of the pt, i.e., the one in evidence from earliest childhood to the onset of the disorder, is periodically supplanted by 1 or more "alternate" or "secondary" personalities. The "switch" from one personality to another is typically abrupt, and each alternate personality is characterized by a different name and identity. Typically, the pt, while in 1 of the alternate personalities, has knowledge of the primary personality; by contrast, when in the primary personality the pt has no direct knowledge of the alternate personalities, and when looking back, encounters blank spaces or "lost time," corresponding to times when alternate personalities were present.

Lab: NC.

Crs: Chronic.

Cmplc: The presence of multiple personalities, often at odds with one another, leads to a chaotic and fragmented life.

Etiol: Often there is a h/o child abuse, typically sexual in nature.

Current speculation implicates dissociation as the mechanism underlying this disorder.

Pts are easily hypnotized.

Some authors believe that most, if not all, cases are induced in suggestible pts by overzealous practitioners.

Ddx: See the discussion for dissociative fugue in 9.2.

Malingering is very difficult to detect, but should be suspected in the presence of potential gain, financial or otherwise.

Rx: Most pts are seen in psychotherapy; hypnosis is advocated by some. Hospitalization is often accompanied by a deterioration and should either be avoided or kept as short as possible.

9.4 DEPERSONALIZATION DISORDER

Am J Psychiatry 1997;154:1107. Br J Psychiatry 1964;110:505. J Clin Psychopharm 1990;10:200.

Epidem: Rare; more common in females.

Sx: Onset in late teenage or early adult years.

Depersonalized pts feel strangely detached from themselves. Although they may continue whatever they were doing, they often feel as if they were watching themselves doing it, as if it were being done by a robot or automaton. Some pts may feel as if they were "floating" over themselves.

Derealization often accompanies depersonalization. Although pts still clearly perceive themselves and their surroundings, they have the uncanny sense that objects and people, including themselves, are not real, that they somehow lack substance.

Lab: NC.

Crs: Chronic, with the intensity of sx waxing and waning, or episodic, with each episode lasting from minutes to hours and fading gradually.

Cmplc: Chronic depersonalization may make it impossible for pts to remain at task.

Etiol: Uncertain; some suggest that depersonalization disorder is a result of dissociation; others suspect that depersonalization disorder is an epileptic disorder characterized solely by simple partial seizures.

Ddx: Panic attacks, as seen in panic disorder, may be accompanied by depersonalization, but are distinguished by the autonomic sx and the severe anxiety.

Intoxication with cannabis or hallucinogens may cause depersonalization (which may also occur as a "flashback") but are distinguished by the other sx of intoxication.

Hypoglycemia may cause depersonalization but is distinguished by tremor, hunger, and relief with sugar.

Simple partial seizures may be very difficult to distinguish. The presence of other seizure types (grand mal, complex partial) is suggestive; in doubtful cases, MRI, EEG, and if necessary, video-EEG monitoring may be required.

Normal individuals may experience depersonalization; however, this typically occurs only in life-threatening situations.

Rx: Inadequately studied. Anecdotally, useful medications include anticonvulsants, neuroleptics, and SSRIs (e.g., fluoxetine (Prozac)). Sequential trials may be justified.

Psychotherapy has also, anecdotally, been successful.

10. Sexual and Related Disorders

10.1 HYPOACTIVE SEXUAL DESIRE DISORDER

J Nerv Ment Dis 1986;174:646. Med Aspects Hum Sex 1977;7:94.
  Psychiatr Clin 1995;18:485.

Epidem: Lifetime prevalence ~20%; female > male.

Sx: Onset from adolescence to old age.

  Both desire for and fantasies or dreams about sex are reduced or absent.

Lab: NC.

Crs: Variable.

Cmplc: Conflict between sexual partners.

Etiol: Hypoactive sexual desire disorder may follow sexual trauma in childhood or adolescence, conflict in a sexual relationship, or reduced frequency of sexual behavior, as may occur secondary to some other sexual dysfunction.

Ddx: Complaints of decreased sexual desire must be evaluated within the pt's personal and cultural context. A pt whose partner had unusually strong desires might, by that comparison, appear to have reduced desire, but when compared to the normal population, may appear to have a quite normal level of desire.

  Depression, as seen in a depressive episode of major depression, is commonly accompanied by decreased libido.

  Decreased sexual desire may be due to a general medical condition, or be substance induced, as noted in Table 10.1-1; in some pts with decreased desire, combined factors may be at work, as for example a pt with hypoactive sexual desire disorder who was placed on an antihypertensive.

Table 10.1-1. Other Causes of Decreased Sexual Desire

General Medical Conditions	Substances
Orbitofrontal lesions	Alcohol
Hypothalamic lesions	Antidepressants (with the exception
Interictal personality syndrome	of nefazodone (Serzone),
Hepatic failure	mirtazapine (Remeron),
Hyperprolactinemia	bupropion (Wellbutrin, Zyban))
Testosterone deficiency	Neuroleptics
	Various antihypertensives
	Anabolic steroids

Rx: Hypoactive sexual desire disorder may respond to a couples or individual approach, often using specific sex therapies.

10.2 SEXUAL AVERSION DISORDER

J Sex Marital Ther 1982;8:3. Psychiatr Med 1992;10:273. Kaplan HS, Sexual aversions, sexual phobias and panic disorders, Brunner-Mazel, New York, 1986.

Epidem: Uncertain.

Sx: Pts find certain kinds of sexual phenomena repugnant or disgusting and actively avoid them. In severe cases, the aversion may encompass all forms of sexual interaction, including holding hands or kissing; most often, however, anxiety arises only at the prospect of genital contact. Pts typically avoid sexual opportunities, and if forced into them, some pts may have anxiety attacks.

Lab: NC.

Crs: Uncertain.

Cmplc: Conflict with partners.

Etiol: Sexual aversion may follow sexual trauma (e.g., rape), or another sexual dysfunction (e.g., dyspareunia), or be related to a distorted view of sexuality.

Ddx: Hypoactive sexual desire is distinguished by, ipso facto, the lack of desire. Pts with sexual aversion may still experience erotic longings.

SEXUAL AND RELATED DISORDERS

Rx: Various forms of psychotherapy and sex therapy, often involving carefully designed desensitization, may help.

10.3 FEMALE SEXUAL AROUSAL DISORDER

J Nerv Ment Dis 1963;136:272. J Neurol Neurosurg Psychiatry 1995; 59:83. J Sex Marital Ther 1993;19:171. NEJM 1978;229:111.

Epidem: Uncertain; isolated cases, with normal sexual desire, may be rare.

Sx: Despite normal sexual desire and adequate foreplay, pts do not experience sufficient vaginal lubrication to allow for satisfactory completion of intercourse.

Lab: NC.

Crs: Early adolescent onset associated with a chronic course.

Cmplc: Dyspareunia may occur; conflict with the sexual partner common.

Etiol: Guilt, sexual ignorance, performance anxiety, and anger at the partner may play a role.

Ddx: Other causes of decreased lubrication include certain general medical conditions and various substances, as noted in Table 10.3-1. By far, the most common cause of decreased lubrication, especially in middle-aged or older women, is estrogen deficiency.

Rx: Sex therapy is indicated; in some pts, lubricants are helpful.

Table 10.3-1. Other Causes of Decreased Lubrication

General Medical Conditions	Substances
Estrogen deficiency (e.g., postmenopause)	Anticholinergics (e.g., atropine, benztropine (Cogentin))
Diabetes mellitus	Antidepressants (esp heterocyclic antidepressants; may also be seen with MAOIs and SSRIs)
Pelvic arteriosclerosis	
Pelvic radiotherapy	Antihistamines
Sacral cord lesions	Various antihypertensives

10.4 MALE ERECTILE DISORDER

J Sex Marital Ther 1991;17:147. NEJM 1989;321:1648. Psychiatr Clin 1995;18:171.

Epidem: Common, with prevalence rising with age, from <10% for adolescents to >50% for those over 55.

Sx: Despite normal desire, pts are unable to obtain or maintain an erection of sufficient quality to allow for satisfactory completion of intercourse.

In male erectile disorder, the difficulty may be selective, occurring only with certain partners, or only intermittently with the same partner. Typically, men with erectile disorder report satisfactory erections at other times, e.g., "wet dreams," upon first awakening, or with self-masturbation.

Lab: Nocturnal penile plethysmography usually, but not always, demonstrates normal erection.

Crs: Varies with mode of onset: Those with an insidious onset without specific precipitants, or those who have never experienced satisfactory erections with sexual partners, tend to have a chronic course; by contrast, pts with a h/o normal erectile functioning who experience an acute onset with a definite precipitant tend to recover spontaneously.

Cmplc: Shame and conflict with sexual partners.

Etiol: Performance anxiety, guilt, shame, anger, or a fear of not being able to please the partner may be operative.

Ddx: Erectile dysfunction must be distinguished from hypoactive sexual desire; furthermore, some pts may confuse erectile dysfunction with premature or retrograde ejaculation, and careful, explicit questioning is in order. Erectile dysfunction may also occur as part of a depressive episode or schizophrenia.

Erectile dysfunction secondary to male erectile disorder must be distinguished from erectile dysfunction that is either substance induced or due to a general medical condition, as noted in Table 10.4-1. For any given case of erectile dysfunction, combined factors are not uncommon; thus, a pt with diabetes mellitus of insufficient severity to cause erectile dysfunction by itself may experience erectile dysfunction after a trivial marital conflict, which by *itself* would not have caused difficulty before the onset of the diabetes.

Table 10.4-1. Other Causes of Erectile Dysfunction

General Medical Conditions

CNS conditions
  Limbic system lesions (infarctions, tumors, MS, neurosyphilis)
  Parkinson's disease
  Spinal cord lesions
Peripheral nervous system lesions
  Polyneuropathy (alcoholism, amyloidosis, diabetes, herpes genitalis)
  Surgical lesions (radical cystectomy, radical prostatectomy)
Peripheral vascular disease
  Large-vessel arteriosclerosis affecting aortoileal vessels (e.g., Leriche's syndrome)
  Arteriolopathy (e.g., diabetes mellitus)
  Pelvic radiation
Testosterone deficiency
  Hypothalamic lesions
  Pituitary lesions (e.g., tumors, esp prolactinomas; hemochromatosis; Cushing's syndrome)
  Primary testicular failure (e.g., mumps orchitis, Klinefelter's syndrome, myotonic dystrophy, lead poisoning, hepatic or renal failure)
Local diseases of the penis
  Peyronie's disease
  Chordee
  Sequela to priapism

Substances

Antidepressants (except nefazodone (Serzone), mirtazapine (Remeron), and bupropion (Wellbutrin, Zyban))
Neuroleptics
Lithium (Eskalith, Lithobid)
Various antihypertensives (propranolol (Inderal), clonidine (Catapres), reserpine, alpha-methyldopa (Aldomet), guanethidine, hydralazine)
Certain diuretics (e.g., hydrochlorothiazide (HydroDIURIL))
Digoxin (Lanoxin)
Cimetidine (Tagamet)
Clofibrate (Atromid)
Various antimetabolites
Alcohol
Stimulants
Opioids
Cannabis

Rx: In acute cases with clear precipitants, sometimes simple reassurance is effective; in other cases, sex therapy may be indicated. Sildenafil (Viagra) is also effective.

Sildenafil (Viagra) is taken in a dose of 25–100 (average 50) mg po ~2 h before anticipated intercourse, no more frequently than once daily. Peak blood levels are obtained within 30–120 min after oral administration, and absorption is delayed and reduced in the presence of a high-fat meal. The peak effect is generally seen 1–2 h after administration. Sildenafil has a half-life of about 3–5 h, and is metabolized in the liver by the cytochrome P450 enzyme 3A4 (CYP450 3A4) to N-desmethyl sildenafil, which is about 50% as potent as the parent compound. Sildenafil should never be given to pts taking nitrates of any kind, those with certain anatomic diseases of the penis (e.g., Peyronie's disease), or those on medications (e.g., trazodone) or with conditions (e.g., sickle cell anemia) that predispose to priapism. SEs include headache, flushing, dyspepsia, rhinitis, and loss of blue-green color discrimination; there are rare reports of cerebrovascular or cardiovascular events in apparently healthy men, and priapism has also been reported. Sildenafil should be given with caution to men with cardiovascular risk factors who are not in appropriate aerobic condition for strenuous intercourse. Fluvoxamine (Luvox) and nefazodone (Serzone) inhibit the CYP450 3A4 enzyme, and although not confirmed, would be expected to increase sildenafil levels. Cimetidine (Tagamet), erythromycin, and ketoconazole (Nizoral), all of which also inhibit the CYP450 3A4 enzyme, increase sildenafil levels up to 2-fold.

10.5 FEMALE ORGASMIC DISORDER

Arch Sex Behav 1975;4:265. Arch Sex Behav 1988;17:463. Arch Sex Behav 1992;21:69. J Consult Clin Psychol 1986;54:158.

Epidem: 5%–10% of females never experience orgasm; in another 30% transient anorgasmia may occur.

Sx: Despite adequate libido, arousal with lubrication, and stimulation, pts persistently and recurrently find themselves unable to achieve orgasm. In some pts, orgasm with self-masturbation is possible,

Table 10.5-1. Other Causes of Anorgasmia

General Medical Conditions	Substances
Spinal cord lesions	Antidepressants (except nefazodone (Serzone),
Hyperprolactinemia	mirtazapine (Remeron), bupropion (Wellbutrin,
Diabetes mellitus	Zyban))
Hypothyroidism	Neuroleptics
Surgery to the vulva or vagina	Various antihypertensives

whereas in others anorgasmia is seen with both intercourse and masturbation.

Lab: NC.

Crs: Pts who never experience orgasm from puberty on tend to have a chronic course.

Cmplc: Shame and dissatisfaction within the sexual relationship.

Etiol: Guilt, anger, and fear of losing control have been cited.

Ddx: Orgasm with intercourse is unlikely if foreplay is inadequate, or if the male has erectile dysfunction or premature ejaculation. Occasional failure to achieve orgasm with otherwise adequate intercourse is not at all uncommon, and should not be a cause for concern, as it typically passes quickly. Some women are concerned that they have orgasm only with clitoral stimulation; however, a lack of "vaginal" orgasm is not considered a disorder.

Depression may be accompanied by anorgasmia.

Orgasmic difficulties may be substance induced or due to a general medical condition, as noted in Table 10.5-1. In some pts, anorgasmia may occur with combined factors, e.g., guilt and use of an antihypertensive medication.

Rx: Sex therapy is often successful; when considerable conflict is present in a couple, couples therapy is often necessary.

10.6 MALE ORGASMIC DISORDER

Am J Psychiatry 1961;118:171. Arch Sex Behav 1979;8:139. Br J Psychiatry 1987;151:107. J Sex Marital Ther 1980;6:234.

Epidem: Rare.

Sx: Despite adequate desire, erection, and stimulation, the man persistently and recurrently fails to experience orgasm, or experiences it only after a very prolonged period; in a variant, orgasm may occur, but is slow and pleasureless. In some cases, the man is able to achieve orgasm with masturbation or fellatio, whereas in others anorgasmia persists in all situations.

Lab: NC.

Crs: Inability to achieve orgasm that begins with puberty is generally chronic.

Cmplc: Both pt and partner are often frustrated, and the partner may feel rejected.

Etiol: Severe guilt and/or hostility toward the partner are common.

Ddx: Hypoactive sexual desire may mimic male orgasmic disorder when the male, simply lacking the desire to consummate intercourse, "gives up."

Older males normally require longer time to achieve orgasm.

Retrograde ejaculation, as may be seen with certain medications (e.g., thioridazine (Mellaril)) or after prostatectomy, is distinguished by the fact that orgasm does occur. All that is lacking is the appearance of the ejaculate, which is directed into the bladder.

Retarded ejaculation may be substance induced or due to general medical conditions, as noted in Table 10.6-1.

Table 10.6-1. Other Causes of Retarded Ejaculation

General Medical Conditions

Sacral cord lesions
Sympathectomy
Polyneuropathy (sensory or autonomic)
Radical prostatectomy
Testosterone deficiency
Hyperprolactinemia

Substances

Antidepressants (esp clomipramine (Anafranil) and SSRIs)
Neuroleptics (esp thioridazine (Mellaril))
Various antihypertensives (esp guanethidine and alpha-methyldopa (Aldomet))
Alcohol
Opioids
Cocaine

Rx: Sex therapy is often successful; when there is considerable hostility, couples or individual psychotherapy is often required.

10.7 PREMATURE EJACULATION

Am J Psychiatry 1994;151:1377. J Clin Psychiatry 1995;56:402. J Clin Psychopharm 1995;15:341.

Epidem: Lifetime prevalence ~30% of men.

Sx: Onset typically in adolescence, with initial intercourse; may also occur after a prolonged period of normal sexual functioning.

Men recurrently experience ejaculation earlier than they wish to, sometimes during foreplay, intromission, or after a few thrusts, and before the woman achieves orgasm.

Lab: NC.

Crs: Early onset tends to be chronic.

Cmplc: Shame, anxiety, and conflict within the relationship.

Etiol: Anxiety, apprehension, guilt, and anger predispose to premature ejaculation.

Ddx: Transient premature ejaculation is the rule in adolescent males, who typically achieve normal functioning with increasing sexual experience.

If the female has female orgasmic disorder (anorgasmia), then, in a sense, ejaculation will almost always be "premature." Considerable clinical judgment is called for here.

Rarely, premature ejaculation occurs with sacral cord lesions or in Parkinson's disease.

Rx: Behavioral treatment, using the "stop and start" or "squeeze" techniques, is very effective.

Sertraline (Zoloft) or paroxetine (Paxil), in doses as used for depression (see 6.1), and clomipramine (Anafranil), at only 50 mg/d, delay ejaculation.

10.8 DYSPAREUNIA (NOT DUE TO A GENERAL MEDICAL CONDITION)

J Nerv Ment Dis 1994;182:264. J Fam Pract 1987;24:66. Psychosomatics 1983;24:1076.

Epidem: Uncertain; although dyspareunia is a common complaint to gynecologists, most cases are due to a general medical condition.

Sx: Pts, male or female, experience pain either during or immediately after intercourse.

Lab: NC, except as noted below under Ddx.

Crs: Uncertain.

Cmplc: Avoidance of intimate situations in males and females; in females, vaginismus may ensue.

Etiol: For dyspareunia not due to a general medical condition, guilt over sexual pleasure often plays a role.

Ddx: See Table 10.8-1. These causes of painful intercourse must be ruled out before tentatively assuming that the dyspareunia is psychologically determined.

Table 10.8-1. Causes of Dyspareunia

General Medical Condition

Female
  Vaginitis
  Postoperative scars
  Hymenal remnants
  Endometriosis
  Allergic reactions to condoms, lubricants, or semen
Male
  Prostatitis
  Urethritis
  Penile rash (e.g., herpes genitalis)
  Peyronie's disease
  Chordee

Substances

Neuroleptics (e.g., thioridazine (Mellaril))
Antidepressants, e.g., amoxapine (Asendin), tricyclics (e.g., imipramine (Tofranil), clomipramine (Anafranil)), SSRIs

SEXUAL AND RELATED DISORDERS

Rx: For dyspareunia of psychological origin, couples therapy is generally required in conjunction with individual approaches; progressive desensitization may be helpful in some women.

10.9 VAGINISMUS

Arch Gen Psychiatry 1979;36:824. Irish Med J 1986;79:59. Irish Med J 1986;79:59.

Epidem: Lifetime prevalence <10% of women.

Sx: Onset often upon first attempted intercourse or during first pelvic examination. Vaginismus following a period of normal sexual functioning may also occur.

Perineal muscular spasm results in tightening or complete closure of the outer third of the vagina, making intromission impossible or very difficult; similar spasm may or may not occur with gynecologic examination.

Lab: NC.

Crs: Generally chronic.

Cmplc: Tension in the sexual relationship almost inevitable; pregnancy and routine gynecologic care may be impossible.

Etiol: Typically seen in women who experience significant guilt or anxiety about intercourse; may follow dyspareunia, or rape or other sexual trauma.

Ddx: Hymenal remnants or surgical scars may make intromission difficult.

Rx: With concurrent couples therapy, pts also undergo graded desensitization to penetration with objects such as dilators.

10.10 PARAPHILIAS

Am J Psychiatry 1981;138:601. Acta Psychiatr Scand 1983;77:199. Br J Psychiatry 1983;142:292.

Epidem: Uncertain; probably vastly underreported. Almost all paraphiliacs are male; exceptions include masochism, pedophilia, and zoo-philia.

Sx: Onset of paraphilic urges typically in adolescence or childhood; an exception might be pedophilia, as some pedophiliacs deny having had urges before middle years.

All the paraphilias share certain common characteristics, namely, that the preferred object of sexual desire is something *other* than mutually enjoyable, nonpainful sexual activity with a postpubertal, consenting partner. Common kinds of paraphilias are as follows:

- *Exhibitionism,* wherein the paraphiliac exposes himself to unsuspecting females, often masturbating during the exposure, or after getting home
- *Fetishism,* wherein the paraphiliac prefers objects, such as shoes, lingerie, locks of hair, etc., to people, and may masturbate to the sight or touch of the fetish
- *Frotteurism,* wherein the paraphiliac selects attractive, unsuspecting females in crowded places (e.g., subway crowds), and insinuates himself through the crowd until he is next to her, whereupon he often rubs his penis or hands on her buttocks or legs
- *Pedophilia,* wherein the pedophile prefers children, in many cases, children of either sex, and may seek employment in day-care centers, elementary schools, etc.
- *Masochism,* wherein the paraphiliac, in order to become aroused and orgasmic, seeks out pain or humiliation
- *Sadism,* wherein the paraphiliac, in order to become aroused and orgasmic, must inflict pain or humiliation on others, sometimes to the point of murder ("lust murder")
- *Transvestic fetishism,* wherein the paraphiliac male, in order to become and stay aroused, must dress as a woman (importantly, such individuals prefer females, and are not homosexually oriented)
- *Voyeurism,* wherein the paraphiliac prefers to surreptitiously watch women as they unclothe or engage in foreplay or intercourse

Other paraphilias, less well studied, include zoophilia (intercourse with animals); coprophilia or urophilia, wherein feces or urine are sexually exciting; necrophilia, wherein dead bodies are preferred; klismaphilia, which involves erotic pleasure from enemas; and asphyxophilia (or hypoxyphilia), wherein pts engage in partial hanging or strangulation for sexual pleasure, activities that may have a fatal outcome.

Some paraphiliacs are married, and capable of normal, nonparaphilic sexual relations. Critically, however, they much prefer the paraphilic activity, and indeed may not be able to engage in intercourse unless they imagine themselves involved in paraphilic activity.

Most paraphiliacs have more than 1 paraphilia; 3–5 are common.

Although some paraphiliacs are ashamed of their behavior, most appear to be comfortable with it, and see nothing wrong. If caught, they may offer elaborate rationalizations.

Concurrent alcoholism, and antisocial and borderline personality disorders are common.

Lab: NC.

Crs: Chronic; although the frequency of paraphilic behavior may decline past age 25, the fantasies remain. An exception is masochism or sadism, wherein age may bring an increase in severity.

Cmplc: If involved with a female who finds out, the paraphiliac may find the relationship over; for others, arrest and incarceration may await.

Etiol: Uncertain; disturbed childhood experiences, subtle central nervous stem abnormalities, hormonal derangements, and heredity have been proposed. In the case of pedophilia, it appears that most of these paraphiliacs were molested as children; and in the case of transvestic fetishism, it appears that a number of these paraphiliacs were forced to cross-dress as young boys.

Ddx: Occasional paraphilic interests are normal in boys, and in men. Most boys occasionally cross-dress, and most men, at times, fantasize about lingerie, dominance, etc. Critically, however, these paraphilic interests are not prominent, and either fade or are used in the service of nonparaphilic sexual behavior (e.g., the man who asks his wife to wear a certain lingerie).

Dementia, personality change, and MR may lead to abnormal sexual behavior; here the accompanying sx indicate the correct dx.

Schizophrenia and mania may lead to bizarre or indiscriminate sexual behavior; here also the accompanying sx indicate the correct dx.

Cross-dressing may occur in situations or conditions other than transvestic fetishism. Effeminate homosexuals may cross-dress to attract other men, in contrast to the transvestic fetishist, whose interest is in women; transsexuals often cross-dress, but this is out of a desire to be a woman, in contrast to the transvestic fetishist, who wishes to remain a man.

Rx: Medroxyprogesterone acetate (Depo-Provera) or leuprolide acetate (Lupron Depot) decrease libido, with a consequent reduction in the frequency of paraphilic acts. Medroxyprogesterone is given as 200–500 mg im q 7 d, with the dose and frequency then titrated to the pt's condition; often it is possible to taper to perhaps 250 mg q 28 d. Leuprolide is given as 7.5 mg im q 28 d; during the first 2 wk there may be an increase in testosterone levels and an exacerbation of the pt's condition, after which testosterone levels fall and remain very low. During the first 2 wk, it may be appropriate to give a testosterone-blocking agent, such as flutamide (Eulexin) 250 mg po bid. Both medroxyprogesterone and leuprolide have considerable SEs, and the risk-benefit ratio must be carefully discussed with the pt.

Sex education and social skills training may enable the pt to develop normal sexual relations to take the place of the paraphilic behavior.

Various behavioral techniques, e.g., imagining adverse consequences, masturbating beyond satiation to paraphilic fantasies, may also be useful.

Alcohol and other disinhibiting drugs must be avoided.

Overall, the treatment of paraphilia is difficult, and many pts drop out of Rx as soon as legally possible; ethical conflicts are common, and difficult cases may be best referred to specialists.

10.11 GENDER IDENTITY DISORDER (TRANSSEXUALISM)

Am J Psychiatry 1980;137:432. Br J Psychiatry 1990;156:894. J Clin Psychiatry 1990;51:57.

Epidem: Probably rare, perhaps 0.00002% of general adult population; probably much more common in males than females.

Sx: Onset may be in early childhood, or delayed until teenage or adult years.

Male transsexuals consider themselves to be females "trapped" within a male body; wish to be rid of facial hair, penis, and testicles; and want to develop breasts and to have a vagina. They typically dress and act like women, and indeed, may be able to pass for women.

Female transsexuals, conversely, consider themselves to be males "trapped" within a female body, wish to be rid of breasts and vagina, and want to develop a penis. Typically, they dress and act like men, and may be able to pass for men.

Esp in male transsexuals, a concurrent borderline personality disorder is often present.

Lab: NC.

Crs: Early, childhood-onset cases tend to be chronic. Delayed-onset cases may exhibit fluctuating sx over time, and such pts at times may exhibit little "gender dysphoria" at all, and be more or less content with their secondary sexual characteristics.

Cmplc: "Discovery" may bring devastating social and personal repercussions; for many male transsexuals, however, the complications of borderline personality disorder are more prominent.

Etiol: Unknown; genetic, endocrinologic, and child-rearing practices have all been suspected.

Ddx: Schizophrenia may cause the delusion that one belongs to the opposite sex. Other sx (auditory hallucinations, looseness of associations, etc.) indicate the correct dx.

Cross-dressing, as may occur in transvestic fetishism or effeminate homosexuality, are fundamentally different from transsexualism. Both the fetishist and the homosexual male value having a penis, whereas the transsexual wants to be rid of it.

Intersex states (e.g., pseudohermaphroditism) are distinguished by the ambiguous genitalia.

Rx: Psychotherapy should be offered to those with delayed onset who are uncertain about their gender.

Patients who are certain about their gender may be offered sex-reassignment treatment. Before surgery, pts are required to live as members of the opposite sex generally at least for a year to see if they are emotionally capable of doing so; those who pass are offered hormonal treatment (and, for males, electrolysis), and if the pt continues to do well, then surgery may be offered. Sex-reassignment treatment should probably be done only at specialized clinics.

11. Eating Disorders

11.1 ANOREXIA NERVOSA

Br J Psychiatry 1992;161:104. Br J Psychiatry 1993;162:452. Psychosomatic Med 1974;36:18. Q J Med 1993;86:791.

Epidem: >95% female; prevalence among teenage and young adult females ~0.5%.

Sx: Onset typically in teenage years, typically 4–5 yr after menarche; onsets in childhood or middle years unusual. Premorbidly, most pts are not overweight.

Hallmark of anorexia nervosa is a persistent conviction that one is fat (or about to become so), coupled with a relentless pursuit of thinness by means of dieting and exercise. The result can be heart wrenching: young women reduced to the appearance of concentration camp survivors by their self-imposed starvation who still insist they are overweight and persist in their refusal to eat. Importantly, at least until starvation-induced inanition sets in, these pts do not lose their appetites; indeed they may be intensely preoccupied with food, reading cookbooks and helping prepare meals that they then refuse to eat. Jogging, running, bicycling, and other "aerobic" exercises are preferred over those that might add mass, such as swimming or weight lifting. Some pts, too weak to stand, may yet continue their aerobics in the hospital bed by doing calisthenics lying down.

In addition to dieting and exercise, some pts may engage in self-induced vomiting or laxative-induced purging in order to rid themselves of calories; a smaller percentage may use diuretics to force more weight off.

The degree of weight loss varies, from as little as 15% to a state of profound emaciation. Most pts experience amenorrhea, and interestingly, this may begin before there is any appreciable weight loss. Constipation is also very common. PE typically reveals findings common to starvation of any cause: decreases in temperature, pulse, and BP, and edema.

The foregoing describes the classic "restricter" anorectic. In about one-fourth of pts, a variant occurs, characterized by episodes of binge eating. As discussed below, under Ddx, in such pts a concurrent dx of bulimia nervosa may be warranted.

Lab: Typical of starvation of any cause: pancytopenia, hypokalemia, prerenal azotemia, elevated liver enzyme levels, hypercarotenemia (which may give a yellowish cast to the skin), and in those with frequent vomiting, elevated amylase levels.

Crs: Death from starvation, suicide, or 1 of the complications noted below, in ~15%. Of survivors, most regain some weight but continue to experience concern over weight and to exhibit peculiarities in eating, and in clothing, often favoring the "baggy" look.

Cmplc: Hypokalemia, which may be quite severe in vomiters or purgers, may precipitate lethal arrhythmias; starvation and pancytopenia predispose to infection; and pts are at risk for pneumonia and septicemia.

Withdrawn, emaciated, and preoccupied with dieting and solitary exercise, pts rarely undergo normal psychosexual maturation.

Etiol: Concordance rises from ~5% for first-degree female relatives to 10% for DZ twins to ~50% for MZ twins.

CSF levels of CRF are elevated, and the ACTH response to CRF is blunted. These findings are *not* typical of starvation, but are similar to those seen in major depression. Furthermore, the prevalence of mood disorders is higher among relatives of anorexia nervosa pts than among relatives of controls.

Early theories of a link between socioeconomic class and anorexia nervosa have not been borne out, and causal links between anorexia nervosa and premorbid family structure are speculative.

Ddx: Multiple other potentially wasting conditions (e.g., depression, cancer, hypothalamic tumors) are ruled out by the absence of intentional dieting.

Schizophrenia, rarely, may be dominated by delusions regarding food, which may prevent pts from eating. Here, other sx, not found with anorexia nervosa, indicate the correct dx: hallucinations, mannerisms, loosening of associations.

Bulimia nervosa is considered when episodes of binge eating occur. In pts in whom the bingeing is infrequent (perhaps less than once monthly) and began only after the onset of anorexia nervosa, an additional dx is not warranted. However, if binges are frequent (e.g., several times per week) and preceded the onset of anorexia nervosa, then one may assume that 2 disorders are present: anorexia nervosa and bulimia nervosa.

Rx: Weight restoration may be accomplished with a behavioral program: failure of outpatient Rx or the presence of inanition or serious complications necessitates admission. Concurrent with weight restoration measures, and afterward, pts must be seen in psychotherapy. Treatment of pts with anorexia nervosa, particularly during weight restoration, is difficult, even in experienced hands. Medications, in general, are not helpful.

11.2 BULIMIA NERVOSA

Am J Psychiatry 1977;134:1249. Am J Psychiatry 1985;142:482. Arch Gen Psychiatry 1992;49:139. J Clin Psychiatry 1990;51:373. J Clin Psychiatry 1998;59(Suppl 15):28. Q J Med 1985;54:177.

Epidem: >90% female; prevalence in female population ~1%–3%.

Sx: Onset from midadolescence to early adult years.

Episodes of binge eating range in frequency from 2 to 50/wk. The urge to binge may appear acutely or gradually; most pts will attempt to resist the urge, generally in vain. Once the binge begins, pts rapidly consume often enormous amounts of food, preferably sweets, cakes, cookies, or ice cream. Most binges last an hour or less; some pts stop out of shame or disgust, others because of bloating, and some because the stomach and esophagus are literally engorged with food. Afterward, most pts feel guilty and anxious over their bingeing and most attempt to undo the damage either by purging or with subsequent diet and exercise. The "purging" type of bulimic may engage in vomiting or laxative abuse. Vomiting is initially self-induced; however, over time it becomes reflexive and automatic; some pts use ipecac. Laxative use at times may be extreme, with up to 50 times the normal therapeutic dose of stimulant laxatives being taken. The "nonpurging" variety of bulimia, which is less common, is characterized by a more or less strict diet and a devotion to aerobic exercise. Such pts may experience substantial fluctuations in weight, with binge-induced gain followed by diet and exercise-induced loss.

In addition to binges, pts also typically have a distorted body image, believing themselves fat, or about to become so.

Other common concurrent disorders include major depression, panic disorder, kleptomania, alcohol abuse, and borderline personality disorder.

Lab: Amylase levels may be elevated, and may show a correlation with the frequency of binges.

Hypokalemia and hypomagnesemia may occur with extensive vomiting and diarrhea.

Crs: Either chronic or episodic (with periods of frequent bingeing alternating with long binge-free intervals) until spontaneous remission in middle years.

Cmplc: Acute gastric dilatation and rupture may occur during a severe binge.

Esophagitis or esophageal rupture may follow vomiting.

Dental erosion and multiple caries may occur secondary to acidic vomitus.

Arrhythmias may occur secondary to hypokalemia, and excessive ipecac use may cause a cardiomyopathy.

Etiol: Serotoninergic transmission disturbed: CSF 5-hydroxyindoleacetic acid levels are low, and tryptophan depletion causes an increased frequency of bingeing. Positive DST result and increased prevalence of mood disorders in pts strongly suggest a link to major depression.

CCK is normally secreted from gut after a meal; in bulimia, both CSF and blood levels of CCK are low, suggesting a disturbance in satiety mechanisms.

The paroxysmal nature of the binge, coupled with the effectiveness of phenytoin, suggests that bulimia, in some pts, may represent a simple partial seizure.

Ddx: Simple overeating is characterized either by constant overeating or by frequent "snacking" and does not involve actual binges.

Hyperphagia, like simple overeating, is chronic and not marked by binges. It may be seen with bipolar disorder, the Prader-Willi syndrome, the Laurence-Moon-Biedl syndrome, and lesions of the thalamus or hypothalamus.

Kleine-Levin syndrome, discussed in 12.3, is distinguished by prolonged (~2 wk) episodes of overeating that are accompanied by somnolence.

Rx: Both cognitive behavior therapy and medications are effective.

Imipramine (Tofranil), desipramine (Norpramin), trazodone (Desyrel), phenelzine (Nardil), and fluoxetine (Prozac) are effective; doses are similar to those used for depression (see 6.1), with the exception of fluoxetine (Prozac), of which doses of 60 mg are generally required. Given the relative lack of SEs, fluoxetine (Prozac) is generally the first choice.

Phenytoin (Dilantin), in 1 double-blind study, was more effective than placebo.

12. Sleep Disorders

12.1 PRIMARY INSOMNIA (PSYCHOPHYSIOLOGIC INSOMNIA AND IDIOPATHIC INSOMNIA)

J Clin Psychiatry 1992;53(Suppl 6):37. Mayo Clin Proc 1990;65:869.
  Sleep 1980;3:59. Sleep 1986;9:38.

Epidem: Uncertain; probably common.

Sx: Onset of the psychophysiologic type generally in early or mid adult years; of the idiopathic type, childhood years.

For at least a month, pts chronically and recurrently have trouble either falling or staying asleep, or commonly, both.

Lab: Polysomnography reveals delayed sleep onset and decreased sleep efficiency.

Crs: Generally chronic, with the exception of psychophysiologic types that begin acutely after a major precipitating event, and may resolve in a matter of months.

Cmplc: Pts often experience drowsiness and poor concentration during the day, and work and personal matters may suffer.

Etiol: The psychophysiologic type typically begins with a major stress (e.g., an illness, divorce, etc.) and becomes self-perpetuating as pts become progressively more anxious and tense about the prospect of not being able to fall asleep. Interestingly, these pts often find it easier to fall and stay asleep when not in their own bed (e.g., on the couch in the living room, at a hotel).

The idiopathic type may represent a disturbance in brain stem mechanisms responsible for sleep.

Ddx: "Short sleepers" are individuals with a reduced need for sleep, and are distinguished by their ability to fall asleep readily and by their wakefulness during the day despite getting 6 h of sleep or less a night.

Table 12.1-1. Causes of Insomnia

Related to Another Mental Disorder

Depressive episode (of major depression or bipolar disorder)
Dysthymia
Schizophrenia
Generalized anxiety disorder
PTSD

General Medical Condition

Circadian rhythm sleep disorder
Sleep apnea
Restless legs syndrome
Syndrome of painful legs and moving toes
Nocturnal myoclonus
Any painful or distressing condition (e.g., GERD, arthritis, CHF)
Dementia (esp fatal familial insomnia)

Substances

Caffeine
Stimulants (e.g., cocaine)
Alcohol withdrawal
Opioid withdrawal

Elderly individuals often simply require less sleep than when they
were younger.

"Sleep state misperception" is said to occur in pts who, despite poly-
somnographically documented adequate sleep, claim insomnia.

Insomnia may be related to another mental disorder, due to a general
medical condition, or substance induced, and examples are provided in Table 12.1-1.

Rx: The bedroom should generally be dark and quiet, and the bed
should be reserved for sleeping or sex (and in cases where sexual
activity is anxiety provoking, it may be prudent to restrict sex to
another room). When pts are unable to fall asleep, they should get
up and do something else, perhaps something boring, until they
feel sleepy again. Wake-up times should be strictly adhered to. In
some pts, relaxation therapy may help, and in pts marked by
excessive worrying, cognitive therapy may also help.

Helpful medications include antihistamines (e.g., hydroxyzine (Vistaril) 50–100 mg), antidepressants (e.g., trazodone (Desyrel)

50–150 mg), and benzodiazepines (e.g., lorazepam (Ativan) 2 mg or zolpidem (Ambien) 10 mg). The benzodiazepines should probably not be used for more than 2 wk, as beyond that tolerance and withdrawal (with "rebound" insomnia) may occur. Neither trazodone (Desyrel) nor zolpidem (Ambien) disturb normal sleep architecture.

12.2 PRIMARY HYPERSOMNIA (IDIOPATHIC HYPERSOMNIA)

Ann Neurol 1992;32:162. Ann Neurol 1996;39:471. Neurology 1991; 41:726.

Epidem: Uncertain; of those who present to a sleep disorders clinic, 5%–10% are diagnosed as having primary hypersomnia.

Sx: Onset is gradual in late teens or early adult years.

In addition to prolonged nocturnal sleep (>8 h, generally 9 h or more) with difficulty waking up, pts also experience excessive daytime sleepiness with frequent naps. The naps may be intentional or not; in any case they come on gradually, are not associated with dreaming, and importantly, are not refreshing.

Lab: Polysomnography reveals a short sleep latency, but is generally otherwise wnl. The multiple sleep latency test fails to reveal any sleep-onset REM during the naps.

Crs: Generally chronic.

Cmplc: Excessive daytime sleepiness and frequent naps may interfere with work and social relations, and may be dangerous (e.g., while driving or operating certain machines).

Etiol: Unknown; in some pts familial.

Ddx: "Long sleepers" may regularly get >8 or 9 h of sleep per night, but here daytime drowsiness and involuntary "naps" are lacking.

"Catch-up" sleep may occur in those who've been sleep deprived, but is only temporary.

Kleine-Levin syndrome, at times referred to as the "recurrent form of primary hypersomnia," is discussed in 12.3.

Primary hypersomnia must be distinguished from hypersomnia related to another mental disorder, hypersomnia due to a general

Table 12.2-1. Other Causes of Hypersomnia

Related to Another Mental Disorder

Depressive episode, as in major depression, or more commonly, bipolar disorder

General Medical Condition

Narcolepsy
Sleep apnea
Circadian rhythm sleep disorder
Pickwickian syndrome
Respiratory failure
Myotonic muscular dystrophy
Hypothyroidism
Posttraumatic (i.e., upon recovery from a closed head injury)
Focal lesions (e.g., tumors, infarcts) in cerebral hemispheres, thalamus, hypothalamus, or brain stem

Substances

Alcohol
Sedative-hypnotics (esp benzodiazepines)
Various antidepressants
Various neuroleptics
Opioids (either during acute use or in withdrawal)
Withdrawal from stimulants or caffeine

medical condition, and substance-induced hypersomnia, as noted in Table 12.2-1.

Narcolepsy may be suggested by the recurrent naps of primary hypersomnia, but is distinguished by the fact that in narcolepsy the "naps" come in discrete sleep attacks, often refreshing, and are typically associated with REM sleep and dreaming.

Sleep apnea is suggested by prominent snoring, and by associated hypertension.

Recurrent hypersomnia is distinguished from primary hypersomnia by its episodic course, and is exemplified by the Kleine-Levin syndrome and menstrual-related (catamenial) sleep disorder.

Rx: Uncertain; proper sleep hygiene is important; unclear if scheduled naps are helpful. Many pts are treated with methylphenidate (Ritalin) or pemoline (Cylert), as described for narcolepsy in 12.4.

12.3 KLEINE-LEVIN SYNDROME (RECURRENT FORM OF PRIMARY HYPERSOMNIA)

Acta Neurol Scand 1990;82:361. Brain 1936;59:494. Brain 1962;85: 627.

Epidem: Rare; almost exclusively seen in males.

Sx: Onset in late childhood or adolescence.

Episodes, lasting usually 1 or 2 wk (range, days to 4 wk), are characterized by hypersomnolence, hyperphagia, and hypersexuality. Pts may sleep 18 h or more per day; when awake, they may consume vast amounts of food, and may engage in unusual sexual behavior, with frequent masturbation, exhibitionism, or unwelcome sexual advances. Pts may also experience affective changes, toward either euphoria or depression, and delusions and hallucinations may also occur.

In between episodes, most pts return to normal; however, some may show some loss of academic ability.

Lab: NC.

Crs: Early on, episodes tend to occur q 3–6 mo; over time episodes become less severe and less frequent, and in most pts cease by the 20s or 30s.

Cmplc: Pts are effectively disabled during the episode.

Etiol: Uncertain; in some pts the initial episode is preceded by a flulike illness or head trauma. Episodic dysfunction of the hypothalamus and related structures is suspected; at some autopsies, damage to the thalamus and brain stem has been noted.

Ddx: The episodic nature of the illness, with the associated hyperphagia and hypersexuality, is distinctive, and not reproduced by any other form of hypersomnia (see 12.2).

Mania of the mixed type (as in bipolar disorder) is distinguished by the absence of hyperphagia.

Bulimia nervosa is distinguished by the absence of somnolence and by the brevity of the attacks of binge eating.

Rx: Lithium (Eskalith, Lithobid) (used as in bipolar disorder), stimulants such as methylphenidate (Ritalin), and some TCAs, anecdotally, have been successful.

12.4 NARCOLEPSY

Arch Neurol 1982;39:164. J Neurol Neurosurg Psychiatry 1995;59:221. NEJM 1990;323:389. Sleep 1994;17(Suppl 8):21.

Epidem: Lifetime prevalence ~0.1%.

Sx: Onset ranges from childhood to 40 yr, typically in late teens or early adult years.

The full syndrome consists of a tetrad of (1) narcoleptic attacks, (2) cataplectic attacks, (3) sleep paralysis, and (4) hypnagogic (or hypnopompic) hallucinations. All pts experience narcoleptic attacks and in the overwhelming majority, the first sx of the illness is a narcoleptic attack; the majority also eventually experience cataplectic attacks and about one-third also experience sleep paralysis or hypnagogic hallucinations. The full tetrad is seen in only ~10%.

Narcoleptic attacks are ushered in by an overwhelming desire to sleep followed by a period of REM sleep that may last from seconds up to a half hour. During the attack pts are easily awakened, by perhaps calling their name or being lightly touched. Upon awakening, most pts feel refreshed and can recall often vivid dreams.

Cataplectic attacks are typically precipitated by a sudden strong emotion, generally mirth, but occasionally anger, or simply being suddenly surprised. The attack itself consists of a sudden weakness. Often the weakness is generalized, and pts fall or slump over; occasionally the weakness may be focal, confined perhaps to the neck or to the hand. Importantly, in all pts, even when the weakness is generalized, diaphragmatic and extraocular muscles remain at full strength and pts remain fully alert. Most attacks clear within a minute; longer attacks may be accompanied by vivid visual hallucinations.

Sleep paralysis may occur upon either falling asleep or awakening. Pts, though fully alert and conscious, experience generalized weakness, which, as with cataplectic attacks, spares the diaphragm and extraocular muscles. Occasionally, there may be visual hallucinations. Most pts, at least initially, find these attacks frightening, but over time, most pts accept them and simply wait them out until strength returns a few minutes later. To an observer, these pts appear peacefully asleep; most pts may be immediately awakened by a touch or calling their name.

Hypnagogic hallucinations are hallucinations (visual > auditory) that occur as the pt is falling asleep; hypnopompic, as they are waking up. The hallucinations are generally quite vivid.

Lab: The multiple sleep latency test reveals sleep-onset REM sleep in most pts. False-negative and false-positive results, however, may occur.

Virtually all pts are positive for the HLA-DR2 antigen; this test is falsely positive, however, in ~20% of the normal population.

Crs: Generally chronic; in a minority there may be long attack-free intervals, and in a small minority, permanent spontaneous remissions may occur.

Cmplc: Narcoleptic attacks may be life-threatening should they occur while driving or operating dangerous machinery; cataplectic attacks pose the same risks, along with the risk of injury through falls.

Etiol: Both sporadic and hereditary cases are seen. Hereditary cases may be autosomal dominant with variable penetrance, or multifactorial; disturbances in brain stem mechanisms for sleep and dreaming are strongly suspected.

Ddx: The combination of narcoleptic attacks and cataplectic attacks is very highly specific for narcolepsy; thus, the ddx question generally only arises with pts who have only sleep attacks, without any of the other elements of the tetrad.

Sleep attacks strongly resembling those seen with narcolepsy may occur in a number of conditions, as listed in Table 12.4-1. The sleep attacks seen with narcolepsy must also be distinguished from the excessive napping seen with primary hypersomnia (see 12.2).

Cataplectic attacks are most commonly produced by narcolepsy; however, they may occur in other conditions, as listed in Table 12.4-2. As noted above, in narcolepsy the first sx generally consists of narcoleptic attacks. Consequently if a pt presents with cataplectic attacks without a h/o narcoleptic attacks, then one of the conditions in Table 12.4-2 should be strongly suspected.

Table 12.4-1. Causes of Sleep Attacks

Brain stem or diencephalic lesions
Temporal lobe lesion
Postencephalitis lethargica
"Idiopathic recurring stupor" (attacks long, from hours to days, and of gradual onset and termination)

Table 12.4-2. Causes of Cataplexy

Idiopathic
Dominantly inherited
Mesencephalic or pontine lesions
Simple partial seizure

Table 12.4-3. Pharmacologic Treatment of Narcolepsy

		Effective for	
	Dose (mg)	Narcoleptic Attack	Cataplectic Attack
Methylphenidate (Ritalin)	20–60	+	−
Pemoline (Cylert)	37.5–150	+	−
Clomipramine (Anafranil)	25–75	+	+
Desipramine (Norpramin)	25–75	+	+
Protriptyline (Vivactil)	10–40	+	+
Phenelzine (Nardil)	30–45	+	+
Tranylcypromine (Parnate)	20–40	+	+

Rx: Until both narcoleptic and cataplectic attacks are controlled, pts
must abstain from driving or using hazardous machines.
Scheduled afternoon naps reduce the frequency of narcoleptic attacks.
Table 12.4-3 lists pharmacologic agents useful for narcolepsy.
Although stimulants (i.e., methylphenidate (Ritalin), pemoline
(Cylert)) are traditional, they are not effective for cataplectic
attacks; antidepressants, effective for both narcoleptic and cataplectic attacks, offer a definite alternative: The MAOIs (phenelzine
(Nardil), tranylcypromine (Parnate)), though effective, are difficult
to use due to dietary restrictions; of the TCAs, clomipramine (Anafranil) tends to be sedating, and thus desipramine (Norpramin) or
protriptyline (Vivactil) may be best to start with. The doses given
are only rough guidelines, and individualization is a necessity.

12.5 SLEEP APNEA (BREATHING-RELATED SLEEP DISORDER)

Ann Int Med 1987;106:434. Lancet 1994;344:653. Lancet 1994;344:
  656. Neurology 1992;42(Suppl 6):53.

Epidem: Lifetime prevalence ~1%–10%, male-female ratio 3:1.
Sx: Onset typically in middle years, in females especially after menopause.

  Apneic episodes last 10–120 sec, and 30–300 may occur each night.
    There are 3 types: obstructive, central, and mixed; obstructive is
    most common, mixed next so, and pure central is rare.

  - Obstructive apneic episodes are characterized by an increasingly
    vigorous inspiratory effort that fails to result in any air inflow
    via the nose or mouth due to closure of the oropharyngeal air-
    way. Eventually, the blockage is interrupted with a loud, gasping
    snort, followed by a brief, partial awakening, lasting only sec-
    onds, after which the pt falls asleep again. Most pts are heavy
    snorers, and rather than complaining of multiple awakenings,
    generally complain of excessive daytime sleepiness.
  - Mixed apneic episodes are biphasic, characterized by an initial
    central apnea, with lack of respiratory effort, followed by an
    inspiratory effort that is blocked by an obstructed oropharyngeal
    airway, which in turn is finally overcome with a gasping snort.
    Mixed apnea pts, like those with obstructive type, generally com-
    plain of excessive daytime sleepiness.
  - Central apneic episodes are characterized by a simple cessation
    of all inspiratory effort. Eventually, diaphragmatic and intercos-
    tal movements occur, and inspiration occurs, often accompanied
    by a brief awakening. Typically these pts complain of multiple
    awakenings, rather than daytime sleepiness.

  In addition to complaints of daytime sleepiness or multiple awaken-
    ings, most pts also experience headaches, difficulty with concentra-
    tion, irritability, or in males, impotence.
Lab: Polysomnography documents the apneic episodes.
Crs: Chronic.
Cmplc: Snoring by obstructive or mixed apneic pts may disturb bed
  partners; daytime sleepiness may lead to accidents or be mis-
  interpreted as "falling asleep at the job," leading to job termina-

Table 12.5-1. Causes of Sleep Apnea

Obstructive

Micrognathia
Tonsillar or adenoidal hypertrophy
Lingual hypertrophy (e.g., hypothyroidism, acromegaly)
Obesity
Defective brain stem respiratory mechanism

Central

Obesity
Defective brain stem respiratory mechanism

tion. Poor concentration and irritability may interfere with most activities.

Apneic episodes may be accompanied by various arrhythmias: sinus bradycardia or tachycardia, sinus arrest, atrial flutter, and ventricular tachycardia.

Hypercapnia occurring during the apnea may eventually lead to pulmonary hypertension; systemic hypertension may also occur.

Etiol: See Table 12.5-1.

Ddx: Normal individuals may have up to 10 apneic episodes/night.

Excessive daytime sleepiness, as noted, is the typical presenting complaint of pts with sleep apnea. Other causes of excessive daytime sleepiness are noted in the Ddx section for primary hypersomnia (see 12.2).

Rx: Correctable etiologies of sleep apnea are attended to; for obese pts weight loss cannot be overemphasized. Instruct pts to sleep on their sides, a position that favors airway patency.

Obstructive sleep apnea may be treated with protriptyline (Vivactil) 20–60 mg/d, and for mild cases, an oral appliance. In moderate or severe cases, continuous positive airway pressure devices are often effective, but many pts find them unacceptable. Surgical approaches include uvulopalatopharyngoplasty or tracheostomy.

Central sleep apnea may be treated with protriptyline (Vivactil), as above, or acetazolamide 250 mg qid. Diaphragmatic pacing may be required in severe cases.

Sedative-hypnotics, alcohol, benzodiazepines, and any medicine likely to reduce respiratory drive should be avoided.

12.6 PICKWICKIAN SYNDROME (CENTRAL ALVEOLAR HYPOVENTILATION SYNDROME)

Am J Med 1956;21:811. Int J Obesity 1992;16(Suppl):37. Neurology 1961;11:950.

Epidem: Uncertain, but a not uncommon problem in pulmonary clinics.

Sx: Onset gradual with severe obesity.

These severely obese pts complain of drowsiness and somnolence during the day; they appear inattentive and lethargic, and in severe cases, confusion may occur.

Lab: Hypercapnia, hypoxemia, erythrocytosis.

Crs: Parallels that of the obesity.

Cmplc: Severe obesity may cause obstructive sleep apnea; pulmonary hypertension may occur.

Somnolence and lethargy impair ability to attend to complex matters.

Etiol: The severe burden of adipose tissue on the chest wall and in the abdomen curtails inspiration, and chronic alveolar hypoventilation occurs. Hypoxemia leads to erythrocytosis and hypercapnia leads to pulmonary hypertension. With severe hypercapnia, intracranial pressure may rise and in some pts papilledema may occur.

Ddx: The triad of somnolence, obesity, and erythrocytosis is an important clue.

Obstructive sleep apnea is distinguished by normal blood gas levels during the day.

Rx: Weight loss is imperative. Oxygen may partially relieve somnolence, but if hypercapnia is severe, may be followed by respiratory failure.

12.7 CIRCADIAN RHYTHM SLEEP DISORDER

NEJM 1990;322:1253. Psychopharmacol Bull 1984;20:566. Science 1982;217:460. Sleep 1990;13:354.

Epidem: Probably common.

Sx: Sx appear when there is a mismatch between the individual pt's endogenous sleep-wake cycle and environmental demands. For example, in the *shift work type,* individuals who normally work during the day and sleep at night who are then transferred to the night shift typically experience some somnolence while working at night, and "insomnia" when attempting to get some sleep during the day. The *jet lag type* typically occurs when individuals fly several time zones eastward. At their new destination they may find themselves very sleepy hours before the new "bedtime" (those who fly westward may find themselves with "insomnia" relative to the new time zone, but most individuals have less trouble with this shift than flying eastward). The *delayed sleep phase type* is a little different, in that it doesn't appear to depend on any change in the pt's schedule or environment. Pts are unable to fall asleep at socially sanctioned times (e.g., before midnight), and unable to awaken (without significant grogginess) at a normal time in the morning; such a "night owl" pattern is not uncommon among adolescents.

Lab: Polysomnography generally is not required.

Crs: Those with the shift work and jet lag types, provided that their new schedule remains constant, typically find their endogenous cycle gradually resetting to the new environmental demands within a week or two. Those with the delayed sleep phase type, in the natural course of events, typically find that after years, or perhaps decades, they gradually come to be able to fall asleep at a "normal" time.

Cmplc: Somnolence can lead to reduced work performance and accidents with cars or machinery; individuals doing shift work whose shifts are changed every 2 wk or so may not have time to recover and have a higher incidence of peptic ulcer and cardiovascular disease.

Etiol: The endogenous sleep-wake cycle is under the control of the hypothalamic suprachiasmatic nucleus and resists change, regardless of environmental demands.

Ddx: The dx is self-evident after the hx is obtained.

Rx: Rx is directed toward "resetting" the endogenous "clock" to bring it into synchrony with environmental demands. Thus, pts should rigidly adhere to the new environmental schedule; exposure to bright light when the environment demands wakefulness may help. With these measures, most individual shift workers find themselves

12.7 Circadian Rhythm Sleep Disorder **233**

"reset" within 2 wk; for those with jet lag, resetting takes a number of days roughly equal to the number of time zones traversed. The delayed sleep phase type may take much longer to "reset." In selected pts, short-acting hypnotics used for a few days may speed the "resetting."

12.8 RESTLESS LEGS SYNDROME (EKBOM SYNDROME)

Ann Neurol 1988;24:455. Neurology 1960;10:868. Sleep 1995;18:681.

Epidem: Uncommon.

Sx: Onset in middle or late years.

Upon sitting, or esp lying down, pts experience an uncomfortable restlessness in the legs, esp the calves (some may complain more of aching, others of formication), that is typically relieved by getting up and walking around. Insomnia is common, as pts are unable to lie down and relax at night, or if they happen to awaken during the night.

Most pts also have nocturnal myoclonus.

Lab: NC, except for the possibility of iron deficiency anemia (see below).

Crs: Chronic, either waxing and waning in intensity or gradually progressive.

Cmplc: Insomnia leaves pts fatigued, irritable, and with difficulty concentrating during the day.

Etiol: Some cases, especially in pts with nocturnal myoclonus, are familial; others are associated with pregnancy, iron deficiency anemia, peripheral polyneuropathy (e.g., uremia), and dialysis.

Ddx: Akathisia secondary to neuroleptics may be clinically indistinguishable, but is suggested by the neuroleptic Rx. A clue is the tendency of pts with neuroleptic-induced akathisia to "march in place" in contrast to pts with restless legs syndrome who tend to rub their feet with their hands; akathisia may also be seen with Parkinson's disease, and is suggested by the accompanying sx, e.g., tremor, bradykinesia.

Rx: Levodopa-carbidopa (Sinemet) (using the prolonged-release preparation to ensure coverage throughout the night), bromocriptine (Parlodel), clonazepam (Klonopin), propranolol (Inderal), carbamazepine (Tegretol), and opioids (e.g., propoxyphene (Darvon), oxycodone, codeine) are useful. Levodopa-carbidopa (Sinemet) is probably a good first choice. Start with low doses and titrate up.

12.9 NOCTURNAL MYOCLONUS (PERIODIC LIMB MOVEMENT DISORDER OF SLEEP)

Arch Neurol 1980;37:119. J Neurol Neurosurg Psychiatry 1953;16:166. Sleep 1986;9:385.

Epidem: Uncommon.

Sx: Onset from adult years to old age, with incidence increasing with age.

The "myoclonus" is typically found in 1 or both lower extremities but may at times affect the upper extremities. It consists of a "triple-flexion" movement, with sudden dorsiflexion of the foot and flexion at the knee, and often, the thigh. Each myoclonic jerk lasts from ½ to 10 sec. Myoclonic jerks tend to appear during NREM sleep and to occur in episodes that may last from minutes to an hour or longer. During the episode, jerks tend to occur every 20–60 sec. Although bed partners may complain of being "kicked" at night, most pts are unaware of the jerks, and complain rather of multiple awakenings and unrefreshing sleep.

A minority of pts will also have restless legs syndrome.

Lab: Polysomnography reveals the typical jerks.

Crs: Chronic.

Cmplc: Fatigue, irritability, and poor concentration may be present the next day.

Etiol: Uncertain; some cases familial.

Ddx: Hypnic jerks, or "sleep starts," are similar to the myoclonic jerks seen in nocturnal myoclonus but appear *only* as individuals are falling asleep.

Myoclonus may occur as a SE to antidepressants or with hepatic or uremic encephalopathy.

Rx: Levodopa-carbidopa (Sinemet) (using the extended-release preparation) or clonazepam (Klonopin) may be used. Start with a low dose and titrate up to effectiveness.

12.10 NIGHTMARE DISORDER (INCUBUS)

Am J Psychiatry 1980;137:1197. J Clin Psychiatry 1983;44:77. Psychiatr Clin 1987;10:667.

Epidem: Uncertain.

Sx: Onset typically in childhood, after an emotionally traumatic event.
Nightmares occur during REM sleep, generally in the latter half of the night. During the nightmare itself, pts tend to be relatively motionless; as anxiety mounts, pts eventually awaken with relatively mild autonomic sx, such as tachycardia, tremulousness, and diaphoresis. Alertness is rapidly attained, and recall of the nightmare is generally good, even vivid; although some pts are able to fall back asleep quickly, some, fearful of having another nightmare, may lay awake for long periods of time.

In nightmare disorder, nightmares recur weekly or more frequently, and may be exacerbated by emotional stress, fatigue, fever, or frightening shows or stories.

Lab: NC.

Crs: Spontaneous remission in most pts by adult years.

Cmplc: Pts unable to get back to sleep may experience daytime fatigue and poor concentration.

Etiol: Unknown.

Ddx: Normal individuals may have occasional nightmares.
Night terrors are distinguished by their occurrence during NREM sleep, prominent autonomic and motor activity, slow attainment of full alertness, and a lack of vivid recall of dream material, if any.

Nocturnal panic attacks are distinguished by their occurrence during NREM sleep, greater autonomic arousal, a lack of dream recall, and in most pts, the occurrence of daytime panic attacks.

Other causes of nightmares are listed in Table 12.10-1.

Rx: Avoidance of the exacerbating factors noted above.

Table 12.10-1. Other Causes of Nightmares

Other Mental Disorders

PTSD
Depression (as in major depression or bipolar disorder)
Schizophrenia
Delirium

Substances

Antidepressants (acutely, or with abrupt discontinuation after chronic use)
Neuroleptics
Reserpine
Alpha-methyldopa (Aldomet)
Clonidine (Catapres)
Levodopa-carbidopa (Sinemet)
Bromocriptine (Parlodel)
Beta-blockers
Benzodiazepines (acutely, or with abrupt discontinuation after chronic use)

In severe cases, REM suppression may be attempted with a tricyclic drug, such as nortriptyline (Pamelor) or imipramine (Tofranil), or a benzodiazepine, keeping in mind that occasionally these agents may paradoxically increase the frequency of nightmares.

12.11 SLEEP TERROR DISORDER (PAVOR NOCTURNUS)

Am J Psychiatry 1979;136:1087. Arch Gen Psychiatry 1973;28:252. J Nerv Ment Dis 1973;157:75.

Epidem: 1%–4% of children; more common in boys.

Sx: Onset typically in childhood, between 4 and 12 yr; rarely onset in early adult years.

Night terror arises from NREM sleep during the first third of the night; pts generally cry out in terror, sit bolt upright in bed, and are very agitated, with abundant tachycardia, mydriasis, and diaphoresis. The episode usually lasts 1–10 min, and attempts to awaken the pt are typically fruitless. At the end of the attack, pts may simply fall back into sleep, without fully awakening, or may come to full alertness. Those that do awaken typically have little or no recall of the terror, and generally fall right back asleep.

Attacks generally appear sporadically every few weeks or months; rarely they occur several nights in succession. Occasionally, "pavor diurnus" occurs, with attacks arising during daytime naps. Exacerbating factors include irregular sleep habits, anxiety, and fever.

Lab: Polysomnography reveals attacks arising from NREM, generally stage 3 or 4 sleep.

Crs: Childhood-onset cases generally resolve by midadolescence; adult-onset cases may be chronic.

Cmplc: There are few direct complications for pts; parents, however, may be very disturbed by the events.

Etiol: Probably familial; there is an association with migraine, enuresis, and possibly, Tourette's syndrome.

Ddx: Nightmares are distinguished by their occurrence during REM sleep, generally in the latter half of the night; the general lack of motor activity; rapid attainment of full alertness; and good recall of the dream.

Nocturnal panic attacks are distinguished by rapid awakening and by the occurrence of daytime attacks.

Nocturnal complex partial seizures are suggested by the occurrence of other seizure types (grand mal, simple partial) at other times.

Rx: Reassuring parents may be sufficient. Imipramine (Tofranil) 25–50 mg hs may prevent attacks, as may diazepam (Valium) 2.5–5 mg.

12.12 SLEEPWALKING DISORDER (SOMNAMBULISM)

Arch Gen Psychiatry 1966;14:586. Arch Gen Psychiatry 1980;37:1406. Neurology 1990;40:749.

Epidem: 1%–6% of all children; more common in boys.

Sx: Onset typically in late childhood; adult onset is rare.

Somnambulistic episodes arise from NREM sleep, typically in the first third of the night. At the onset of the episode, pts typically sit up in bed and fumble with the sheets or their pajamas; if the eyes are opened, a blank stare is seen. Although the episode may terminate at this point, most pts get out of bed and wander about in a semiautomatic manner. Some avoid obstacles, whereas others trip or overturn furniture. Some pts use the bathroom, some get something to eat, and some pts climb out windows or leave through the door. Rarely, pts engage in complex activity, such as writing or even driving a car. Attempts to awaken the pt are generally fruitless; some pts say a few words, but the speech is usually mumbled or inarticulate. Most episodes last 15–30 min; at the end of the episode, pts, without regaining full consciousness, either return to bed or simply lie down, perhaps on a couch or the floor. If, as is rarely the case, it is possible to awaken the pt, a brief period of confusion is usually observed before full consciousness is gained, after which the pt has little or no memory of what happened.

The frequency of episodes is increased by irregular sleep habits, fever, or emotional stress.

Lab: Polysomnography with audiovisual capacity reveals the episode to arise from NREM, often stage 3 or 4 sleep.

Crs: In childhood-onset cases, remission typically occurs by midadolescence; in some pts, however, relapses may appear in the 20s or 30s. Late-adolescent- or early-adult-onset cases generally pursue a chronic course.

Cmplc: Injury may occur with falls, or if the pt climbs out a window or attempts to use hazardous materials (e.g., knives, cars).

Etiol: Clearly familial.

Ddx: Nocturnal complex partial seizures are suggested by the occurrence of other seizure types, e.g., grand mal or simple partial.

Sleep-drunkenness is distinguished by its appearance upon morning awakening.

Sleepwalking may occur as a SE to antidepressants, neuroleptics, and sedative-hypnotics, such as chloral hydrate.

Rx: Windows and door generally should be locked, and potentially dangerous items removed. Imipramine (Tofranil) 25–50 mg hs or diazepam (Valium) 5–10 mg hs may prevent episodes.

12.13 REM-SLEEP BEHAVIOR DISORDER

Am J Psychiatry 1989;146:1166. Neurology 1989;39:1519. Neurology 1996;46:385. Neurology 1997;49:523.

Epidem: Uncertain; probably rare.

Sx: Onset typically in the late 50s; most pts are male.

Episodes arise during REM sleep as muscle atonia is lost and pts, without awakening, act out their dream role while in the bedroom. One pt, dreaming of football, tried to tackle a dresser; another, dreaming of trying to break a deer's neck, tried to choke his wife. If awakened, pts, although typically able to recall the dream, have no recall of what actually happened in the bedroom. Injuries are not uncommon, and some pts, after learning of their behavior, may tie themselves to the bed to prevent future damage.

Lab: Polysomnography reveals the sudden loss of atonia during REM sleep.

Crs: Uncertain.

Cmplc: Injuries include bruises, fractures, and head trauma.

Etiol: There is a strong association with parkinsonism, either as Parkinson's disease, diffuse Lewy body disease, or the striatonigral variant of MSA. In some pts, REM sleep behavior disorder may be the presenting sx of 1 of these conditions.

Ddx: Somnambulism is distinguished by its appearance during NREM sleep and by the absence of any dream recall.

Nocturnal complex partial seizures are distinguished by the occurrence of other seizure types, e.g., grand mal or simple partial.

Rx: Clonazepam (Klonopin) 1–2 mg hs may prevent episodes; carbamazepine (Tegretol) may also be effective.

12.14 SLEEP PARALYSIS (ISOLATED SLEEP PARALYSIS)

Arch Neurol 1962;6:228. J Nerv Ment Dis 1942;45:153. J Nerv Ment Dis 1957;125:140.

Epidem: Uncertain.

Sx: Either upon falling asleep (hypnagogic or predormital) or upon awakening (hypnopompic or postdormital), pts, although fully conscious and alert, are, with the exception of the diaphragmatic and extraocular muscles, paralyzed, and remain so for up to a minute. Occasionally, pts may also experience dreamlike visual hallucinations. Importantly, although pts are motionless and unable to move, they may be restored to full strength simply by being touched.

Lab: NC.

Crs: Uncertain.

Cmplc: None.

Etiol: Both familial and sporadic cases occur.

Ddx: Narcolepsy (accompanied by sleep paralysis in approximately one-third of pts) is distinguished by the presence of sleep attacks, which are not seen with isolated sleep paralysis.

Rx: Reassurance.

13. Impulse-Control Disorders Not Classified Elsewhere

13.1 INTERMITTENT EXPLOSIVE DISORDER

Am J Psychiatry 1971;127:1473. J Clin Psychiatry 1998;59:203. Mayo Clin Proc 1987;62:204.

Epidem: Rare; more common in males.

Sx: Onset in late teens or early 20s.

Episodes of explosiveness generally preceded by an uneasy tension, followed by a paroxysmal onset of anger and aggression. Other persons may be assaulted or property may be destroyed. The episode resolves in usually less than an hour and afterward pts typically have only a patchy recall of what happened, and feel true remorse and guilt over what they've done. Episodes may or may not be preceded by some precipitating factor. When a precipitant is present, however, it appears trivial in light of the violence of the episode.

Critically, in between episodes pts are neither violent, irritable, nor short-tempered.

Lab: NC.

Crs: Long-term course uncertain; frequency of explosive episodes varies widely among pts.

Cmplc: Strained relations with others; jail.

Etiol: Subtle developmental malformations of the CNS may play a part, and the prevalence of postprandial hypoglycemia is higher than expected.

Some speculate that intermittent explosive disorder is a kind of complex partial epilepsy.

Ddx: Occasional unprovoked violence may be seen with mania (as in bipolar disorder), cyclothymia, schizophrenia, schizoaffective disorder, antisocial or borderline personality disorder, dementia, and as part of a personality change. In all these disorders, however, characteristic sx are present in between the episodes, in contrast with intermittent explosive disorder, where the intervals between episodes are sx free.

Typical complex partial seizures are suggested by a brief motionless stare, automatisms such as lip smacking, and the presence of other seizure types, e.g., grand mal seizures. In doubtful cases, MRI and video-EEG monitoring may be appropriate, along with measurement of postepisode prolactin and neuron-specific enolase levels.

Malingering is suggested when legal charges are pending.

Rx: Propranolol (Inderal), in high doses (for otherwise healthy young men, 600–800 mg/d) is the best-studied Rx; other drugs found useful include divalproex (Depakote), carbamazepine (Tegretol), phenytoin (Dilantin), and lithium (Eskalith, Lithobid). Sequential trials may be required.

Benzodiazepines and alcohol must be avoided.

13.2 KLEPTOMANIA

Am J Psychiatry 1991;148:652. Am J Psychiatry 1991;148:986. Br J Psychiatry 1981;138:346.

Epidem: Apparently rare, but may be underreported; more common in females.

Sx: Onset in late teens or early 20s.

Kleptomania is characterized by recurrent shoplifting, which in turn is motivated *not* by a desire for gain but rather by an irrational and often irresistible impulse to steal. Little or no planning goes into the theft, and most pts have enough money to purchase the item in any case. Afterward, the stolen item is typically either thrown away or perhaps hidden in the car or the house.

Major depression and borderline personality disorder are commonly present.

Lab: NC.
Crs: Uncertain; probably chronic.
Cmplc: Apprehension and legal consequences.
Etiol: A link with obsessive-compulsive disorder is suspected.
Ddx: Simple theft, as seen in common criminals or those with antisocial personality disorder, is motivated by gain and often preceded by planning.

Mania (as in bipolar disorder) may be associated with unlawful taking, but as far as manic pts are concerned, they own it anyway, so there's nothing illegal going on.

Dementia or MR may be characterized by unlawful taking, but here pts fail to recognize the unlawfulness of what they're doing.

Personality change, esp of the frontal lobe type, may be accompanied by disinhibited taking.
Rx: Fluoxetine (Prozac) may dramatically reduce the urge to steal in kleptomania.

13.3 PYROMANIA

Arch Gen Psychiatry 1970;22:63. Br J Psychiatry 1982;140:357. Med J Aust 1969;1:579.

Epidem: Rare; more common in males.
Sx: Onset in late childhood or early teens.

Pyromaniacs are fascinated with and repeatedly set fires. Often, considerable planning goes into the arson, and pts typically stick around to watch their flaming handiwork. Some may become firefighters to feed their fascination. Importantly, these pts seek neither financial gain nor revenge; their motive springs solely from their fascination.
Lab: NC.
Crs: Uncertain.
Cmplc: Apprehension and imprisonment.
Etiol: Not known.
Ddx: The overwhelming majority of arson is committed for gain or revenge.

Schizophrenia may be accompanied by voices that command arson. Demented or MR pts may accidentally set fires.

Rx: Inadequately studied; behavior therapy may help some.

13.4 PATHOLOGIC GAMBLING

Acta Psychiatr Scand 1991;84:113. Can J Psychiatry 1998;43:43. J Clin Psychiatry 1996;57(Suppl 8):80.

Epidem: Lifetime prevalence ~1%–2%; more common in males.

Sx: Onset of the restless urge to gamble generally in the late teens or early 20s, and may be insidious or acute, as for example after a chance "big win" awakens the pt's thirst for gambling.

There is a restless and at times intoxicating fascination with gambling and chasing after a "big win" with ever-larger bets. Bills go unpaid, and pts may embezzle or steal money to feed their habit; some may truly "bet the farm," waging their house on 1 more attempt to score big. Large losses may bring depression and remorse; however, these restraining affects rarely last long.

Mood disorders and alcoholism are common accompaniments.

Lab: NC.

Crs: Chronic, waxing and waning in intensity.

Cmplc: Bankruptcy, divorce, and imprisonment.

Etiol: Familial, and associated with a fhx of alcoholism.

Disturbances in serotoninergic transmission strongly suspected.

Ddx: "Social" gamblers, unlike pathologic gamblers, can prospectively set (and stick to) a loss limit, and after some losses, can "walk away from it" without being troubled by a restless urge to try their luck just 1 more time.

Manic pts (as in bipolar disorder, or to a less severe degree, cyclothymia) may exultantly gamble away all they have at breathtaking speed; here, however, one finds other manic sx and an absence of excessive gambling in the intervals between manic episodes.

Rx: Both Gamblers Anonymous and behavioral treatments have had success.

Fluoxetine (Prozac) may reduce the urge to gamble.

IMPULSE-CONTROL DISORDERS

13.5 TRICHOTILLOMANIA

Am J Psychiatry 1991;148:365. J Clin Psychiatry 1996;57(Suppl 8):42. NEJM 1989;321:497.

Epidem: Lifetime prevalence <1%; more common in females.

Sx: Onset in late childhood or early teens.

There is a recurrent and generally irresistible urge to engage in hair pulling with significant hair loss, most often on the scalp, but also at times on the eyebrows, eyelashes, pubic area, axillary area, and beard. Hair loss on the scalp occurs in patches, which are often ragged with irregular borders. Close inspection reveals no scarring or inflammation and in most pts some "leftover" normal hair may be seen. Most pts deny pulling their hair and most will attempt to cover up the evidence with hats, wigs, scarves, etc.

Lab: NC.

Crs: Varies; permanent remission, episodic, and chronic courses have been reported.

Cmplc: Embarrassment is common and some may give up jobs and social contact to avoid discovery.

Rarely, in pts who eat the pulled hair, bezoars form.

Etiol: A relationship with obsessive-compulsive disorder is suspected.

Ddx: Normal children and adolescents occasionally pull hairs out, but the practice is temporary and does not result in a "moth-eaten" appearance.

MR pts may, as a stereotypy, pull out large amounts of hair.

Schizophrenic patients, in response to voices, may pull out great quantities of hair.

A variety of other conditions possibly confused with trichotillomania are listed in Table 13.5-1.

Table 13.5-1. Other Causes of Hair Loss

Generalized Hair Loss	Patchy Hair Loss
Hypothyroidism	Secondary syphilis
Lithium	Tinea capitis
Vitamin A	Systemic lupus erythematosus
Thallium poisoning	
	Alopecia Areata

Generalized hair loss is unusual in trichotillomania; the patchy hair loss seen with syphilis, tinea, and systemic lupus erythematosus is accompanied by inflammation, not present in trichotillomania. Alopecia areata may cause either generalized or patchy hair loss. When patches occur, they are sharply bounded and lack any normal hairs, in contrast to the patches of trichotillomania, which are ragged and do contain some (albeit broken) normal hairs.

Rx: Clomipramine (Anafranil), given as described in 6.1, reduces the urge to pull hair out.

14. Personality Disorders

14.1 PARANOID PERSONALITY DISORDER

Br J Psychiatry 1961;107:687. J Pers Disord 1993;7:53. Shapiro D, Neurotic styles, Basic Books, New York, 1965.

Epidem: Lifetime prevalence ~0.5%–2.5%; more common in males.
Sx: Onset in adolescence.

Pts present a seamless fabric of mistrust, guardedness, and more or less thinly veiled hostility; others are typically perceived as malevolent and untrustworthy. Pts are quick to see insults and slights where none were intended, and prone to harbor long-standing grudges. Mutually intimate relations are virtually impossible. Such pts rigidly maintain their autonomy and rarely let their guard down.

Under great stress, these pts temporarily may have delusions of persecution and reference.

Lab: NC.
Crs: Chronic.
Cmplc: Satisfactory relations with others almost impossible; some pts may engage in violence as they "protect" themselves or exact "justified" revenge.
Etiol: Probably a "forme fruste" of paranoid schizophrenia.
Ddx: Delusional disorder, persecutory subtype, is distinguished by the chronicity of delusions and by the absence of persistent mistrust and guardedness.

Paranoid schizophrenia is marked not only by chronicity of delusions, but also by other sx, such as auditory hallucinations, mannerisms, loosening of associations, etc.

Rx: There are no controlled Rx trials; pts rarely remain in Rx, as they see no need for it and mistrust the physician in any case. Studied politeness and a nonconfrontational stance are necessary; neuroleptics, such as olanzapine (Zyprexa) or risperidone (Risperdal), may be useful during stressful periods.

14.2 SCHIZOID PERSONALITY DISORDER

J Pers Dis 1991;5:135. J Pers Dis 1993;7:43. Beck A, Freeman A, Cognitive therapy of personality disorders, Guilford, New York, 1990.

Epidem: Uncertain; lifetime prevalence <1%; more common in males.
Sx: Onset in late childhood or early teens.

Pts are characteristically detached, aloof, and isolated; take little pleasure and show little interest in social relations (including sexual relations); and tend to engage in solitary activities, often involving machines or more or less mechanical routines. Others find these pts to be cold and lacking in emotional display; when forced to be in company, pts are awkward and socially inept, and typically fail to respond appropriately to the nuances and subtle cues of normal social interchange.

Lab: NC.
Crs: Probably chronic.
Cmplc: Pts typically fail in any endeavor that requires social give-and-take.
Etiol: Possibly a "forme fruste" of simple schizophrenia.
Ddx: Schizotypal personality disorder is distinguished by the presence of peculiarities of thought and speech.

Avoidant personality disorder is distinguished by the presence of a strong desire for social interaction in contrast to the pervasive indifference seen with schizoid personality disorder.

Simple schizophrenia is distinguished by its "downhill" course with progressive deterioration; the other subtypes of schizophrenia are distinguished by associated sx, such as auditory hallucinations, delusions, etc.

Autism is distinguished by an onset in early childhood and by the presence of such signs as gaze avoidance, "fascinations," pronominal reversals, etc.

Personality change, esp the interictal personality syndrome, is distinguished by the premorbid presence of a normal personality.

Rx: Supportive psychotherapy with an emphasis on the gradual assumption of more social activities is often offered on a chronic basis; some pts are placed in group psychotherapy. Neither of these approaches has been proved effective.

Neuroleptics of the typical type do not appear effective; it is unclear whether atypical neuroleptics (e.g., olanzapine (Zyprexa) or risperidone (Risperdal)) would be helpful.

14.3 SCHIZOTYPAL PERSONALITY DISORDER

Acta Psychiatr Scand 1996;94:303. Am J Psychiatry 1986;143:1222. Arch Gen Psychiatry 1986;43:680.

Epidem: Lifetime prevalence ~3%; more common in males.

Sx: Onset in late childhood or early adolescence.

Uncomfortable and ill at ease in social situations, such pts generally remain aloof and distant; peculiar thinking is typical, and pts may express odd or bizarre beliefs, e.g., concerning clairvoyance, supernatural powers, or mystical, metaphysical issues. Speech may be circumstantial, tangential, or stilted, and overall behavior is often eccentric.

Under great stress, transient delusions, often referential or somatic, may appear.

Lab: NC.

Crs: Chronic.

Cmplc: Marriage, friendship, or cooperative work with others is often impossible.

Etiol: Probably a "forme fruste" of schizophrenia. The prevalence of schizotypal personality disorder is increased in the biologic, but not adoptive, relatives of pts with schizophrenia. Furthermore, as in schizophrenia, pts with schizotypal personality disorder display deficits in smooth pursuit eye movements and an increased ventricle-brain ratio.

Ddx: Schizoid personality disorder is distinguished by an absence of peculiarities in thought and speech.

Schizophrenia is distinguished by the chronic presence of delusions and other sx, such as auditory hallucinations, looseness of associations, etc.

Autism is distinguished by an onset in early childhood and by the presence of such signs as gaze avoidance, "fascinations," pronominal reversals, etc.

Female carriers of the fragile X gene may display schizotypal traits; here, the fhx is critical, and genetic testing may be appropriate.

Rx: Supportive psychotherapy with gentle guidance may be helpful.

Neuroleptics in low doses (e.g., haloperidol (Haldol) 2.5–5 mg, olanzapine (Zyprexa) 5–7.5 mg) may alleviate some of the peculiarities.

14.4 ANTISOCIAL PERSONALITY DISORDER

Am J Psychiatry 1983;140:887. Am J Psychiatry 1990;147:173. Comp Psychiatry 1995;36:130.

Epidem: In the general population, ~5% of males and ~1% of females.

Sx: Onset in childhood, with the full picture evident by late teenage years.

Sociopaths experience little sympathy or compassion for others, and lack respect for law and authority. Their selfish interests thus unchecked, these individuals repeatedly and persistently violate the rights of others and fail to live up to their own obligations. True remorse and guilt are absent; if caught, a sociopath might profess remorse, but such manipulative contrition rings false.

Predictably, the lives of sociopaths are marked by lying, infidelity, and irresponsibility. Some may progress to "pathologic lying" wherein any statement is as likely to be a lie as the truth. Divorce and abandonment of friends and children are common; bills and other financial obligations go unpaid.

Most sociopaths have a long h/o arrests and incarceration; however, an absence of such a hx does not rule out the dx. Indeed, some otherwise gifted sociopaths are so cunning and charming that they "get away with it." Some successful politicians are good examples of "successful" sociopaths.

Abuse or dependence on alcohol or other substances, such as cocaine, is common.

Lab: NC.

Crs: Although the disorder is chronic, most sociopaths "burn out" by their mid-40s. Although the sociopathic view of the world persists, the actual frequency of antisocial acts falls. Eventually, some socio-paths become delightful raconteurs; others drift into a misery of self-pity and hypochondriacal concerns.

Cmplc: Imprisonment and violent death are common.

Etiol: Antisocial personality disorder is familial and adoption studies implicate both genetic and environmental factors. Being aban-doned as a child appears particularly important.

Childhood attention-deficit disorder with hyperactivity is often found in the h/o these pts.

Nonspecific EEG changes are commonly present.

Ddx: Dementia and MR may, in some pts, be accompanied by illegal activities; however, here the pt isn't aware of the illegal nature of the act.

Personality change (esp of the frontal lobe type) may be characterized by disinhibition with resulting illegal behavior; however, here the pt's behavior represents a change from the premorbid personality, whereas in antisocial personality disorder the antisocial traits may be traced back to early childhood.

Mania (as in bipolar disorder) may be accompanied by a riotous pro-fusion of criminal, irresponsible, and irrepressible behavior, but is distinguished by a normal premorbid personality structure and by the presence of typical manic sx, such as pressured speech, etc.

Alcoholism and certain other addictions (cocaine, amphetamines, opi-oids) may be marked by recurrent antisocial acts, such as theft, lying, and abandonment, all in the service of ongoing substance use. Here, one finds a normal premorbid personality structure, or if the substance use began in childhood or early teenage years, one finds that with abstinence, the antisocial activity gradually fades.

Simple criminality is suggested by finding evidence for loyalty, sympa-thy, and responsibility in other areas of the criminal's life. Some "professional" criminals may sacrifice themselves for their loved ones. By contrast, sociopaths would never sacrifice themselves for anyone.

Rx: Psychotherapy is not effective. In some cases, long-term incarcera-tion until the sociopath "burns out" is the best alternative.

If impulsivity is prominent, lithium or carbamazepine (Tegretol) (as described in 6.6) may be helpful. Such Rx, however, is pointless in the cold-blooded predatory type.

14.5 BORDERLINE PERSONALITY DISORDER

Acta Psychiatr Scand 1994;89(Suppl 379):12. Am J Psychiatry 1975; 132:1. J Clin Psychiatry 1997;58(Suppl 14):48.

Epidem: Lifetime prevalence ~2%–3%; male-female ratio 1:3.

Sx: Onset in early teens.

Borderline personality disorder pts have been aptly characterized as "stably unstable." Their opinions of themselves and of others, their affects, and their relationships lack firm grounding and are prone to rapid and disturbing shifts. Pts tend to think in "black or white," "all good or all bad" terms. Others may be idealized, and seen as gratifying and nurturing, but if others engage in 1 significant misstep, perhaps a slight, or a missed appointment, then as far as the pts are concerned, the others' images are tarnished, even blackened, and pts typically devalue them with enraged criticism. A similar instability may be seen in pts' own attitudes toward themselves: Although at times pts may experience a sense of self-sufficiency, such experiences are precarious and liable to sudden disintegration, leaving pts with a sense of worthlessness, despair, and most importantly, emptiness. These shifting visions of themselves and others are accompanied by often similarly dramatic changes in mood and affect. Idealized relationships may be accompanied by a brittle sense of bliss and security; conversely, a devalued relationship may provoke some of the most intense rage seen in clinical practice. Such shifts in mood are at times so intolerable to pts that as a protective move, they may retreat from human contact, perhaps allowing themselves to interact with others only in highly structured, relatively "safe" environments, such as work.

Relationships, predictably, are very unstable. Others, perhaps initially flattered by pts' idealization, often soon find pts' demands for "ideal" attention overwhelming, and begin to withdraw. Pts, ever alert to any sign of withdrawal or rejection, typically either become more dependent, even clinging, or become enraged. Few relationships can stand such strains, and a h/o "stormy" relationships is common.

Recurrent, even frequent, suicide attempts or gestures are common. In some pts, self-injury is also an outstanding feature. Some may slash their wrists and forearms so many times as to present a virtual "ladder" of scar tissue up the arm.

PERSONALITY DISORDERS

Psychotic sx, such as auditory hallucinations and delusions of persecution or reference, may appear during times of great personal stress, but resolve spontaneously when the stress passes.

Alcohol abuse or dependence is not uncommon, and one may also see concurrent panic disorder, major depression, or dysthymia.

Lab: NC.

Crs: Chronic, with a gradual diminution in intensity of sx by middle years.

Cmplc: Marriage and friendship rarely survive.

Suicide in ~10%.

Etiol: Borderline personality disorder appears to derive from a failure of normal maturation of a stable "good enough" self-image and a capacity to modulate affects. Although borderline personality disorder is clearly familial, the relative contribution of genetic and environmental influences is not clear. On the one hand, there might be a genetically determined maturational disability; on the other hand, an otherwise normal maturation may be prevented by childhood abuse or abandonment.

Ddx: Schizophrenia may be suggested by psychotic sx, but is distinguished by the persistence of psychotic sx in times of low stress, and by the presence of other sx, such as loosening of associations, mannerisms, etc.

Dysthymia, of early onset, may cause significant defects in self-esteem and self-image and leave the pt with a desperate dependency on others. Here, however, the persistent affect is one of depression, in stark contrast to the sense of emptiness experienced by borderline personality disorder pts. Furthermore, dysthymia is not accompanied by the mercurial shifts seen in the lives of borderline personality disorder pts.

Cyclothymia, if of early onset, may create a life as stormy as that seen with borderline personality disorder; here, however, one also finds heightened mood, rather than emptiness.

"Identity crises," common in mid to late adolescence, may be very difficult to distinguish from borderline personality disorder; however, identity crises resolve by the late teens, whereas the personality disorder does not.

Rx: Alcoholism or other addictions must be treated first, and some pts, with heavy involvement in AA, in fact experience some stabilization of their personality.

Hospitalization, if necessitated by suicidal risk, should be highly structured, practically oriented, and brief. Long hospital stays are almost inevitably accompanied by deterioration.

Psychotherapy may be helpful, but few pts can tolerate it. A recent specific form of psychotherapy, "dialectical behavior therapy," may constitute an exception as it appears to reduce the frequency of suicidal acts.

Fluoxetine (Prozac) in doses of 80 mg/d may reduce anger, dysphoria, and impulsivity. Both carbamazepine (Tegretol) and lithium (Eskalith, Lithobid) (used as described in 6.6) also reduce impulsivity. Low-dose neuroleptics (e.g., haloperidol (Haldol) 2.5–5.0 mg, risperidone (Risperdal) 4 mg, olanzapine (Zyprexa) 5.0–7.5 mg) may be required for psychotic sx, and also appear to reduce dysphoria. Amitriptyline (Elavil) may worsen sx, and benzodiazepines, such as alprazolam (Xanax), may be followed by disinhibition. Overall, although fluoxetine (Prozac), carbamazepine (Tegretol), lithium (Eskalith, Lithobid), and neuroleptics have shown short-term effectiveness, long-term benefit (e.g., years) has not been demonstrated yet.

14.6 HISTRIONIC PERSONALITY DISORDER

Am J Psychiatry 1974;131:518. Arch Gen Psychiatry 1974;30:325. Br J Psychiatry 1987;150:241.

Epidem: Lifetime prevalence ~2%–3%; more common in females.
Sx: Onset around puberty.

Pts characteristically act as if they were starring in their own melodrama: They insist on being the center of attention, and if the "spotlight" is directed to others, pts may create a "scene" to steal it back. Typically, pts are "colorful" and overemotional, sometimes gushingly so, but their emotions are shallow and may rapidly change with a change in the social setting. Dress is often flamboyant and jewelry often excessive. Females are typically sexually provocative and males favor the tough, "macho" image. Although others may initially be attracted to such pts, usually the histrionics eventually wear thin and others, finding the pts shallow and lacking in true feeling or warmth, learn to keep a distance.
Lab: NC.

Crs: Probably chronic.

Cmplc: Intimate, mutually satisfactory, relationships are often beyond the pt's grasp.

Etiol: Not known.

Ddx: Borderline personality disorder is distinguished by pervasive loneliness, emptiness, and instability.

Narcissistic personality disorder is distinguished by a lack of "histrionics." Although narcissists do like the spotlight, they would never deign to engage in theatrics to get it.

Rx: Individual, group, and marital psychotherapy are all offered, but there is no proof of their effectiveness.

14.7 NARCISSISTIC PERSONALITY DISORDER

Am J Psychiatry 1982;139:12. Am J Psychiatry 1990;147:918. Arch Gen Psychiatry 1990;47:676.

Epidem: <1% of general population; more common in males.

Sx: Onset typically in teenage years.

Pts characteristically vain and self-important. Convinced of their exalted position in the world, they expect admiration and feel entitled to special privileges. Other "ideal" types are sought out, but quickly abandoned if their radiance should dim, or worse, outshine the pts. Haughty with "less than perfect" persons, narcissists may either disdain their presence, or conversely, allow them to offer fawning adoration, as long as their imperfections do not reflect poorly on the narcissist's own shining self. Criticism and humiliation are not borne well, as self-esteem is actually quite brittle, and pts may either lash out at critics or affect a lofty disdain. Some pts may retreat into fantasies of impossibly romantic love or grand personal successes. Others often find such pts exploitative, arrogant, and at bottom, cold and incapable of true emotional reciprocity.

Lab: NC.

Crs: Chronic; in later years narcissists often are unable to adapt to the inevitable decline with age, and many become depressed.

Cmplc: Intimate, emotionally satisfying relationships simply do not form.

Etiol: Unknown.

Ddx: Histrionic personality disorder is distinguished by frequent theatrical displays, which narcissists would never allow.

Antisocial personality disorder is distinguished by the purpose of the pts' exploitativeness. Sociopaths exploit for material gain; narcissists, for admiration and esteem.

Obsessive-compulsive personality disorder is distinguished by a smugness and arrogance based on rectitude and accomplishment, in contrast to the often shining emptiness of the narcissist.

Rx: Individual and group psychotherapy are offered, with only anecdotal reports of success.

14.8 AVOIDANT PERSONALITY DISORDER

Comp Psychiatry 1989;30:498. J Pers Dis 1991;5:353. J Clin Psychopharm 1992;12:62.

Epidem: Lifetime prevalence 0.5%–1%; equally common in males and females.

Sx: Onset typically in childhood.

Pts characteristically view themselves as socially inept and awkward; although desirous, even at times desperate, for intimate relations, pts are so fearful of embarrassing or humiliating themselves in social situations that they remain withdrawn and often self-effacing. In situations where others offer strong reassurances of acceptance, such pts may be willing to venture into a relationship, but once there they remain tense and inhibited, unwilling to relax for fear of taking a misstep or doing something embarrassing. Tragically, the conviction these pts have that they will be criticized and rejected often becomes a self-fulfilling prophecy. Others, spotting their painful timidity, may either avoid them or hold them up to ridicule.

Lab: NC.

Crs: Probably chronic; however, with age sx may partially remit.

Cmplc: Pts typically have trouble sustaining intimate relationships and work that may require social interactions.

Etiol: Uncertain; possibly represents a very-early-onset generalized social phobia.

Ddx: Generalized social phobia, as defined, has a later age at onset, and these pts generally do not have as well elaborated a sense of personal inadequacy as do pts with avoidant personality disorder.

Dependent personality disorder is distinguished by the pt's reaction to being "under the wing" of another. Avoidant types do not relax, whereas the dependent types relax, and may even function well.

Schizoid personality disorder is distinguished by the absence of a desire for intimacy.

Dysthymia is distinguished by the presence of fatigue, anhedonia, and other mild vegetative sx.

Rx: Social skills training, combined with cognitive behavioral therapy, appears to hold promise.

Some may benefit from phenelzine (Nardil) 60 mg/d, fluoxetine (Prozac) 20 mg, or clonazepam (Klonopin) 1–4 mg/d.

14.9 DEPENDENT PERSONALITY DISORDER

Br J Soc Clin Psychol 1977;16:317. J Pers Dis 1991;5:135. Beck A, Freeman A, Cognitive therapy of personality disorders, Guilford, New York, 1990.

Epidem: Uncertain prevalence in general population; may be common in clinical population and appears to be more common in females.

Sx: Onset in childhood or early adolescence.

Characteristically, these pts view themselves as incapable of pursuing any endeavor successfully unless they are acting under the direction of another. Although often otherwise quite capable of tasks, these pts shrink from situations where they might have to act independently, and look for others to take responsibility. Their indecisiveness, however, typically rapidly dissolves when given direction by others; indeed, such pts, when they feel themselves acting under another's aegis, may be capable of quite determined, even courageous behavior. The "loneliness of command" is not for these pts and they may go to any length to retain someone who will act as "captain" of their lives. Some pts will never disagree with the other (even though they know the other is wrong) and some will put up with abuse, at times extreme abuse, rather than risk having to navigate life on their own.

Lab: NC.

Crs: Uncertain; probably chronic.

Cmplc: Opportunities for advancement that entail independent action may be foregone, and pts may remain in abusive relationships.

Etiol: Possibly familial.

Ddx: Avoidant personality disorder is distinguished by the avoidant type pt's reaction to being under the aegis of another. The avoidant type pt does not relax and become more capable, but remains tense and ill at ease.

Rx: Individual (including cognitive behavioral therapy), group, and couples therapy have been offered, with some reports of success.

14.10 OBSESSIVE-COMPULSIVE PERSONALITY DISORDER (COMPULSIVE PERSONALITY DISORDER, ANANKASTIC PERSONALITY DISORDER)

Am J Psychiatry 1986;143:317. Am J Psychiatry 1993;150:1226. Arch Gen Psychiatry 1990;47:826. J Pers Dis 1991;5:363.

Epidem: Lifetime prevalence ~1%.

Sx: Onset in teenage years.

These pts exercise a rigid control over themselves, and often attempt to regiment others' lives also. They are often perfectionists and overly concerned with details in a quest to set all things in their right and proper places. Schedules, regimens, and routines are very important. Spontaneity is frowned on and pts keep a tight control over their emotions, maintaining a constricted affect; money is also typically tightly held, and such pts may be quite frugal, even miserly. Making decisions or completing projects is typically very difficult. The importance of recurrently weighing and reweighing the pros and cons, or of polishing each aspect of a project until a perfect product appears, is often paralyzing.

Lab: NC.

Crs: Although chronic, some pts undergo some relaxation in middle years.

Cmplc: Marriage and friendship rarely flourish under the sterile, humorless guidance of these pts.

Although pts with mild cases may do well in some occupations that demand orderliness and precision (e.g., accounting), career advancement is often precluded by the pt's inability to produce a final product.

Etiol: Familial; more likely in firstborn.

Ddx: Obsessive-compulsive disorder must be clearly distinguished from obsessive-compulsive personality disorder. The near identity of the names of these 2 separate disorders is very unfortunate as it suggests a similarity, in either sx or etiology, whereas in fact no such similarity exists. Obsessive-compulsive disorder is characterized by obsessions and compulsions, which are not part of obsessive-compulsive personality disorder. Further, although it was once thought that obsessive-compulsive disorder developed from the "soil" of obsessive-compulsive personality disorder, it is now clear that pts with obsessive-compulsive disorder are no more likely to also have obsessive-compulsive personality disorder than any other personality disorder.

Rx: Most pts are seen in psychotherapy, with anecdotal reports of success.

14.11 PASSIVE-AGGRESSIVE PERSONALITY DISORDER

Am J Psychiatry 1970;126:97. J Pers Disord 1988;2:170. J Nerv Ment Dis 1982;170:164.

Epidem: Uncertain; probably uncommon.

Sx: Onset in late childhood or early teenage years.

Characteristically, these individuals find any demands or expectations to be unfair, unjust, and unduly burdensome; they are often sullen and resentful, and although prone to complain to peers about the injustices done to them, it is rare for them to complain openly to superiors. Rather, by all manner of procrastination, inefficiency, "forgetting," and more or less subtle sabotage, they seek to bring their superiors to failure, dismay, and frustration. If taken to task by superiors, these pts may blame others, or claim to have "forgotten" some critical item, or protest that they were never told clearly what to do in the first place.

Importantly, this pattern of passive-aggressiveness, although most evident at work, is pervasive, and shows up at home and in the neighborhood.

Lab: NC.

Crs: Chronic.

Cmplc: Lack of advancement at work, or outright dismissal, is not uncommon; significant others, likewise fed up with the pt's sullen obstructionism, often leave.

Etiol: Uncertain.

Ddx: Transient passive-aggressive behavior is not uncommon, and in some situations may even be praiseworthy. Prisoners of war, forced to work in enemy factories, may receive high praise for their sabotage. The critical difference here is that when the situation passes, so does the passive-aggressiveness.

Paranoid personality disorder is distinguished by the overt, direct expression of the pt's resentment.

Catatonia of the stuporous type may present with negativism but is distinguished by the presence of a normal premorbid personality and by the presence of other catatonic sx, e.g., muteness, waxy flexibility.

Rx: Pts rarely stay in any form of Rx, seeing it as just another unfair burden; it is unclear whether any currently available Rx would be effective.

15. Other Conditions

15.1 PARKINSONISM (INCLUDING NEUROLEPTIC-INDUCED PARKINSONISM)

Arch Neurol 1995;52:294. J Neurol Neurosurg Psychiatry 1988;51:850.
J Neurol Neurosurg Psychiatry 1996;60:213. Lancet 1974;2:928.
Neurology 1995;45:2183.

Epidem: Neuroleptic-induced parkinsonism occurs in >50% of pts taking high-potency typical neuroleptics; the incidence is much lower in pts taking atypical neuroleptics and those taking low-potency typical neuroleptics.

Sx: Classic triad of rigidity, bradykinesia, and tremor:
- Rigidity generally of the cogwheel type, but "lead pipe" rigidity may also be seen. In cogwheel rigidity, upon passive extension (e.g., at the elbow joint), a "ratcheting" may be appreciated (placing the pt's elbow in the palm, with the thumb of your hand on the biceps tendon, and then using your other hand to extend the forearm facilitates appreciation of the cogwheeling).
- Bradykinesia is evident in a generalized slowness of movement and thought.
- Tremor is usually rhythmic, of moderate amplitude, and most evident at rest. Typically, when the hands are involved, the tremor has a "pill-rolling" quality, as if the pt were rolling a pill between the thumb and fingers.

Other features include a flexion posture, festination, postural instability (with retropulsion and propulsion), masked facies, hypophonia, drooling, and micrographia.

Lab: Reflects etiology.

Crs: Determined by etiology; in the pt with neuroleptic-induced parkinsonism sx generally appear gradually, over days to several weeks after starting a neuroleptic or increasing the dose, then worsen over a few days to a plateau that is generally maintained until the dose is reduced or the drug is stopped. With drug discontinuation, the parkinsonism should gradually recede over a matter of days to several weeks, or rarely, several months (in the case of depot preparations, i.e., haloperidol (Haldol Decanoate) and fluphenazine (Prolixin Decanoate), the parkinsonism may take many months, even up to a year, to fully resolve).

Cmplc: Activities requiring fine-motor control or swift movement are hindered; at its worst, parkinsonism may render pts bed bound and helpless.

Etiol: Causes of parkinsonism are listed in Table 15.1-1.

Of the drugs capable of causing parkinsonism, neuroleptics are by far the most common; parkinsonism secondary to other agents is often very subtle.

Of the toxins, MPTP, a contaminant of "street" meperidine, is perhaps most important. Manganese poisoning is rare in the USA.

Of the gradually progressive parkinsonian conditions, Parkinson's disease (see 3.9) and diffuse Lewy body disease (see 3.10) are the most common.

Ddx: Isolated "lead pipe" rigidity may be part of catatonia, which is distinguished by mutism, waxy flexibility, etc.

Isolated bradykinesia may resemble psychomotor retardation of a depressive episode, which is distinguished by the presence of other depressive sx (e.g., depressed mood, tearfulness, fatigue, insomnia).

Rx: Neuroleptic-induced parkinsonism is generally treated either by a dose reduction, by a change to a neuroleptic less likely to cause parkinsonism, or by the addition of an anticholinergic antiparkinsonian agent, such as benztropine (Cogentin) 2–4 mg/d. Amantadine (Symmetrel) may also be used, in doses of 200–300 mg/d. The antiparkinsonian agent should be continued until the dose of the neuroleptic is substantially reduced, or the drug stopped, at which point the antiparkinsonian agent may be gradually tapered. Levodopa-carbidopa (Sinemet) and direct-acting dopaminergic agents (e.g., bromocriptine (Parlodel)) are not required.

Table 15.1-1. Causes of Parkinsonism

Drugs or Toxins

Neuroleptics
Lithium (Eskalith, Lithobid)
Fluoxetine (Prozac) and paroxetine (Paxil)
Divalproex (Depakote)
Calcium channel blockers
Phenelzine (Nardil)
Disulfiram (Antabuse)
MPTP
Methanol
Manganese
Diquat

Chronic, Gradually Progressive Parkinsonism

Parkinson's disease
Diffuse Lewy body disease
MSA ("striatonigral" variant)
Dementia pugilistica
Vascular or "arteriosclerotic" parkinsonism
Progressive supranuclear palsy
Cortico–basal ganglionic degeneration
Alzheimer's disease
Westphal variant of Huntington's disease
Hallervorden-Spatz disease
Calcification of the basal ganglia (e.g., Fahr's disease)

Others

Posthypoxic
Postencephalitic (e.g., von Economo's disease)
Focal lesions of the basal ganglia
Pellagra ("encephalopathic" form)
Rapid-onset dystonic parkinsonism

15.2 DYSTONIA (INCLUDING ACUTE NEUROLEPTIC-INDUCED DYSTONIA)

Am J Psychiatry 1978;135:1414. Br J Psychiatry 1994;164:115. Brain 1974;97:793. Neurology 1991;41:1088.

Epidem: Acute neuroleptic-induced dystonia commonly occurs with Rx with high-potency typical neuroleptics.

Sx: Dystonic movements are sustained, rigid, abnormal postures that may be focal (involving only 1 muscle group), segmental (involving 1 or more adjacent groups), or generalized.

Focal dystonias include
1. Cervical dystonia, which may manifest with torticollis with the head turned to 1 side or the other; lateralcollis, with the head bent down to 1 side or the other; and either anterocollis or retrocollis, with the head bent, respectively, forward or backward (extraocular muscle dystonia, producing an "oculogyric crisis" is distinctive, and is discussed in 15.3)
2. Cranial dystonia (e.g., blepharospasm, lingual dystonia, pharyngeal dystonia)
3. Dystonia affecting only 1 limb, or a part thereof (e.g., "writer's cramp").

Segmental dystonia often involves ipsilateral muscle groups, e.g., the upper extremity and the ipsilateral cervical musculature.

Generalized dystonia typically begins focally, and may be dramatic, literally contorting the pt into a "pretzel."

Lab: Reflects the etiology.

Crs: Reflects the etiology. In acute neuroleptic-induced dystonia, sx generally appear fairly acutely within hours to days of either starting or increasing the dose of a neuroleptic, and are most often seen with high-potency, typical neuroleptics. Generally, acute neuroleptic-induced dystonias resolve spontaneously over several hours. Recurrences, though, with continued neuroleptic Rx, are common.

Cmplc: Although most acute neuroleptic-induced dystonias are not painful (with the exception of oculogyric crises), they are very alarming to pts and may provoke noncompliance. Lingual dystonia ("thick tongue") may cause dysarthria, and pharyngeal dystonia may lead to aspiration or respiratory embarrassment.

Etiol: Table 15.2-1 lists the various causes of dystonia. Tardive dystonia is considered with tardive dyskinesia in 15.7.

OTHER CONDITIONS

Table 15.2-1. Causes of Dystonia

Drugs

Neuroleptics (including both acute neuroleptic-induced dystonia, described in 15.2,
    and "tardive dystonia" described in 15.7)
MDMA ("Ecstasy")
Cocaine (during withdrawal)
Flunarizine

Idiopathic

Focal
  Cervical
  Cranial (Brueghel's syndrome, Meige's syndrome)
  Limb (e.g., "writer's cramp")
Generalized
  Dystonia musculorum deformans

Paroxysmal

Epileptic
Idiopathic paroxysmal dystonia (kinesigenic or nonkinesigenic)

Secondary to Focal Lesions

Basal ganglia
Thalamus
Brain stem

As Part of a More Widespread Disorder

Cortico–basal ganglionic degeneration
Hallervorden-Spatz disease
Dopa-responsive dystonia
Wilson's disease

Others

Head injury
Anoxia
Cyanide poisoning
Postencephalitic

Ddx: Catatonic posturing is distinguished by the presence of other catatonic sx, e.g., muteness, waxy flexibility.

Rx: Acute neuroleptic-induced dystonia may be treated acutely with diphenhydramine (Benadryl) 50–75 mg im or if required, 50 mg iv; benztropine (Cogentin) 2 mg po or im may also be used, but is somewhat slower acting. If the neuroleptic is continued, then prophylactic treatment with benztropine (Cogentin) 2–4 mg/d should be continued for as long as the neuroleptic is used at that dose, with the dose of benztropine (Cogentin) gradually reduced if the neuroleptic is stopped or the dose substantially reduced. Other neuroleptics less likely to cause acute dystonia (i.e., atypical neuroleptics and low-potency typical neuroleptics) may also be used.

15.3 OCULOGYRIC CRISIS

Brain 1987;110:19. J Neurol Neurosurg Psychiatry 1981;44:670. Mov Disord 1993;8:93.

Epidem: Oculogyric crises are a common form of acute neuroleptic-induced dystonia.

Sx: Onset is acute, generally over seconds or minutes.

There is a sustained, conjugate deviation of the eyes, upward, downward, or to the side. In neuroleptic-induced oculogyric crisis, the eyes generally deviate upward and to 1 side or the other. As noted in 15.2, this is the only dystonia that is routinely uncomfortable, even painful. Interestingly, in pts with schizophrenia treated with neuroleptics, oculogyric crises are often accompanied by a transient exacerbation of psychotic sx, such as voices.

Lab: Reflects the etiology.

Crs: Reflects the etiology; in the case of neuroleptic-induced oculogyric crisis, the forced deviation may persist for many hours before resolving. Subsequent to its resolution, however, recurrences are the rule with continued Rx.

Cmplc: With upward deviation, pts may fall while attempting to walk down stairs.

Etiol: High-potency typical neuroleptics are the most common cause; in the past, however, oculogyric crises were commonly seen as part of postencephalitic parkinsonism (importantly, although no new

OTHER CONDITIONS

epidemics of encephalitis lethargica have appeared, sporadic cases still occur).

Ddx: Vertical gaze palsy, as may be seen in progressive supranuclear palsy or with midbrain lesions, is distinguished by gradual onset, chronic course, and the fact that pts with vertical gaze palsies complain only of an inability to look up or down (as the case may be) and not of a painful sense of "forced" looking 1 way or the other.

Rx: Neuroleptic-induced oculogyric crisis is treated in same way as other acute neuroleptic-induced dystonias (see 15.2).

15.4 AKATHISIA (INCLUDING ACUTE NEUROLEPTIC-INDUCED AKATHISIA)

Am J Psychiatry 1994;151:763. Arch Gen Psychiatry 1994;51:963. Comp Psychiatry 1075;16:43. J Clin Psychiatry 1991;52:491.

Epidem: Among pts receiving high-potency typical neuroleptics, acute akathisia may occur in ~50%.

Sx: Akathisia may appear in 1 of 2 types, either "motor" or "cognitive," and these may or may not coexist in the same pt.

Motor akathisia presents with a very uncomfortable sense of restlessness, often felt most acutely in the legs, accompanied by an urge to walk or pace. The restlessness is typically worse when the pt is lying down or seated, and is partially relieved by getting up. Pts may pace about or stand in 1 place, often rocking back and forth from 1 foot to the other, or "marching in place." If seated, pts may rock back and forth in the seat, or restlessly swing their legs.

Cognitive akathisia may present with "restless" thoughts, and pts may complain that their thoughts are "jumbled" or "crowded" or "racing." In pts being treated with neuroleptics for schizophrenia or other psychotic conditions, the akathisia may present with an exacerbation of their psychotic sx, such as hallucinations, delusions, or loosening of associations. Interestingly, in pts with schizophrenia, such an akathisia-mediated exacerbation, rather than being accompanied by any restlessness, may be accompanied by withdrawal and muteness.

Lab: Reflects the etiology.

Table 15.4-1. Causes of Akathisia

Drugs

Neuroleptics (including both acute neuroleptic-induced akathisia, described in 15.4, and "tardive akathisia," discussed in 15.7)
SSRIs (e.g., fluoxetine (Prozac))
Nefazodone (Serzone)
Prochlorperazine (Compazine)
Metoclopramide (Reglan)

Others

Parkinson's disease
Uremia

Crs: Reflects the etiology; in the case of acute neuroleptic-induced akathisia, sx generally appear within a week or more after starting the neuroleptic or substantially increasing its dose; rarely an acute akathisia is delayed for up to 8 wk. Although the severity of acute neuroleptic-induced akathisia may wax and wane, it remains chronic until the dose is substantially reduced or the drug stopped.

Cmplc: An acute akathisia-induced exacerbation of psychotic sx may be mistaken for an exacerbation related to the underlying schizophrenia, and in such cases, the dose of the neuroleptic may be increased, setting the stage for a vicious cycle that can end up with very high doses and ever-worsening psychosis.

In the midst of an akathisia, pts may become irritable, agitated, violent, or suicidal.

Etiol: Various causes of akathisia are listed in Table 15.4-1. Tardive akathisia is discussed with tardive dyskinesia, in 15.7.

Ddx: Restless legs syndrome is distinguished by the tendency of these pts to rub their legs or calves and to pace around, in contrast with pts with acute neuroleptic-induced akathisia who rarely rub their legs and tend to march in place.

Rx: Acute neuroleptic-induced akathisia is best treated with propranolol (Inderal), in doses ranging from 60 to 240 mg/d. In otherwise healthy adults, one may begin with a single daily dose of the long-acting preparation of propranolol (Inderal) at 60 mg, with the dose increased as tolerated and as dictated by the pt's condition. In frail or elderly pts, or those with hepatic failure, begin with short-acting propranolol (Inderal) at 10–40 mg/d in divided doses.

OTHER CONDITIONS

Benztropine (Cogentin) 2–4 mg/d may also be used, but is less effective. Acute neuroleptic-induced akathisia should always be suspected in a neuroleptic-treated psychotic pt whose condition inexplicably worsens. In such pts, a "diagnosis by treatment response" to propranolol (Inderal) is appropriate. Acute neuroleptic-induced akathisia may also be approached by reducing the dose of the neuroleptic or stopping it.

15.5 TREMOR (INCLUDING MEDICATION-INDUCED POSTURAL TREMOR)

Acta Psychiatr Scand 1988;78:434. Ann Neurol 1994;35:717. J Clin Psychiatry 1995;56:283.

Epidem: Medication-induced postural tremor is common with certain psychopharmacologic agents, such as lithium (Eskalith, Lithobid), tricyclic and tetracyclic antidepressants, and stimulants.

Sx: Tremor consists of a rhythmic alternating contraction of agonist and antagonist muscles and is characterized according to (1) frequency (e.g., rapid or slow, or if possible, timed, e.g., 3 cps)); (2) amplitude (e.g., fine or coarse); and (3) whether postural, rest, or intention (postural tremor best seen with the hands held extended, with fingers spread apart; rest tremor best seen when the hands are at rest, as for example in a seated pt's lap; intention tremor best seen when the pt is intentionally doing something with the hand, e.g., as in the "finger-to-nose" test). Other characteristics, if present, may be added to the description (e.g., "rubral," "wing-beating," "flapping"). Thus, the tremor seen with lithium (Eskalith, Lithobid) at therapeutic blood level is a rapid, fine *postural* tremor; that with Parkinson's disease is classically a 3-cps coarse *rest* tremor of the "pill-rolling" type; and that with cerebellar lesions is an *intention* tremor of variable frequency and amplitude.

Lab: Reflects the etiology.

Crs: Reflects the etiology.

Cmplc: Medication-induced postural tremor may interfere with handwriting or any activity that demands fine-motor control, and is often embarrassing to the pt.

Etiol: See Table 15.5-1.

Table 15.5-1. Causes of Tremor

Postural

Medications
  Divalproex (Depakote)
  Lithium (Eskalith, Lithobid)
  Carbamazepine (Tegretol)
  Neuroleptics
  SSRI antidepressants
  Nefazodone (Serzone)
  Venlafaxine (Effexor)
  Stimulants (methylphenidate (Ritalin), pemoline (Cylert), dextroamphetamine
    (Dexedrine), cocaine)
  Caffeine
  Theophylline
  Sympathomimetics (e.g., pseudoephedrine)
  Tricyclic and tetracyclic antidepressants
Other
  Alcohol or sedative-hypnotic (e.g., benzodiazepine) withdrawal
  Generalized anxiety disorder
  Hyperthyroidism
  Panic attack
  Hypoglycemia
  Pheochromocytoma
  Essential tremor

Rest

Parkinsonism
"Rabbit" syndrome

Intention

Cerebellar lesions
Wernicke's encephalopathy

Other

Rubral (seen, e.g., in Benedikt's syndrome with lesion of the midbrain tegmentum)
Wing-beating (e.g., as seen in some cases of Wilson's disease)
Flapping (as in autism)

Ddx: Myoclonus is distinguished by the "shocklike" contraction of ago-nist muscles, followed not by a contraction of antagonistic muscles but rather by a slightly slower relaxation of the agonist muscula-ture.

Rx: Medication-induced postural tremor often lessens with dose reduc-tion; if this is not possible owing to a loss of therapeutic effect, and the tremor is bothersome, propranolol (Inderal) or another beta-blocker (e.g., nadolol (Corgard)) is generally effective. The required daily dose of propranolol (Inderal) varies widely, from as little as 20–40 mg up to 240 mg or more, and thus the physician should start with a low dose and titrate up gradually, switching, when possible, to a long-acting form of the beta-blocker to facili-tate compliance.

15.6 NEUROLEPTIC MALIGNANT SYNDROME

Am J Psychiatry 1989;146:717. Am J Psychiatry 1998;155:1113. Biol Psychiatry 1987;22:1004. J Neurol Neurosurg Psychiatry 1995;58: 271. Neurology 1985;35:258.

Epidem: Rare.

Sx: Onset is typically within a day or 2 of an abrupt diminution in dopa-minergic tone; exceptionally onset may be within an hour or con-versely, after several weeks. As noted below, this diminution in dopaminergic tone is usually due to a neuroleptic.

The full syndrome usually evolves over 1–3 d, and is characterized by delirium, rigidity, fever, and autonomic instability. The rigidity is generalized, and may be severe; it is often accompanied by a coarse tremor and rarely by chorea or dystonia. Fever may range up to 103°F. Autonomic instability manifests with tachycardia, dia-phoresis, and labile BP. Some pts may develop a stuporous cata-tonic state. There may be tachypnea; however, this appears to be secondary to severe rigidity of the chest wall.

Lab: Leukocytosis (often up to 15,000/mm^3), elevated CPK (likewise up to 15,000 units/L), and when rhabdomyolysis occurs, myoglobin-uria.

Crs: Untreated, fatal in 10%–20%; once dopaminergic tone is normal-ized, sx spontaneously resolve within 1–2 wk.

Cmplc: Renal failure, pulmonary emboli, aspiration pneumonia, respiratory failure, and disseminated intravascular coagulation.

Etiol: Neuroleptic malignant syndrome occurs in a small minority of pts in whom there is an abrupt diminution in dopaminergic tone in the striatum and hypothalamus. The most common cause is Rx with a neuroleptic, either at its initiation or with a substantial dose increase. Although high-potency typical neuroleptics (e.g., fluphenazine (Prolixin), haloperidol (Haldol)) are most often responsible, low-potency typical agents (e.g., chlorpromazine (Thorazine)) or atypical neuroleptics (e.g., risperidone (Risperdal) or clozapine (Clozaril)) have also been reported to be causative. Metoclopramide, a dopamine blocker, may also cause the syndrome.

Dopaminergic tone can be reduced by discontinuation of long-term Rx with dopaminergic agents, such as levodopa-carbidopa (Sinemet), bromocriptine (Parlodel), and amantadine (Symmetrel).

Ddx: The triad of delirium, rigidity, and autonomic instability is distinctive, and whenever any one of these sx appears in the setting of decreased dopaminergic tone, the suspicion of neuroleptic malignant syndrome should be high.

Stauder's lethal catatonia (see 3.19) is distinguished by preexisting excited catatonia. When a pt with excited catatonia is treated with a neuroleptic and then develops fever and prostration, the ddx may be difficult. One clue is that in neuroleptic malignant syndrome, the rigidity is often severe and accompanied by tremor, whereas in Stauder's lethal catatonia, the rigidity is often mild and is not accompanied by tremor.

Rx: Hospitalization, generally in an ICU, is appropriate.

Neuroleptics must be discontinued. Bromocriptine (Parlodel) may be given, po or per nasogastric tube, in doses of 2.5–20 mg tid.

If discontinuation of a dopaminergic agent is at fault, that agent should be restarted.

Dantrolene (Dantrium) 1–2 mg/kg iv may provide relief, especially of rigidity, and may be repeated prn up to a total dose of 10 mg/kg/24 h.

Fever is treated with cooling blankets, and hydration is ensured with iv fluids. Pressor agents and respiratory support may be required.

OTHER CONDITIONS

15.7 TARDIVE DYSKINESIA

Am J Psychiatry 1993;150:498. Am J Psychiatry 1994;151:925. Arch
  Gen Psychiatry 1979;36:585. Can J Psychiatry 1995;40(Suppl 2):49.

Epidem: 2%–3% of pts treated chronically with neuroleptics.
Sx: Neuroleptic Rx for 1 yr or longer precedes tardive dyskinesia in
  most pts; occasionally it may occur after only a half year, and
  rarely, after only a month of Rx. Tardive dyskinesia may appear
  suddenly, if the dose of the neuroleptic is reduced acutely, or only
  gradually with ongoing Rx.

  Dyskinesia is most commonly of the choreic type; athetoid and dystonic types are much less common. In some pts, one may see an
  akathisia rather than a dyskinesia.

  Chorea of tardive dyskinesia most commonly affects the face, less
  commonly the upper or lower extremities, and rarely the trunk.
  Facial chorea, importantly, affects only the lower half of the face,
  sparing the forehead. There may be tongue thrusting, lip smacking, puckering, blepharospasm, or facial grimacing. Upper-
  extremity involvement may manifest with shoulder shrugging or
  "piano-playing" movements of the fingers, and lower-extremity
  involvement may show with foot tapping. Truncal involvement
  may appear with a rocking to-and-fro movement or with pelvic
  thrusting. Rarely, the diaphragm may be involved, producing irregular, grunting respirations.

  Athetosis and dystonia of tardive dyskinesia rarely appear in isolation, but are generally accompanied by chorea. Dystonia may manifest with torticollis, retrocollis, upper-extremity dystonia, facial
  dystonia, or rarely, generalized dystonia.

  Akathisia of tardive dyskinesia presents in a manner quite similar to
  acute neuroleptic-induced akathisia that occurs shortly after the
  neuroleptic is started or the dose is increased. Pts may complain
  of a sense of restlessness, march in place, or experience restless,
  chaotic thoughts.

Lab: NC.
Crs: If the neuroleptic is stopped, the severity of the dyskinesia will temporarily increase, and then after a matter of weeks, will progressively decrease in severity over several weeks or months. In about
  one-third of pts, this diminution of sx will gradually continue until
  the dyskinesia resolves; in the other two-thirds, however, the sever-

ity of the dyskinesia stabilizes and remains more or less stable indefinitely.

If the neuroleptic is continued, in most pts the dyskinesia will increase in severity until it reaches a certain plateau, which then persists.

If the dose of the neuroleptic is increased, the dyskinesia will be more or less completely "masked." With continued Rx, however, the underlying dyskinesia worsens, and eventually resurfaces.

Cmplc: May range from simple embarrassment to an inability to perform simple motor tasks.

Etiol: Disturbances in dopaminergic or GABAergic transmission are suspected.

Of the neuroleptics, high-potency typical neuroleptics (e.g., fluphenazine (Prolixin), haloperidol (Haldol)) are the most common cause; low-potency typical neuroleptics and atypical neuroleptics are far less common causes. Metoclopramide (Reglan) and prochlorperazine (Compazine) may also cause tardive dyskinesia.

Ddx: Acute neuroleptic-induced dystonia and acute neuroleptic-induced akathisia are distinguished by their occurrence early in the course of neuroleptic Rx and their resolution with a substantial dose reduction or discontinuation of the neuroleptic.

Other causes of chorea are listed in Table 15.7-1; of them, Huntington's disease is most often the ddx. In Huntington's disease, however, there is often forehead chorea and a "dancing and prancing" gait, neither of which is seen with tardive dyskinesia. Furthermore, whereas in Huntington's disease the chorea moves, lightning like, from 1 body part to the other, in tardive dyskinesia the choreiform movements are often repetitive in the same spot.

Other causes of chronic dystonia, noted in Table 15.2-1, must also be considered.

Rx: Prevention is accomplished by avoiding chronic use of neuroleptics for disorders (e.g., major depression, bipolar disorder) that can be treated effectively in other ways.

When chronic neuroleptic Rx is necessary (e.g., for schizophrenia), the dose should be as low as possible and consistent with adequate sx relief. "Drug holidays," rather than reducing the risk of tardive dyskinesia, may actually increase it.

Vitamin E 400 IU tid substantially reduces the severity of sx.

ECT may also be effective in some pts, regardless of whether the pt is depressed or not.

Table 15.7-1. Causes of Chorea

Drugs

Chronic neuroleptic Rx (tardive dyskinesia)
Levodopa-carbidopa (Sinemet)
Phenytoin (Dilantin)
Lithium (Eskalith, Lithobid)
Stimulants (methylphenidate (Ritalin),
  dextroamphetamine (Dexedrine),
  pemoline (Cylert), cocaine)
Divalproex (Depakote)
Gabapentin (Neurontin)
Oral contraceptives
Baclofen (Lioresal)

Heredodegenerative Conditions

Huntington's disease
Neuroacanthocytosis
Benign hereditary chorea
Senile chorea
Dentatorubropallidoluysian atrophy
Acquired hepatocerebral degeneration
Wilson's disease

Focal Lesions

Basal ganglia
Associated with proprioceptive sensory
  loss

Others

Postanoxic encephalopathy
Post–carbon monoxide poisoning
Hyperthyroidism
Polycythemia vera
Mercury poisoning

Anticholinergic drugs (e.g., benztropine (Cogentin)) generally worsen tardive dyskinesia and, if possible, should be avoided.

15.8 SEROTONIN SYNDROME

Am J Psychiatry 1982;139:954. Am J Psychiatry 1991;148:705. J Clin Psychiatry 1990;51:222. Neurology 1995;45:219.

Epidem: Rare.
Sx: Onset is within hours to days after a pharmacologically induced enhancement of serotoninergic tone, as for example by a combination of an SSRI and an MAOI.

Pts present with varying combinations of delirium, restlessness, and myoclonus; common associated findings include shivering, coarse tremor, and diaphoresis. On PE, DTRs may be increased with

Table 15.8-1. Causes of the Serotonin Syndrome

MAOI plus	Tryptophan plus
SSRI	MAOI
Clomipramine (Anafranil)	SSRI
TCA	Clomipramine (Anafranil)
Venlafaxine (Effexor)	Trazodone plus
SSRI plus	Bupropion (Wellbutrin, Zyban)
MAOI	Single agent (rare)
TCA	SSRI
	Clomipramine (Anafranil)

ankle clonus and bilateral Babinski signs. In severe cases, convulsions, rhabdomyolysis, and renal failure may supervene.

Lab: Rhabdomyolysis may cause elevated CPK levels and myoglobinuria.

Crs: Fatalities may occur; however, with restoration of normal serotoninergic tone, recovery occurs gradually, without sequelae, within several days.

Cmplc: Complications of delirium are discussed in 3.1.

Etiol: Pharmacologic manipulations capable of causing the serotonin syndrome are listed in Table 15.8-1.

By far the most common cause is a combination of an MAOI with another serotoninergic agent, as listed in Table 15.8-1. The combination of an SSRI and a TCA is a rare cause of the serotonin syndrome, and it is exceptionally rare to see the serotonin syndrome secondary to Rx with an SSRI or clomipramine alone. In the past, the combination of tryptophan with serotoninergic agents was a common cause. Tryptophan was removed from the market; however, it is now appearing in health food supplements or herbal combinations, and this may at times *not* be reflected in the labeling.

Ddx: Delirium or myoclonus appearing in the context of one of the pharmacologic measures listed in Table 15.8-1 should arouse immediate suspicion.

Other causes of delirium and myoclonus include hyponatremia, hypomagnesemia, and uremia.

Rx: In addition to supportive care and general measures for delirium (see 3.1), cyproheptadine (Periactin), in doses of 8–32 mg/d, may reverse the syndrome.

Best Rx is prevention, and an MAOI and an SSRI should never be

OTHER CONDITIONS

used together. If one wishes to switch from an MAOI to an SSRI, one must wait at least 2 wk after stopping the MAOI in order to allow a new "crop" of MAO to appear; conversely, if one switches from an SSRI to an MAOI, one must wait at least 5 half-lives after stopping the SSRI (e.g., 1 wk for paroxetine (Paxil) or sertraline (Zoloft), and at least 7 wk for fluoxetine (Prozac) given its long-half-life active metabolite).

15.9 POSTCONCUSSION SYNDROME

J Nerv Ment Dis 1992;180:683. J Neurol Neurosurg Psychiatry 1983; 46:1084. Neurology 1995;45:1253.

Epidem: Approximately one-third of pts who suffer a concussion will go on to develop the postconcussion syndrome.

Sx: Within hours to a day after recovering from the concussion, sx of the postconcussion syndrome appear.

Concussions are caused by head trauma, usually of the acceleration-deceleration type, as may occur during a motor vehicle accident or upon being struck on the head. Pts either appear dazed, or more commonly, experience a transient loss of consciousness, recovering generally in a matter of minutes. Upon recovery of consciousness, there is both anterograde and retrograde amnesia, which clears fairly rapidly, leaving the pt with a permanent "island" of amnesia covering events from just before to a variable period of time after the head trauma.

The postconcussion syndrome is characterized by difficulty with memory and concentration (pts often seem forgetful, and have difficulty completing tasks, especially those that are novel or complex); fatigue, irritability, depressed, or anxious mood, and in some pts, insomnia; headache, which may be either dull or throbbing; light-headedness or vertigo (which is often precipitated by sudden movements of the head); and in some, photophobia, hyperacusis, and hyperhidrosis (which may be severe). Alcohol often exacerbates sx.

Lab: Typically wnl. Although some abnormalities have been found on brain stem evoked potential studies and SPECT scans, these tests are not diagnostically reliable here. MRI occasionally reveals evidence of scattered, old petechial hemorrhages; here again, though, this test is not useful in routine dx of the postconcussion syndrome.

Crs: Gradual recovery occurs over weeks to months, and most pts recover completely. In a minority, recovery may drag out much longer, up to 3 yr. Sx present beyond 3 yr generally remain chronic.

Cmplc: Difficulty with memory and concentration generally impair work; irritability and affective changes cause strain in personal relations.

Etiol: Probably secondary to a mild degree of DAI (discussed more fully in 3.8).

Ddx: Malingering is suspected when pts gain, or stand to gain, from their sx, e.g., either by being released from work or by winning a lawsuit. Atypical sx suggest the dx of malingering; some sx, such as hyperhidrosis, point away from it, as most laypeople are simply not aware of this as a sx.

Dementia due to head trauma (see 3.8) is distinguished by the severe cognitive deficits.

Subacute subdural hematoma and delayed intracerebral hemorrhage are suggested by a deteriorating course often accompanied by focal findings.

Communicating hydrocephalus, as may occur after a traumatic subarachnoid hemorrhage, is suggested by deteriorating course, and findings such as ataxia and incontinence.

Rx: Reassurance.

Antidepressants, such as nortriptyline (Pamelor), may relieve irritability, affective sx, and insomnia.

Antihistamines may relieve vertigo.

Acetaminophen or an NSAID is appropriate for headache.

Alcohol is forbidden until the syndrome resolves.

15.10 ADJUSTMENT DISORDERS

Am J Psychiatry 1978;135:660. Am J Psychiatry 1980;37:1166. Arch Gen Psychiatry 1987;44:567.

Epidem: Thought to be common, but probably overdiagnosed.

Sx: Shortly after a significantly stressful event (or upon the accumulation of a number of relatively minor stresses), pts experience a disturbance in their emotions and/or conduct that is greater than would be expected from the stress in question or that impairs their ability to function to a greater degree than would be seen in otherwise normal persons. The emotional changes may tend either to depression or to anxiety and the change in conduct is generally characterized by misconduct of the "acting out" type, with vandalism, fights, or reckless behavior.

Lab: NC.

Crs: Most pts come back to normal within a half year; in pts in whom the stress is ongoing, or has ongoing consequences, however, the adjustment disorder may persist for much longer.

Cmplc: Some decrement in ability to sustain relationships or work; rarely, suicide may occur.

Etiol: Uncertain; some suspect an as yet poorly understood inability to respond adaptively to stressful situations.

Ddx: The dx of adjustment disorder is problematic, and represents a gray area in psychiatric nosology. In many cases, the dx is admittedly given to avoid stigmatizing a pt. Especially among adolescents, the disturbance in emotion or conduct, over time, proves to be a prodrome to an illness such as major depression or schizophrenia, and thus the dx should always be tentative.

The dx of adjustment disorder is not given when the disturbance represents a stress-induced exacerbation of another disorder (e.g., a pt in a depressive episode who gets fired and feels more depressed, or a pt with a histrionic personality disorder who, upon being rejected by a lover, embarks upon a siege of lamentations and tears).

PTSD is distinguished by the characteristic sx of numbing to the environment and involuntary reexperiencing of the stressful event in dreams, unwanted memories, etc.

Rx: Short-term psychotherapy is generally offered.

15.11 BEREAVEMENT

Am J Psychiatry 1944;101:141. J Clin Psychiatry 1990;51:34. J Clin Psychiatry 1993;54:365.

Epidem: Normal, uncomplicated bereavement is the rule after the death of a spouse, parent, child, or significant other.

Sx: Onset of bereavement begins shortly after the death.

Normally, individuals initially enter a stage of *shock and denial,* which can last from days to weeks. During this time they may feel numb and express disbelief that the death could have occurred; often yearning for the dead and anger and protest over the death are intermingled. Subsequently, individuals enter what is often termed *acute grief.* There may be waves of despair; individuals may withdraw from others, become preoccupied with the dead, and give up former activities. During this state of acute grief, depressive sx are common, with depressed mood, fatigue, anhedonia, some agitation or anxiety, guilt over not having done enough before the death, and insomnia. Suicidal ideation may occur, often expressed as a wish to join the deceased. This stage of acute grief eventually resolves, and is followed by a stage of *resolution,* wherein individuals reintegrate into life, forming new attachments.

Lab: NC.

Crs: In most individuals, bereavement is substantially resolved by 3–6 mo, and in almost all, it is over by about a year.

Cmplc: If depressive sx are severe, individuals may be unable to function, and may lose jobs and friendships.

Suicide may occur, and the mortality rate (esp from cardiovascular and infectious causes) is higher, esp in older men.

Alcohol abuse or dependence may occur.

Etiol: Bereavement is a normal life experience.

Ddx: Bereavement that persists beyond a year is often referred to as "chronic grief," and appears to be more likely when the relationship with the deceased was marked by dependency or substantial ambivalence.

Depressive sx normally present during bereavement must be distinguished from a depressive episode of major depression. A h/o depressive episodes earlier in life is suggestive. The presence of certain sx, very uncommon in normal bereavement, should also suggest the dx; these include psychomotor retardation, guilt (not over

OTHER CONDITIONS

not having done enough, but over having, in some way, directly caused the death), a profound sense of worthlessness or self-condemnation, and delusions of sin or guilt. Transient hallucinations of seeing or hearing the deceased may occur in normal bereavement, but frequent or constant hallucinations, esp if they have a persecutory or bizarre aspect, are not. Finally, a persistence of prominent depressive sx beyond 1 yr is unlikely in bereavement, and suggests a major depression.

Rx: The vast majority of individuals survive bereavement with the help of family, friends, and clergy; in some cases, referral to a support group (such as compassionate friends for those whose children have died) is appropriate. When depressive sx are severe, consideration should be given to using an antidepressant, as outlined in 6.1. Antidepressants do not interfere with the normal work of grieving, and indeed may make it possible. Cognitive behavioral therapy may also be helpful in such cases.

15.12 SUICIDAL BEHAVIOR

Acta Psychiatr Scand 1982;65:221. Br J Psychiatry 1974;125:355. Br J Psychiatry 1987;150:78. Br J Psychiatry 1992;161:749.

Epidem: USA lifetime prevalences: suicidal *ideation* ~10%; suicide *attempts* ~0.3%; *completed* suicide ~0.012%. Overall, for *completed* suicide, male-female ratio 2–7:1.

Approximately two-thirds of all suicide completers had seen their personal physician in the month prior to killing themselves.

Approximately 70%–90% of all suicide completers had a psychiatric illness that was potentially treatable; in the majority of cases this was a depressive illness and/or alcoholism.

Sx:

Predicting *Completed* Suicide: Although there is no foolproof way to predict who among those with suicidal ideation will go on to a suicide attempt or to completed suicide, certain risk factors do exist, as noted in Table 15.12-1.

Age increases the risk, especially after 45 yr, with the risk rising even higher >60 yr.

Table 15.12-1. Risk Factors for Completed Suicide

	Suicide Attempts	Completed Suicide
Age	Younger, <45 yr	Older, >45 yr
Sex	Female > male	Male > female
Race	Black	White
Psychiatric dx	Adjustment disorder	Depression, alcoholism
General health	Good	Poor
Recent losses	Absent	Present
Social ties	Present	Minimal or absent
Religious affiliation	Catholic, Jewish	Protestant
Hope for future	Present	Absent
Lethality of intended method	Low	High
Probability of rescue	High	Low
H/o prior attempts	None, or >2 yr prior	Within 2 yr

Sex is a strong predictor. Males are more likely than females to complete suicide at all ages.

Race becomes increasingly important, for males, after age 40 yr. Before age 40 the risk of completed suicide is only slightly higher for white males than black males; after 40 it is much higher. The risk for white females remains only slightly higher than for black females at all ages. Native Americans are at higher risk than white males.

Psychiatric dxs of depression and/or alcoholism (or mixed substance dependence) greatly increases the risk of completed suicide, whereas a dx of adjustment disorder is associated with a lower risk of completion.

In depression, the risk is further increased when psychotic features (e.g., delusions of sin, nihilistic delusions) are present. Furthermore, the risk, paradoxically, may be higher as pts start to recover from their depression. During the depth of a depression, pts may be so anergic that they simply cannot act; when they begin to improve, however, they have enough energy to do what they wanted to do all along (in this regard, one may see a sudden brightening of mood in some pts with depression who now find themselves with the energy to end their suffering).

Schizophrenia also increases the risk, but in unusual ways. In schizophrenia, the risk is higher among younger than older pts; furthermore, the risk in schizophrenia is highest *not* during a period characterized by an exacerbation of psychotic sx, but

OTHER CONDITIONS

rather in the partial remission that follows. A unifying hypothesis here is that completed suicide in schizophrenics is associated with the barren sense of hopelessness experienced by pts as, while in the depressive aftermath of an exacerbation, they realize that they will never be able to attain their life goals; conversely, older "burnt out" schizophrenics, having come to some terms with the illness, seem less devastated by each new exacerbation.

Other disorders associated with higher risk include a mixed-manic episode of bipolar disorder, anorexia nervosa, antisocial personality disorder, and borderline personality disorder. Pts with borderline personality disorder, although at higher risk for completed suicide than those, say, with an adjustment disorder, are far more notable for their incredibly high risk for repeated suicide attempts. Indeed, certain borderline personality disorder pts make so many attempts that they gain a certain local notoriety.

General health status influences the risk, with pts having serious, esp chronic conditions being at higher risk. Examples include those with cancer, AIDS, and MS. The risk is also higher in pts suffering from chronic complex partial seizures.

Recent losses that increase risk include the death of a loved one, divorce or separation, job loss, and bankruptcy.

Social ties, such as with spouses, children, and friends, reduce the risk; conversely, those who lead isolated lives are at higher risk.

Religious affiliation with the Roman Catholic church or Judaism decreases the risk, but only if the pt feels bound by the religious teachings of these faiths.

Hope for the future reduces the risk of completed suicide; conversely a sense of hopelessness is a strong predictor of suicide.

Lethality of the intended method naturally bears on whether any attempt will lead to a completed suicide. A pt who intends on overdosing on vitamins or penicillin is at far lower risk than one who plans on hanging or shooting.

Probability of rescue also has an obvious bearing on risk. A pt who intends on overdosing in front of family members is much more likely to be rescued than someone who plans on the same method, but plans to do it in a deserted building.

Hx of prior attempts is generally irrelevant if the attempt occurred more than 2 yr earlier. Attempts within 2 yr generally increase the risk, except if the attempt just occurred. It appears that in the immediate aftermath of an attempt, the risk of a pt going on to completing suicide is low.

Other factors that are associated with increased risk include akathisia (as may occur in a depressed pt given an SSRI), intoxication with alcohol, phencyclidine use, and perhaps, LSD use.

Examples of high-risk and low-risk pts would be (1) a 55-yr-old white, divorced, recently fired man, suffering from alcoholism, depression, and cirrhosis of the liver, with no friends and no hope, who planned on taking his pistol and a bottle of whiskey to an abandoned warehouse, getting drunk, and then shooting himself in the head; and (2) a 23-yr-old white, married female store clerk with a histrionic personality disorder, but otherwise good health, who, after her husband failed to buy her the ring she wanted, threatened to run upstairs, get her bottle of vitamins, and take a "handful."

Clinical Judgment: This *must prevail* when it conflicts strongly with the above risk factors. No rating scale, computer program, or algorithm has successfully balanced and weighted these various risk factors such that they should *ever* be construed as necessarily taking precedence over good judgment. For example, consider a 24-yr-old white, married female nurse who lived at home with her husband and children, had many friends, was a strong Catholic, and was in otherwise good health who had a mixed-manic episode of bipolar disorder and heard voices telling her to kill herself before she murdered her children. Although such a pt "scores" low on risk factors, an experienced psychiatrist would have no hesitation in hospitalizing her immediately.

Rx: If the risk of suicide appears high, hospitalize pt (involuntarily, if necessary), preferably on a locked ward. Search pt for any potentially dangerous items, and arrange for close observation; in certain situations, 1:1 observation is appropriate. Compliance with medications should be ensured. Pts may "cheek" pills and stockpile them, and in some pts it is appropriate to use liquid concentrates or suspensions.

If the risk appears low, outpatient Rx may be attempted. Visits should be relatively frequent, and if possible, pts should be supervised at home. Firearms and potentially lethal medications should be removed. Medications of low lethality (e.g., an SSRI rather than a tricyclic for depression) are preferable, and if a potentially lethal medicine is required, always limit the number of pills to a sublethal amount. Pts should be instructed to call if they feel like they are about to lose control.

The "*No Suicide Contract,*" currently popular, may be more of an assessment tool than a preventive measure. After some rapport has been established, pts with suicidal ideation are asked to say the following: "I will not hurt myself in any way, no matter what happens, until [provide the time of day, day of the week, month, date, year, e.g., 1 PM, Monday, December 28, 1999]." Gently stress with the pt that "in any way" means exactly that, as does "no matter *what*," and insert a date (this may be the following day the pt is seen on rounds, or if an outpatient, the next appointment). Pts who are in good control will have little difficulty saying this with a straight face; those who are bent on self-destruction either will refuse to say it or will mouth the words with obvious insincerity. Those who are in the gray area and struggling may or may not be shored up by making such a commitment, and a lot of clinical judgment must come into play in assessing the answers of these pts.

Treatment of the underlying illness should be aggressive. For depressed or mixed-manic pts judged at high risk, consideration for ECT should be given.

15.13 VIOLENT BEHAVIOR

Acta Psychiatr Scand 1977;55:269. Am J Psychiatry 1982;139:1346. Am J Psychiatry 1983;140:1356. Arch Gen Psychiatry 1992;49:493.

Epidem: Violence is ubiquitous, and in the overwhelming majority of cases, violence is committed by people who are not psychiatrically ill. Such people fall under the purview of the law, not of medicine. Some psychiatric disorders, however, are associated with violence, and these are noted below.

Sx:

Predicting Violent Behavior: Of all the risk factors for violence noted in Table 15.13-1, the current mental status is generally the most important.

Current Mental Status Findings: These are very helpful in pre-

Table 15.13-1. Risk Factors for Violence

Current Mental Status Findings

Hostile, irritable
Agitation
Victim(s) apparently picked out
Weapons available

Disorders

Mania (when characterized by prominent irritability), as in bipolar disorder or
   schizoaffective disorder, bipolar type
Paranoid schizophrenia
Anabolic steroid abuse
Personality change (with disinhibition, e.g., frontal lobe syndrome)
Dementia
Delirium
MR
Paranoid personality disorder
Antisocial personality disorder
Borderline personality disorder
Alcohol intoxication
Phencyclidine intoxication
Stimulant intoxication (cocaine, amphetamines)
Intermittent explosive disorder
Delusional disorder

Personal History

H/o violent behavior in similar circumstances
H/o being physically abused in childhood
Growing up in a family where parents were violent toward each other
Childhood h/o enuresis, cruelty to animals, and fire setting (the "triad")

Demographic

Male ≫ female
Young (late teens or early 20s) > older

dicting immediate violence. An irritable, hostile, progressively more agitated pt who has begun threatening specific people and who has a weapon (e.g., a knife, or simply balled fists) at hand requires immediate intervention. When an experienced nurse reports that a pt is about to "go off," rapid action is generally required.

Disorders: Mania of the irritable type (whether occurring in bipolar disorder or schizoaffective disorder, bipolar type) may lead to a very rapid escalation to violence, and should be treated as rapidly as possible.

Paranoid schizophrenics are typically on guard and suspicious and may abruptly and irrationally attack others in "self defense."

Anabolic steroid abuse may create a bulked-up, hostile male who feels invulnerable and won't tolerate anyone standing in his way.

Personality change (especially if accompanied by disinhibition, as in the frontal lobe syndrome), by robbing pts of the capacity for self-control, may set them up for violence whenever things don't go their way.

Delirium, dementia, and MR may similarly impair the capacity for self-control. This is particularly problematic when pts are, for any reason, agitated (e.g., in a "noisy" delirium).

Paranoid personality disorder, like paranoid schizophrenia, leaves pts guarded and ready for "counterattack"; here, however, pts are often able to keep their hostility in check, and it is only when they seem about ready to lose control that one must be worried.

Antisocial personality disorder may or may not present a threat of immediate danger, depending on the level of self-control, impulsivity, and agitation. Some sociopaths (the "successful" ones) exercise remarkable restraint, and engage in violence only when it is necessary, and never when there is a high risk of apprehension. Such sociopaths pick their victims with care, and only those on the "list" generally need be concerned. On the other extreme are the sociopaths with such little self-control that they immediately do what they want, hurting anyone who stands in their way, even if they are likely to get caught in the act. The danger with this latter type is obviously increased when there is a considerable amount of agitation or impulsivity.

Borderline personality disorder may be associated with considerable impulsivity and anger, esp when the pt feels acutely rejected or abandoned. Threats or impulsive assaults may follow.

Alcohol, by its disinhibiting effect, is strongly associated with violence. The "mean drunk" is a common sight in the ER.

Phencyclidine intoxication may be associated with unpredictable, at times bizarrely aggressive behavior.

Stimulant intoxication, when accompanied by agitation and

delusions of persecution, may leave pts precipitously on the brink of counterattack.

Intermittent explosive disorder is characterized by paroxysmal explosive anger, which can occur spontaneously or after trivial precipitants. Pts with this condition should be carefully monitored.

Delusional disorder generally poses a danger only to those individuals who have been incorporated into the pt's delusional system. Thus, the erotomanic type may pose a danger only to the object of his or her love (or to that person's current "significant other"), and the jealous type only to his or her lover. The "target" of the persecutory type may be harder to predict, and may change over time. Usually, upon hospitalization, the pt with delusional disorder, persecutory subtype, presents little or no danger to people in the hospital; over time, however, if someone in the hospital is incorporated into the delusional system, then danger exists.

Personal Hx: Hx of violence may be very helpful. Hx tends to repeat itself, and if the pt is in a situation similar to one wherein violence occurred in the past, then violence is more likely in the present.

Children who were abused or who grew up with parents who were violent toward each other, or who had the "triad" of enuresis, cruelty to animals, and fire setting are more likely to be violent as adults. It is not clear whether these findings are useful in predicting immediate dangerousness.

Demographics: Although young men are more likely to be violent than females or older men, this risk factor should not be used in isolation, but only in combination with one of the earlier risk factors; i.e., for a given condition (e.g., irritable mania), the risk of violence is higher if the pt is a young male than a female or an older man.

Clinical Judgment: This must be exercised in using most of the risk factors to predict violence; the only exception would be a current mental status indicative that a pt is about to "go off." With regard to the various disorders, some, like irritable mania, almost universally pose a very high risk, whereas others seem to increase the risk only if the pt with that condition is irritable or frustrated (e.g., pts with MR who pose no threat unless someone takes something, such as a toy or some food, away from them).

Rx: If the risk of immediate violence appears high, several alternatives may be considered: verbal intervention, prn medication, and seclusion and/or restraints.

Verbal Intervention: Generally not attempted with pts who have lost control and are "going off."

Calm pts, or those who are struggling to retain control and seem to be succeeding for the time being, may often benefit from a talk. In the presence of a physician who is calm in voice, manner, and posture and who is able to talk with the pt without authoritarianism or anger, many pts will calm down, sometimes dramatically. The setting for such talks should vary depending on the pts' condition. Those in good control may be interviewed in an office with the door closed; those in somewhat less control may be seen alone, but with the door open, with or without a guard posted outside. In either case, pt and physician should be seated, the door should be readily accessible to each, and there should be no potential weapons in reach (knives, scissors, etc.). Pts close to losing control may be seen in a public area, but at enough distance from others that they don't feel the necessity to salvage their pride by making good on their threats in front of the "audience."

Verbal intervention should not be relied on when the disorder makes it impossible for the pt to cooperate (e.g., a florid psychosis, severe dementia).

Prn Medications: Should be considered for pts who are "going off" or about to do so, and may include either a neuroleptic or a benzodiazepine.

Neuroleptics are a mainstay: chlorpromazine (Thorazine) 50–100 mg or haloperidol (Haldol) 5–10 mg, with either given qh (if im) or q 2 h (if po—always use concentrate) until the pt is calm, limiting SEs occur, or a maximum dose of ~1000 mg chlorpromazine or ~50 mg haloperidol is reached. Chlorpromazine (Thorazine) is more sedating and more likely to cause hypotension, whereas haloperidol (Haldol) carries a greater risk of extrapyramidal SEs such as dystonia, akathisia, and parkinsonism. All things being equal, chlorpromazine (Thorazine) may have an edge. Lower doses and longer dosing intervals are indicated for the elderly, debilitated, or those with impaired hepatic function.

Benzodiazepines may be useful in selected pts, but carry a risk of further disinhibition; some manics, however, do well with lorazepam (Ativan) 2 mg im qh until the pt is calm, limiting SEs occur, or a maximum dose of ~12 mg is attained. As for neuroleptics, lower doses are required for the elderly or debilitated (lorazepam (Ativan), dosage adjustment is not required with impaired hepatic function unless the impairment is severe).

Seclusion and/or Restraints: For those who have lost control and either don't respond to prn medications or for whom control is required before the prn medication can become effective, seclusion and/or restraints should be considered. For some pts, the dramatic reduction in stimulation entailed by the seclusion room may be enough to let them calm down; in others, restraints may be necessary.

Hospitalization is generally appropriate when immediate violence threatens; exceptions include situations wherein the risk of violence is likely to rapidly fall (e.g., with resolution of alcohol intoxication). When violence is not imminent, outpatient treatment may be considered.

Treat the Underlying Condition: If this is not possible, or ineffective, and the condition itself is likely to persist, consider symptomatic Rx.

Symptomatic Rx: Rxs likely to reduce the risk of violence regardless of the underlying condition include lithium (Eskalith, Lithobid), carbamazepine (Tegretol), and divalproex (Depakote) (all used as described in 6.6 for mania). Propranolol (Inderal) in doses up to 640 mg may be helpful, esp in cases of personality change due to a traumatic brain injury; provided there are no contraindications, begin with ~60 mg/d of propranolol (Inderal), increasing at intervals long enough to allow for an adequate assessment (given the frequency of violent behaviors) in increments of ~60 mg; most pts require doses of 240 mg or more, and the "time-release" preparation should be used.

Duty to Warn: A legal *duty to warn* exists in every state of the USA. If the intended victim is known (regardless of whether the pt is hospitalized or not), then notification must be made to the intended victim and to the police (both to police in whose jurisdiction the pt is and to those in whose jurisdiction the intended victim is).

16. Psychopharmacology and Electroconvulsive Treatment

16.1 PSYCHOPHARMACOLOGY

Bloom FE, Kupfer DJ, eds, Psychopharmacology: the fourth generation of progress, Raven Press, New York, 1994. Schatzberg AF, Nemeroff CB, eds, The American Psychiatric Association textbook of psychopharmacology, American Psychiatric Press, Washington, DC, 1998.

INTRODUCTION

Table 16.1-1 provides data regarding most psychopharmacologic agents in routine use. The drugs are grouped as follows: mood stabilizers, neuroleptics, antiparkinsonian medications, antidepressants, selected benzodiazepines, stimulants, antihistamines, and others.

For each drug, there are entries regarding generic (and trade) name; how supplied (tablets and capsules are listed by milligram sizes; if liquid forms are available, they are listed as mg/mL; and if an injectable form is available, the initial "I" is added); time to peak blood level after oral administration, in hours; protein binding; and for some agents, pertinent facts regarding metabolism (i.e., when active metabolites are present, they are noted; also, if a significant percentage of the drug is excreted in the urine in unchanged form, the initial "U" is added, followed by an estimate as to the percentage excreted unchanged).

In the following sections, further information is provided regarding indications, metabolism, SEs, drug-drug interactions, and therapeutic use.

Table 16.1-1. Psychopharmacology

Generic (Trade) Name	Supplied	Peak	Protein Binding	Half-life	Metabolism
Mood Stabilizers					
1. Divalproex (Depakote)	125, 250, 500	3–8	93%[a]	14 h	2-Propyl-2-pentenoic acid
2. Lithium[b] (Eskalith)	300; 8 mEq/mL[c]	1–2	0	18–24 h	U: >90%
3. Carbamazepine[d] (Tegretol)	200	4–8	75%	25–65 h[e]	10,11-Epoxide
Neuroleptic					
Typical					
Low Potency					
4. Chlorpromazine (Thorazine)	10, 25, 50, 100, 200; 100/mL; I	2–4	95%	12–30 h	>50 active
5. Thioridazine (Mellaril)	10, 25, 50, 100, 200	2–4	90%	10–30 h	Mesoridazine
6. Mesoridazine (Serentil)	10, 25, 50, 100; 25/mL; I	2–4	90%	10–30 h	?
High Potency					
7. Trifluoperazine (Stelazine)	1, 2, 5, 10; 10/mL; I	2–4	90%	10–30 h	?
8. Perphenazine (Trilafon)	2, 4, 8, 16; 16/5 mL; I	2–4	90%	10–30 h	?
9. Thiothixene (Navane)	1, 2, 5, 10, 20; 5/mL; I	2–4	90%	10–30 h	?
10. Pimozide (Orap)	2	6–8	99%	50–100 h	?
11. Fluphenazine (Prolixin)	1, 2.5, 5, 10; 2.5/5 mL; I	2–4	>90%	10–30 h	?
12. Haloperidol (Haldol)	0.5, 1, 2, 5, 10, 20; 2/mL; I	2–4	>90%	18 h	Reduced haloperidol (half-life = 67)
Medium Potency					
13. Loxapine (Loxitane)	5, 10, 25, 50; 25/mL; I	2–4	90%	4 h	?
14. Molindone (Moban)	5, 10, 25, 50, 100; 20/mL	1.5	90%	10–30 h	?
Atypical					
15. Risperidone (Risperdal)	1, 2, 3, 4; 1/mL	1–2	90%	3 h	9-Hydroxyrisperidone (half-life = 20)
16. Olanzapine (Zyprexa)	2.5, 7.5, 10	6	93%	30 h	?
17. Clozapine (Clozaril)	25, 100	1–6	95%	8–12 h	Desmethylclozapine

Table 16.1-1. (Continued)

Generic (Trade) Name	Supplied	Peak	Protein Binding	Half-life	Metabolism
Neuroleptic (cont.)					
Possibly Atypical					
18. Quetiapine (Seroquel)	25, 100, 200	1.5	83%	6 h	?
Antiparkinsonian					
Anticholinergic					
19. Benztropine (Cogentin)	0.5, 1, 2; I	?	?	?	?
20. Trihexyphenidyl (Artane)	2, 5; 2.5/5 mL	1–2	?	4–12 h	?
Dopaminergic					
21. Amantadine (Symmetrel)	100; 50/5 mL	2–4	67%	16 h	U: >>50%
Antidepressants					
SSRI					
22. Citalopram (Celexa)	20, 40	1–6	80%	33 h	Desmethylcitalopram
23. Sertraline (Zoloft)	25, 50, 100	4–8	98%	25 h	?
24. Fluoxetine (Prozac)	10, 20; 20/5 mL	6–8	95%	48–72 h	Norfluoxetine (half-life = 168–240)
25. Paroxetine (Paxil)	10, 20, 30, 40	3–8	95%	20–26 h	?
26. Fluvoxamine (Luvox)	25, 50, 100	2–8	80%	15 h	?
Tricyclic					
Secondary Amine					
27. Nortriptyline (Pamelor)	10, 25, 50, 75; 10/5 mL	2–6	92%	20–50 h	10-Hydroxynortriptyline
28. Desipramine (Norpramin)	10, 25, 50, 75, 100, 150	2–6	82%	10–30 h	2-Hydroxydesipramine
29. Protriptyline (Vivactil)	5, 10	6–12	92%	78 h	
Tertiary Amine					
30. Amitriptyline (Elavil)	10, 25, 50, 75, 100, 150; I	6–12	94%	15–30 h	Nortriptyline
31. Imipramine (Tofranil)	10, 25, 50	6–12	90%	15–30 h	Desipramine
32. Clomipramine (Anafranil)	25, 50, 75	2–6	95%	19–40 h[f]	Desmethylclomipramine
33. Doxepin (Sinequan)	10, 25, 50, 75, 100, 150; 10/mL	2–6	?	10–25 h	Desmethyldoxepin

Tetracyclic

34. Maprotiline (Ludiomil)	25, 50, 75	8–12	?	25–50 h	7-Hydroxyamoxapine[g]; 8-hydroxyamoxapine
35. Amoxapine (Asendin)	25, 50, 100, 150	1–2	90%	5–10 h	

MAOI

36. Phenelzine (Nardil)	15	0.5–4	?	3 h[h]	
37. Tranylcypromine (Parnate)	10	1.5	?	2–3[h]	
38. Selegiline (Eldepryl)	5	0.5–4	94%	2–10 h[h]	N-Desmethylselegiline

Other

39. Mirtazapine (Remeron)	15, 30	2	85%	20–40 h	
40. Nefazodone (Serzone)	100, 150, 200, 250	1	99%	2–4 h	Hydroxynefazodone
41. Bupropion[i] (Wellbutrin)	75, 100	2	85%	12–14 h	Hydroxybupropion (half-life = 24), threobupropion (half-life = 24)
42. Venlafaxine[j] (Effexor)	25, 37.5, 50, 75, 100	1.5	27	5 h	O-Desmethylvenlafaxine (half-life = 11)
43. Trazodone (Desyrel)	50, 100, 150, 300	1–2	93%	6 h	

Selected Benzodiazepines

44. Lorazepam (Ativan)	0.5, 1, 2; I	2	85%	12 h	[k]
45. Diazepam (Valium)	2, 5, 10; I	1	99%	40 h	[k]
46. Chlordiazepoxide (Librium)	5, 10; I	1–5	97%	10 h	
47. Alprazolam (Xanax)	0.25, 0.5, 1, 2	1–2	80%	12 h	Alpha-hydroxyalprazolam
48. Clonazepam (Klonopin)	0.5, 1, 2	1–4	86%	23 h	

Stimulants

49. Methylphenidate[l] (Ritalin)	5, 10, 20	2	15%	1–3 h	U = 50%
50. Pemoline (Cylert)	18.75, 37.5, 75	2–4	50%	5–7 h	U = 30%–80%[m]
51. Dextroamphetamine (Dexedrine)	2	?	?	10 h[m]	

Antihistamines

52. Diphenhydramine (Benadryl)	25, 50; I	2	78%	8 h	
53. Hydroxyzine (Vistaril)	25, 50, 100; 25/mL; I	8	?	20 h	

Table 16.1-1. (Continued)

Generic (Trade) Name	Supplied	Peak	Protein Binding	Half-life	Metabolism
Others					
54. Propranolol[n] (Inderal)	10, 20, 40, 60, 80; I	1–1.5	90%	4 h	U = 50%
55. Clonidine (Catapres)	0.1, 0.2, 0.3	3	20%	10–16 h	l-Pyrimidynylpiperazine
56. Buspirone (BuSpar)	5, 10, 15	0.5–1.5	95%	2.5 h	
57. Donepezil (Aricept)	5, 10	3–4	96%	70 h	
58. Disulfiram (Antabuse)	250, 500	1–2	?	[o]	[o]
59. Naltrexone (ReVia)	50	1	20%	3 h	
60. Naloxone (Narcan)	I	N/A	?	0.5–1.5 h	
61. Flumazenil (Romazicon)	I	N/A	50%	1 h	
62. Zolpidem (Ambien)	5, 10	1.5	92%	2.6 h	

I = injectable form available; U = excreted in urine in unchanged form (percentage).

[a] Protein binding drops significantly as blood level rises through the therapeutic range.

[b] Also available as Eskalith CR 450, peak level rises in 4 h.

[c] As lithium citrate, with 8 mEq = 300-mg tablet.

[d] Also available as Tegretol XR, 100, 200, 400; peak level in 4–12 h.

[e] Over ~21 d, autoinduction occurs with half-life falling to 12–17 h.

[f] Half-life increases with doses >150.

[g] 7-Hydroxyamoxapine is a neuroleptic.

[h] As all these MAOIs are irreversible inhibitors of MAO, the half-life, clinically, is irrelevant; more important is the fact that it takes ~14 d for a new "crop" of MAOs to appear.

[i] Also supplied as Wellbutrin SR 100, 150; with peak in 3 h; half-life = 21 h.

[j] Also supplied as Effexor XR 37.5, 75, 150.

[k] Diazepam metabolizes to desmethyldiazepam (half-life = 73); chlordiazepoxide metabolizes to desmethylchlordiazepoxide (half-life = 100), which is then metabolized to desmethyldiazepam.

[l] Also supplied as Ritalin SR, 20 mg; with peak in 2–4 h; half-life = 12.

[m] Urinary excretion of unchanged dextroamphetamine increases with urinary acidity; half-life = ~30 h in alkaline urine and ~8 h in acidic urine.

[n] Also available as Inderal LA, 60, 80, 120, 160; with peak in 6 h; half-life = 10 h.

[o] Disulfiram very rapidly metabolized to active metabolites; overall the *clinical* effect of disulfiram may last up to 14 d.

The doses supplied are for otherwise healthy adults with normal hepatic and renal function. Doses must be adjusted for the elderly, debilitated, or those with hepatic or renal failure that might significantly affect elimination of the drug.

MOOD STABILIZERS

The most common indication for a mood stabilizer is bipolar disorder; others include schizoaffective disorder, bipolar type, and cyclothymia. Of the 3 agents listed in Table 16.1-1, divalproex (Depakote), by virtue of its ease of use and overall tolerability, is preferred. Other agents currently undergoing trials as mood stabilizers include lamotrigine (Lamictal) and gabapentin (Neurontin); initial reports are favorable.

Divalproex (Depakote) is a coordination compound of sodium valproate and valproic acid in an enteric-coated capsule. Once absorbed, valproic acid is converted to valproate. Valproate is almost completely metabolized in the liver, and the active metabolite noted in Table 16.1-1 is almost twice as potent. SEs include gastrointestinal distress (nausea, vomiting, cramping, diarrhea), sedation, ataxia, tremor, weight gain, and hair loss; rare SEs include pancreatitis, hepatitis, thrombocytopenia, hyperammonemia (presenting with delirium or coma *without* elevated liver enzymes), and very rarely, a dementia (accompanied by cortical atrophy and reversible upon discontinuation of the drug).

Drug-drug interactions include the following: With phenytoin (Dilantin), valproate level increases, and whereas the level of *free* phenytoin increases, the *total* (free and bound) level of phenytoin may increase or decrease; with carbamazepine (Tegretol), valproate level falls, and the level of the active 10,11-epoxide of carbamazepine (Tegretol) rises; with lamotrigine (Lamictal), valproate level falls and lamotrigine (Lamictal) level rises; with aspirin, valproate is displaced from plasma proteins, and the resulting rise in free level may prove toxic. The combination of clonazepam (Klonopin) and valproate in pts with petit mal epilepsy may lead to status. When used as a mood stabilizer, divalproex may be "loaded" the first day with a total daily dose of 15–20 mg/kg, with subsequent adjustments based on SEs and blood level. The recommended therapeutic range is 50–100 mcg/mL.

Lithium (Eskalith, Lithobid) is generally supplied as lithium carbonate, which contains ~8 mEq of lithium/300 mg. In addition to the above indications, is also useful for Rx-resistant depression (where it is used adjunctively), for postpartum psychosis (when manic sx are prominent), and in impulsively violent pts or those with intermittent explosive disorder. Lithium is freely filtered at the glomerulus, and competes with sodium for reabsorption in the renal tubule.

SEs include gastrointestinal distress (nausea, vomiting, diarrhea), fine postural tremor, incoordination (often very subtle), hair loss, weight gain, exacerbation of acne or psoriasis, lassitude, nephrogenic diabetes insipidus, and primary hypothyroidism (before this is *clinically* apparent, there is a fall in the free thyroxine index and a rise in the TSH level; importantly, this is *not* an indication to stop lithium, and may be easily corrected with exogenous thyroxine; in any case it is fully reversible with discontinuation of the drug). With lithium toxicity, gastrointestinal distress is prominent, ataxia is quite apparent, and tremor becomes coarse. Renal toxicity secondary to chronic Rx with lithium does not seem to occur (although an interstitial nephropathy may be seen in such pts, it appears to be of no clinical consequence unless the pt has concurrent renal failure from some other cause).

Drug-drug interactions include the following: With thiazide (and to a lesser degree, loop) diuretics, ACE inhibitors, and NSAIDs (with the notable exception of sulindac (Clinoril)), lithium levels rise, sometimes to toxic range; with fluvoxamine (Luvox), seizures may occur.

In pts with normal renal function, lithium may be started at 900–1200 mg/d (divided tid or qid), with subsequent adjustments based on SEs and the goal of a therapeutic level of 0.6–1.2 mEq/L. This therapeutic range is a rough guide only; some pts require higher levels (e.g., 1.2–1.8) for a therapeutic effect and tolerate it without SEs. Once the optimum dose is achieved, consider switching to a time-release preparation, which may be given all in 1 dose (often hs). Over time, it is appropriate to periodically check thyroid profile with measurements of TSH, BUN, creatinine, and electrolytes.

Carbamazepine (Tegretol), in addition to the indications already noted, is also useful for the alcohol withdrawal syndrome, impulsively violent pts, and intermittent explosive disorder. As noted in Table 16.1-1, carbamazepine induces its own hepatic metabolism, and with this autoinduction, the dose must be increased to keep the blood level within the therapeutic range.

SEs include sedation, ataxia, dizziness, nausea, dry mouth, blurry vision, and constipation. Rashes are not uncommon, and typically appear within the first 2 wk of Rx. Mild leukopenia develops in ~10%; rarely, agranulocytosis may occur. A transient, benign elevation of transaminases occurs in 5%–10%. Occasionally an SIADH may occur with hyponatremia; this may be treated with demeclocycline (Declomycin) 600 mg. Free thyroxine index may fall slightly, and this may be accompanied by either a rise or a *fall* in TSH level.

Drug-drug interactions include the following: With phenytoin (Dilantin), both carbamazepine and phenytoin levels fall; with divalproex (Depakote), valproate levels fall, and levels of the 10,11-epoxide of carbamazepine rise (at times with significant sedation); with lamotrigine (Lamictal), lamotrigine levels fall; carbamazepine reduces the levels of TCAs, haloperidol (Haldol), theophylline, doxycycline, warfarin (Coumadin), and oral birth control pills (dosages must be increased to maintain contraception). Carbamazepine levels are increased by verapamil (Calan), diltiazem (Cardizem), isoniazid (INH), propoxyphene (Darvon), and erythromycin. Clonidine (Catapres) decreases the anticonvulsant effect of carbamazepine; given that it is unknown if the mechanism whereby carbamazepine stabilizes mood is the same as that whereby it prevents convulsions, it is prudent to avoid this combination.

For otherwise healthy adults with normal hepatic function, the average dose falls between 600 and 1200 mg/d, with a therapeutic range from 4 to 12 mcg/mL. In acute situations (e.g., mania, alcohol withdrawal), one may begin with 800 mg/d, in 3 or 4 divided doses; in nonurgent situations, the dose may be increased gradually, in 200-mg weekly increments (often, in nonacute conditions where there is not much agitation, increasing the dose any faster leads to unacceptable sedation). Once the dose is stabilized, switch to the time-release preparation, which may be given on a bid schedule. Blood levels should be checked periodically until autoinduction is complete. One or more dose increases may be required to keep the level within the therapeutic range.

NEUROLEPTICS

These versatile medications are useful for schizophrenia, schizophreniform disorder, schizoaffective disorder, delusional disorder, brief
psychotic disorder, postpartum psychosis, alcoholic paranoia and
alcoholic hallucinosis, secondary psychoses, delirium and dementia,
borderline personality disorder, mania, depression (when accompanied by psychotic features, as discussed in 6.1), autism, Tourette's syndrome, Huntington's disease, and others. Neuroleptics are most
usefully divided into 2 groups: typical (or "classical") and atypical.
Typical neuroleptics are, by and large, therapeutically equivalent;
where they differ is in their SE profiles. Atypical neuroleptics are therapeutically superior to the typical neuroleptics and of the 3 atypical
neuroleptics, 2 of them, risperidone (Risperdal) and olanzapine
(Zyprexa), have, overall, fewer SEs than any of the typical neuroleptics. Clozapine (Cloazaril), although clearly therapeutically superior
to any other neuroleptic (including risperidone and olanzapine), has
so many SEs (including agranulocytosis) that it is held in reserve. Quetiapine (Seroquel) is the newest neuroleptic to become available in the
USA, and it is currently not clear whether it should be classified as
typical or atypical. All of the neuroleptics are metabolized in the
liver; unfortunately, with the exception of chlorpromazine (Thorazine), haloperidol (Haldol), risperidone, and clozapine, little is known
of their metabolites. It is safe to assume, however, that all the neuroleptics have active metabolites.

The SEs of neuroleptics are discussed in 5.1, and summarized in
Table 5.1-2. Additional SEs, common to almost all neuroleptics,
include weight gain (more common with clozapine and low-potency
typical neuroleptics; molindone (Moban) generally does not cause
weight gain), elevated prolactin levels (with the exception of quetiapine), sexual dysfunction, and photosensitivity. Some neuroleptics
have unique SEs: Thioridazine (Mellaril) may cause nasal stuffi-
ness, pigmentary retinopathy (if the dose is chronically >800 mg);
pimozide (Orap) may prolong the QT interval with cardiac syncope
and sudden cardiac death; risperidone is prone to cause orthostatic
hypotension, esp if the dose is increased rapidly. Clozapine may
cause agranulocytosis, seizures, increased salivation, tachycardia, and
during the first few weeks of Rx, a transient temperature elevation,
and during the 3rd–5th weeks of Rx, a transient, benign eosino-
philia.

Drug-drug interactions involving most neuroleptics include increasing TCA levels, and reducing the effectiveness of dopaminergic agents such as levodopa-carbidopa (Sinemet) and direct-acting dopaminergics such as bromocriptine (Parlodel). Some neuroleptics with unique aspects here are as follows: Haloperidol levels, when combined with carbamazepine, fall, sometimes by as much as 50%; olanzapine (Zyprexa) levels, when combined with INH, rifampin, or carbamazepine, fall; quetiapine levels, when combined with phenytoin (Dilantin), fall, and when combined with cimetidine (Tagamet), rise. Clozapine, exceptionally among the neuroleptics, does not appear to antagonize dopaminergic agents, and indeed may allow for a dose reduction of these agents in pts with Parkinson's disease. Quetiapine (Seroquel) levels may be substantially reduced by phenytoin and thioridazine; cimetidine may increase quetiapine levels.

The therapeutic use of these agents is discussed in 5.1; the algorithm for their use in schizophrenia presented in Figure 5.1-1, in general, is useful for most conditions treatable with neuroleptics; however, the specific chapter should be consulted for the condition in question. Some students are overwhelmed by the number of neuroleptics to choose among, and appropriately so. Start by familiarizing yourself with the following: chlorpromazine (Thorazine), fluphenazine (Prolixin), haloperidol (Haldol), risperidone (Risperdal), and olanzapine (Zyprexa).

ANTIPARKINSONIAN AGENTS

Those considered here are useful for controlling extrapyramidal SEs to neuroleptics. Levodopa-carbidopa (Sinemet) and direct-acting dopaminergics, as used in Parkinson's disease, are not useful in this regard.

Anticholinergics include a large number of agents, 2 of which, benztropine (Cogentin) and trihexyphenidyl (Artane), are in most common use, and between these, benztropine, despite the dearth of knowledge about its pharmacokinetics, is the one in most common use. SEs include dry mouth, blurry vision, mydriasis, urinary hesitancy (esp with prostatic hypertrophy), and decreased sweating (which may predispose to heat stroke). Drug-drug interactions of concern include additive effects with any other medicines with anticholinergic effects, e.g., cyclic antidepressants and low-potency typical neuroleptics. Benztropine is given in doses from 2 to 4 mg/d, and in most pts, once-daily dosing suffices. Doses above 6 mg generally only cause further SEs. Benztropine may be given 2 mg im in emergency situations; iv administration does not appear to be appreciably faster acting.

Amantadine (Symmetrel) is generally a second-choice agent for controlling extrapyramidal SEs. It may not be as effective as anticholinergics and, furthermore, it appears to lose its effectiveness in some pts after ~6 mo. Given that the majority of the drug is excreted unchanged in the urine, the dose must be substantially reduced in those with renal failure. SEs include poor concentration, light-headedness, lethargy, insomnia, and esp in females, livedo reticularis. Drug-drug interactions include the following: With thiazide diuretics or triamterene, urinary excretion is reduced; with anticholinergics or levodopa, there is a risk of delirium. For otherwise healthy pts, begin with 100 mg bid; doses above 300 mg/d are generally not more helpful.

ANTIDEPRESSANTS

Like neuroleptics, these are versatile medicines. The most common indication is a depressive episode (of major depression, bipolar disorder, or schizoaffective disorder); others include dysthymia, "postpsychotic" depression in schizophrenia, premenstrual syndrome, postpartum depression, secondary depression, PTSD, panic disorder, and bulimia. Certain antidepressants are also very useful in migraine prophylaxis, chronic pain (e.g., diabetic polyneuropathy), attention-deficit/hyperactivity disorder, separation anxiety disorder, enuresis, obstructive sleep apnea, and pseudobulbar palsy. All of the antidepressants are metabolized in the liver; interestingly, 2 of the tertiary amine tricyclics, amitriptyline (Elavil) and imipramine (Tofranil), have secondary amine metabolites, namely, nortriptyline (Pamelor) and desipramine (Norpramin), which are themselves commercially available. Importantly, as pointed out in Table 16.1-1, one of amoxapine's metabolites, 7-hydroxyamoxapine, has neuroleptic activity and can cause tardive dyskinesia; given this, there is little justification for using it chronically.

SEs are discussed in 6.1 and common ones are summarized in Table 6.1-1. Importantly, when used for bipolar disorder or schizo-affective disorder, bipolar type, all antidepressants are liable to pre-cipitate a manic episode. Some antidepressants have unique SEs: SSRIs may cause weight loss, akathisia, and bradycardia; tricyclic and tetracyclic antidepressants may slow cardiac conduction (with increased PR interval, QRS duration, and QT interval) with possible atrioventricular block and bundle-branch block; MAOIs phenelzine (Nardil) and tranylcypromine (Parnate) (and selegiline (Eldepryl), when dose is >10 mg/d) may cause a hypertensive crisis in pts who consume tyramine-containing foods or who take any of a large num-ber of medicines; consequently, MAOI Rx should only be under-taken by a physician thoroughly familiar with them; venlafaxine (Effexor) may increase supine BP; trazodone (Desyrel) may cause priapism.

Drug-drug interactions between antidepressants and between antidepressants and selected other drugs, are summarized in Table 16.1-2. Other interactions of note include the following: Combina-tion of SSRIs and cyproheptadine (Periactin) may negate antidepres-sant effect of SSRI; combination of fluvoxamine (Luvox) and lithium (Eskalith, Lithobid) may lead to seizures; combination of TCA and either clonidine (Catapres) or guanabenz (Wytensin) not only negates effect of clonidine and guanabenz but also may negate the antidepres-sant effect of the TCA; combination of TCA and class I antiarrhyth-mic (i.e., quinidine, disopyramide (Norpace), or procainamide) may lead to quinidine toxicity with arrhythmias; combination of TCA with sedatives may lead to enhanced sedative effect, and combination of TCA with anticholinergic (e.g., benztropine (Cogentin)) may lead to enhanced anticholinergic effect; combination of MAOI with tyra-mine-containing foods (e.g., aged cheeses) or certain medicines (pseu-doephedrine, ephedrine, cocaine, phenylpropanolamine, fenfluramine, reserpine, alpha-methyldopa, and guanethidine) may cause a hyperten-sive crisis; and combination of bupropion (Wellbutrin, Zyban) with a dopaminergic agent (levodopa-carbidopa (Sinemet) or bromocriptine (Parlodel)) may be followed by dyskinesia and delirium. The general use of antidepressants is discussed in 6.1.

Table 16.1-2. Antidepressant Drug-Drug Interactions

	SSRIs	Fluvoxamine	TCAs	MAOIs	Mirtaz-apine	Nefazodone	Bupro-pion	Venlafaxine	Trazo-done
Neuroleptics	↑ hpd, ↑ cloz	hpd → ↑ flv; flv → ↑ olz, cloz	↑ TCAs						
SSRIs			↑ TCAs[a]	SS		↑ cit			
Fluvoxamine			↑ tertiary amines; cmi → ↑ flv	SS					
TCAs	↑ TCA[a]	↑ Tertiary amines; cmi → ↑ flv		htn crisis		↑ TCAs		↑ TCAs	
MAOIs	SS	SS	htn crisis		SS	SS	?	NMS-like syn-drome	
Benzodiazepines (diazepam, des-methyldiazepam, alprazolam, tri-azolan)		↑ bz				↑ alpr, triaz			

Methylphenidate, dextroamphetamine			↑ TCA	htn crisis		
Propranolol		↑ prop		↓ prop		
Buspirone				htn		↑ SGPT
Cimetidine		↑ TCA			↑ vlx	↑ pht
Phenytoin		↑ pht				
Warfarin	↑ war	↑ war				
Digoxin				↑ dig		↑ dig
Astemizole, cisapride		↑ astem, cisa[b]		↑ astem, cisa[b]		

alpr = alprazolam; astem = astemizole; bz = benzodiazepine; cisa = cisapride; cit = citalopram; cloz = clozapine; cmi = clomipramine; dig = digoxin; flv = fluvoxamine; hpd = haloperidol; htn = hypertensive; MAOI = monoamine oxidase inhibitor; NMS = neuroleptic malignant syndrome; olz = olanzapine; pht = phenytoin; prop = propranolol; SS = serotonin syndrome; SSRI = selective serotonin reuptake inhibitor (including fluoxetine, paroxetine, sertraline, and citalopram); TCAs = tricyclic and tetracyclic antidepressants; triaz = triazolam; vlx = venlafaxine; war = warfarin.

[a]This interaction is dependent on the inhibition of cytochrome P450 2D6 enzyme system, and of the 4 SSRIs, the potential for doing this ranges as follows: fluoxetine>>>paroxetine>sertraline>citalopram; thus fluoxetine tends to elevate TCA levels the most, whereas sertraline and citalopram have minimal effect.

[b]Elevations in astemizole and cisapride levels may cause a fatal torsades de pointes.

SELECTED BENZODIAZEPINES

Five commonly used benzodiazepines are discussed here; for the most part, the rest are "me too" drugs, with little unique to recommend them. The indications for benzodiazepines are noted in Table 16.1-3; in each case, the reader should refer to the appropriate chapter, as in many instances, a benzodiazepine is *not* the first choice. With the exception of lorazepam (Ativan), all of these benzodiazepines have intermediary metabolites, which in some cases are active. Lorazepam, however, undergoes direct glucuronidation prior to being excreted in the urine. Given that glucuronidation is generally not affected by mild to moderate degrees of hepatic failure, lorazepam generally may be given safely to pts with such degrees of hepatic failure, without fear of drug accumulation. For diazepam (Valium) and chlordiazepoxide (Librium), the long half-life of their active intermediary metabolites ensures a long "benzodiazepine" effect.

SEs include sedation, light-headedness, ataxia, and disinhibition. With chronic use, tolerance and dependence may occur, and this appears particularly likely with alprazolam (Xanax). Drug-drug interactions of clinical significance do not occur with lorazepam; with the other 4, however, blood levels may rise with fluvoxamine (Luvox) and fall with carbamazepine (Tegretol); nefazodone (Serzone) may increase alprazolam levels. Therapeutic use of these benzodiazepines is discussed in the respective chapters; for agitation, lorazepam 2 mg po q 2 h or im q 1 h may be given until the pt is calm, limiting SEs have occurred, or a total dose of ~12 mg is reached.

STIMULANTS

These are indicated for attention-deficit/hyperactivity disorder and narcolepsy. Both methylphenidate (Ritalin) and dextroamphetamine (Dexedrine) have considerable abuse potential; pemoline (Cylert) has little. The high urinary excretion of pemoline and dextroamphetamine argues for care in their use in pts with renal failure. SEs include insomnia, anorexia, increased BP and heart rare (with possible palpitations), and tics. Both dextroamphetamine and methylphenidate may exacerbate sx of schizophrenia and mania, and in children, may slow linear growth (with, however, a "catch-up" if the drug is discontinued in adolescence). Drug-drug interactions are generally absent

Table 16.1-3. Indications for Selected Benzodiazepines

	Lorazepam (Ativan)	Diazepam (Valium)	Chlordiazepoxide (Librium)	Alprazolam (Xanax)	Clonazepam (Klonopin)
Catatonia	X				
Alcohol withdrawal	X	X	X		
Premenstrual dysphoric disorder					X
Panic disorder				X	X
Social phobia (generalized type)				X	
Generalized anxiety disorder		X	X	X	
Secondary anxiety		X	X		
Primary insomnia	X				
Restless legs syndrome					X
Nocturnal myoclonus					X
Nightmare disorder		X			
Sleep terror disorder		X			
Sleepwalking disorder		X			
REM sleep behavior disorder					X
Agitation	X				

for pemoline; both dextroamphetamine and methylphenidate elevate tricyclic and tetracyclic antidepressant levels and in combination with an MAOI, may cause a hypertensive crisis. Methylphenidate may also elevate phenytoin (Dilantin) and warfarin (Coumadin) levels. Therapeutic use is discussed with attention-deficit/hyperactivity disorder (see 2.12) and narcolepsy (see 12.4).

ANTIHISTAMINES

These may be given for insomnia, anxiety, or agitation, and are particularly useful in situations where one wishes to avoid medicines, such as benzodiazepines, that may lead to dependence or lend themselves to abuse. Diphenhydramine (Benadryl) is also dramatically effective in relieving neuroleptic-induced acute dystonia, as discussed in 15.2. Although hydroxyzine (Vistaril) has a long half-life, its pharmacologic effect generally lasts no longer than that of diphenhydramine. SEs include sedation, dizziness, nausea, and anticholinergic effects (dry mouth, blurry vision, constipation). In some females, vaginal dryness, with possible dyspareunia, may occur, and in some pts with COPD, bronchial secretions may become so dried that they cannot be cleared. In children, diphenhydramine, rather than sedation, may cause a paradoxical restlessness. Drug-drug interactions are limited to a potentiation of other drugs with sedative or anticholinergic effects. Therapeutic doses for anxiety are 25–50 mg diphenhydramine and 25–75 mg hydroxyzine, both po, given tid or qid; for insomnia, the dose is 50–100 mg diphenhydramine and 50–150 mg hydroxyzine, both po at hs.

OTHER MEDICATIONS

Propranolol (Inderal) is indicated for social phobia (of the circumscribed type), generalized anxiety disorder (when autonomic sx are prominent), some cases of impulsive violence, neuroleptic-induced acute akathisia, medication-induced postural tremor, essential tremor, and migraine prophylaxis. SEs include bradycardia, prolonged atrioventricular conduction time (making it dangerous in pts with 2nd- or 3rd-degree atrioventricular block, those with the Wolff-Parkinson-White syndrome, or those in atrial fibrillation or flutter), a negative inotropic effect (worsening congestive heart failure), hypotension, bronchospasm (contraindicating its use in pts with asthma or COPD), vasospasm (contraindicating its use in pts with vasospastic angina and Raynaud's phenomenon), fatigue, vivid dreams, impotence, and apparently rarely, exacerbation of depression. Drug-drug interactions include the following: The combination of chlorpromazine (Thorazine) and propranolol is followed by elevations of blood levels of both agents; fluvoxamine (Luvox), nefazodone (Serzone), and cimetidine (Tagamet) may increase propranolol levels; both nefazodone and phenytoin (Dilantin) may decrease propranolol levels; aluminum hydroxide, as found in certain antacids, may bind with propranolol in the gut. The therapeutic use of propranolol is discussed for each indication in the respective chapter. Despite the significant SEs, propranolol is very useful, esp for social phobia, akathisia, and tremor.

Clonidine (Catapres) is indicated for attention-deficit/hyperactivity disorder, Tourette's syndrome, autism, and opioid withdrawal. SEs include sedation, dry mouth, hypotension (with possible dizziness), impotence, and uncommonly, depression. Drug-drug interactions are few; notably, however, clonidine may antagonize the antidepressant effect of tricyclic and tetracyclic antidepressants. Therapeutic use is discussed in the respective chapters.

Buspirone (BuSpar) is indicated for major depression and generalized anxiety disorder. SEs include sedation, dizziness, nausea, and occasionally, an akathetic-type restlessness. Drug-drug interactions include the following: Combination with MAOI may cause hypertension; with trazodone (Desyrel), an elevated SGPT; and with haloperidol (Haldol), increased haloperidol levels. Therapeutic doses for depression are ~60 mg, and for generalized anxiety disorder, ~25 mg: In each case begin with 5 mg tid and increase by 5–10-mg increments q 3–4 d.

Donepezil (Aricept) is indicated for mild-moderate Alzheimer's disease. It is *not* useful for other dementias. SEs include nausea, diarrhea, vomiting, insomnia, fatigue, anorexia, and muscle cramping. Drug-drug interactions are as follows: The effect of succinylcholine (Anectine) is increased; anticholinergics blunt the effectiveness of donepezil. Therapeutic use is discussed in 3.3.

Other Medications, continued

Disulfiram (Antabuse) has only 1 indication, namely, alcoholism, and is discussed in 4.1.

Naltrexone (ReVia) is indicated for both opioid dependence and alcoholism. SEs include fatigue, dysphoria, and nausea; there is also a dose-related hepatotoxicity that becomes quite significant at doses >300 mg. Drug-drug interactions are with other opioids, including diphenoxylate (Lomotil). Therapeutic use is discussed in 4.1 and 4.13.

Naloxone (Narcan) is indicated for the Rx of opioid overdose, and in non-opioid-dependent pts, has no effects. There are no known drug-drug interactions. Therapeutic use is discussed in 4.13.

Flumazenil (Romazicon) is indicated for the Rx of benzodiazepine overdose. SEs include nausea, vomiting, flushing, headache, diaphoresis, dizziness, and agitation; those with panic disorder may have a panic attack precipitated. There are no known drug-drug interactions. Therapeutic use is discussed in 4.15.

Zolpidem (Ambien), although structurally different from benzodiazepines, is functionally quite similar to them. It is indicated for insomnia. SEs include drowsiness, dizziness, nausea, diarrhea, and unsteadiness. Tolerance and dependence may occur. Drug-drug interactions are apparently limited to potentiation of other sedative agents, such as alcohol, other benzodiazepines, etc. Therapeutically, it is given 10 mg po hs.

16.2 ELECTROCONVULSIVE THERAPY

Am J Psychiatry 1983;140:463. Am J Psychiatry 1994;151:1637. Arch Gen Psychiatry 1975;32:1557. NEJM 1984;311:163.

INTRODUCTION

The most common indication for ECT is severe depression, and in this case it is the *safest* and *most effective* treatment in the world. This is the only place in this book I will editorialize, but I feel compelled to here. I have seen ECT bring pts back from the brink of death, and have been reminded of the miracle of Lazarus. The only scoffers at ECT are those who have not seen pts before and after a course of Rx. Too many residents and medical students are finishing their training without ever seeing ECT, and this is a tragedy. If you have not seen it, see it, and see it in more than 1 pt. You will never forget it, and if you learn how to do it, you will save lives.

INDICATIONS

ECT is indicated for any of the disorders in the list below, provided that one or more of the following conditions are met: (1) imminent risk of death; (2) inanition or malnutrition to the point where survival for long enough to allow other Rxs to be successful is not ensured; (3) resistance to other treatments; (4) inability to tolerate other treatments; or (5) pt preference (some pts, for a variety of sound reasons, do not wish to take a chance on Rx with medications that might fail, but prefer to proceed immediately to the most effective treatment available).

- Depression, either a depressive episode of major depression, bipolar disorder, or schizoaffective disorder, or a secondary depression (e.g., poststroke depression).
- Mania, either a manic episode of bipolar disorder or schizoaffective disorder.
- Catatonia (esp Stauder's lethal catatonia).
- Schizophrenia during either acute onset or exacerbation when accompanied by prominent perplexity or affective sx. "Negative" sx do *not* respond to ECT.
- Neuroleptic malignant syndrome.
- Delirium (e.g., DTs, phencyclidine delirium).
- Parkinson's disease (ECT is effective for the motor sx of Parkinson's disease *regardless* of whether pt is depressed or not).

There are no absolute contraindications to ECT, and the risks posed by these relative contraindications must be weighed against the potential benefits of ECT.

Cardiovascular Conditions
- Myocardial infarction within 3 mo.
- Severe CHF.
- Aortic aneurysm.

Pacemakers are *not* a contraindication provided that the pacemaker is converted to a fixed mode and that the pt is carefully grounded during stimulation.

Intracranial Lesions
- Tumors. ECT may enlarge any area of perilesional edema, leading to possible herniation; thus, tumors lacking edema (e.g., slow-growing meningiomas or calcified lesions) pose little risk; furthermore, if there is only a small amount of edema, it may be treated with dexamethasone allowing one to proceed with ECT.
- Subdural hematoma, when accompanied by edema, is a relative contraindication; old, calcified hematomas, however, are not.
- MS, when active. Edema surrounds expanding plaques, and if the plaques are quite large, significant mass effect could occur. It is not clear whether dexamethasone would be effective here. When inactive, MS probably is not a contraindication.
- Infarction. As with tumors, the risk is created by perilesional edema; thus, old infarcts pose no risk.
- Aneurysms and arteriovenous malformations potentially could hemorrhage with the surge in BP that occurs with ECT. In such cases, pretreatment with labetalol (Normodyne) or other antihypertensive may allow ECT to proceed.
- Nonlesional increased intracranial pressure (e.g., NPH, "benign" intracranial hypertension) must be relieved by Rx of the underlying condition first.

Other Relative Contraindications
- Retinal detachment.
- Untreated glaucoma.
- Pheochromocytoma.
- Extensive muscle damage (e.g., active *and* extensive lower motor neuron disease, muscular dystrophy, myotonia dystrophica, recent crush injuries, recent extensive burn injuries). Here, the fascicula-

tions seen with the use of succinylcholine (Anectine) for muscle relaxation may be followed by severe, potentially fatal, hyperkalemia. In such conditions, a nondepolarizing relaxant must be substituted.

Uncomplicated pregnancy is generally *not* a contraindication. Pregnant women tolerate ECT well, and fetal monitoring has failed to reveal any significant distress during ECT.

PRE-ECT EVALUATION

At a minimum, should include
- *General PE* with a detailed neurologic examination
- *Routine pre-ECT labs*
    CBC
    Chem survey, including electrolyte and calcium levels
    Magnesium level
    Chest xray
    EKG
- *Further labs, as indicated*
    If intracranial lesion suspected, MRI
    With osteoporosis (e.g., postmenopausal females) or in elderly, lumbosacral spine films
- *Preanesthetic evaluation by an anesthesiologist*

PREPARATION

Obtain informed consent.

Rx medical conditions, e.g., hypertension (must be fully controlled), glaucoma, electrolyte or calcium abnormalities, dental abnormalities (loose teeth should generally be extracted).

Review all medications that might adversely affect ECT, as in Table 16.2-1.

Lithium, heterocyclic agents, and MAOIs generally should be discontinued.

Beta-blockers may be continued, but only if the vagally mediated bradycardia is prevented by a substantial dose of atropine.

Table 16.2-1. Pre-ECT Medication Review

Increased Post-ECT Delirium
   Lithium[a]
Increased Risk of Arrhythmia
   Heterocyclic antidepressants[a]
Increased Risk of Hypertension
   MAOI antidepressants[a]
Increased Risk of Bradyarrhythmia and Asystole
   Beta-blockers
Potentiation of Succinylcholine
   Donepezil (Aricept)
   Tacrine (Cognex)
   Pyridostigmine (Mestinon)
   Neostigmine (Prostigmin)
   Echothiophate
   Isofluorophate
   Cimetidine (Tagamet)
   Loop diuretics
   Aminoglycosides
Increased Seizure Threshold
   Anticonvulsants
   Benzodiazepines
Decreased Seizure Threshold
   Theophylline
   Clozapine (Clozaril)
   Bupropion (Wellbutrin, Zyban)

[a]Should generally be discontinued before ECT (in the case of MAOIs, at least 2 wk before ECT).

Drugs that potentiate succinylcholine (Anectine) may be continued, but will necessitate a lower dose of succinylcholine.

Drugs that increase the seizure threshold may, if necessary, be continued. Epileptics may continue on anticonvulsants, but when these drugs have been unsuccessful in controlling mania, they should probably be discontinued. Benzodiazepines, ideally, should be discontinued, but for those who are at risk for withdrawal sx, tapering may take so long as to be impractical. If drugs that increase the seizure threshold are continued, then a higher stimulus intensity is generally required.

Drugs that decrease the seizure threshold may, if necessary, be continued, but lower stimulus intensities may be required, and one must be on guard for prolonged seizures. Continuing bupropion (Wellbutrin, Zyban) is generally not necessary.

1. Personnel include the psychiatrist, an anesthesiologist (or in uncomplicated cases, an anesthetist), and a nurse experienced with ECT.
2. Familiarize yourself thoroughly with the ECT machine to be used.
3. Schedule ECT for early morning, and on the previous night, the pt should clean the scalp and avoid using any creams or lotions on the scalp or hair.
4. NPO for at least 6 h before ECT.
5. On the morning of ECT, have pt use the commode and dress in a loosely fitting hospital gown.
6. Clean scalp area where electrodes will be placed with an alcohol-soaked rough piece of gauze, then dry thoroughly.
7. Remove dentures.
8. Place a BP cuff on the right arm and measure pressure.
9. Attach EKG leads.
10. Attach EEG leads. If there is only 1 active lead apply it in the Fp1 position, about 1 inch above the midpoint of the left eyebrow, with the indifferent lead attached to the left mastoid area; if a second active lead is possible, apply it in the Fp2 area, about 1 inch above the midline of the right eyebrow, with the indifferent lead applied to the right mastoid.
11. Start an iv line in the left forearm.
12. Apply a generous amount of electrode paste in the desired positions, and apply the 2 ECT electrodes. *Before* beginning ECT, decide whether to use unilateral (nondominant) placement or bilateral placement. In bilateral ECT, the first lead is placed 1 inch above the midline of a line drawn between the right tragus and the right external canthus, and the second is placed 1 inch superior to the midpoint of a line drawn between the left tragus and the left external canthus. In unilateral ECT, the left-sided placement is not used, and the second electrode is placed instead 1 inch to the right of the vertex. Unilateral placement results in less postictal delirium; however, it appears to be somewhat less effective overall. Conversely, although generally causing more postictal delirium, bilateral placement is clearly more effective therapeutically. In practice, for depression, many psychiatrists start with unilateral ECT, and continue with it unless there is no significant improvement after 4 Rxs, at which point they switch to bilateral treatment. Imminent suicide constitutes an exception, and in such cases most psychiatrists would

begin Rx of depression with bilateral ECT. For mania and other indications, it appears most prudent to start with bilateral placement.

13. Test impedance. Very low impedance suggests a "short circuit" (e.g., electrodes too close together; widely spread electrode gel bridging the space between electrodes); very high impedance must also be corrected (e.g., not enough electrode gel; electrodes too loosely applied).

14. Give atropine 0.6–1.0 mg iv; some prefer glycopyrrolate (Robinul) (0.2–0.4 mg iv) on the belief that because glycopyrrolate does not cross the blood-brain barrier, it is less likely to contribute to postictal confusion (this belief is unconfirmed, and given the decades of experience with atropine, it is generally preferable). These anticholinergic medications diminish the vagally mediated bradycardia seen with ECT.

15. Give methohexital (Brevital) (a short-acting barbiturate anesthetic) 0.75–1.0 mg/kg iv.

16. Insert airway and begin ventilating pt with 100% O_2.

17. Inflate the BP cuff on the right arm to at least 10 mm Hg above *systolic* to prevent succinylcholine from reaching the right forearm.

18. Give succinylcholine (Anectine) 0.5–1.0 mg/kg iv and observe for fasciculations. Fasciculations usually evident in <60 sec, beginning in the face and proceeding gradually to the toes; when fasciculation in the toes stops, relaxation is complete.

19. Insert a soft bite block; if front teeth in danger of cracking, use a semicircular block to spread the pressure around.

20. Gently hold the jaw closed, and apply the stimulus. As soon as possible, remove the bite block and resume ventilations.

21. Stimulation is applied, according to a previously determined plan. Stimulus intensity should exceed the seizure threshold by about 50%–200% for unilateral ECT (it appears that unilateral ECT is even less effective unless the stimulation is well above the seizure threshold). Some clinicians will estimate the seizure threshold, while others will attempt to determine it by beginning with a subthreshold intensity and then "titrating" up (by about 50% with each step) until a seizure occurs (if unilateral placement is being used, the intensity of the *second* treatment is then 50%–200% above this initially determined level).

22. Observe seizure activity not only on the EEG readout but also by tonic and then clonic activity observed in the right forearm.

Electrical seizure activity, evident on the EEG, is generally 30%–40% longer than the motor activity. Motor seizures lasting <25 sec are generally not therapeutically effective.

23. If a seizure does not occur within 20 sec of the stimulation (a "missed" seizure), rapidly check ECT electrodes to be sure they are properly applied, and then immediately restimulate at an intensity 25%–100% higher than the initial intensity (a 50% increase is generally adequate). This process may be repeated until a total of 4 stimulations have been used. Further stimulation is generally fruitless. Be sure to distinguish between a seizure and the intense contraction of the masseter muscles that occurs secondary to local spread of the stimulus, regardless of whether a seizure is induced or not.

24. If the seizure is too brief, wait 60–90 sec after the end of the seizure, then restimulate using the same procedure as for a "missed" seizure.

25. Carefully record ictal events, noting seizure duration, both by EEG and by "cuff" method, and note changes in BP and pulse, and any arrhythmias. Immediately after stimulation, a vagally mediated bradycardia may evolve into an asystole lasting up to 7 sec; moments later, there is an ictal surge of sympathetic activity with a substantial rise in systolic and diastolic pressure and a sinus tachycardia, which may be accompanied by arrhythmias, generally PVCs.

26. Postictally, continue ventilation until spontaneous respirations are fully reestablished. For at least 15 min, monitor pulse and BP, continue the iv line, and keep the pt in the "postop" position.

27. Postictal delirium is typical, and usually lasts 15–30 min after the first treatment, with the severity and duration of the delirium progressively worsening with successive treatments, often extending up to several hours or more. Once the pt is comfortable and ambulatory, he or she may be returned to the ward. The ward should be locked, and until the delirium is fully cleared, the pt should be under 1:1 observation, with phone calls and visitors restricted.

COURSE

Administer Rx 3 times per week (usually Monday, Wednesday, Friday).
During a course of Rx, the seizure threshold increases, and the stimulus
  intensity must be commensurately increased. When the maximum
  stimulus intensity is unable to produce a sufficiently long seizure, any
  one of the following maneuvers may be tried: hyperventilation;
  sodium benzoate caffeine 350–750 mg iv 2–5 min before stimulation
  (this carries a risk, however, of tachycardia and ventricular ectopy);
  decreasing the dose of methohexital (Brevital); decreasing the dose (or
  discontinuing, if possible) of any medications that increase the seizure
  threshold.
Discontinue Rx when any one of the following occurs: (1) Pt recovers
  (in general: for depression, after 6–12 treatments; for mania after 8–
  20; for schizophrenia after 17–20; for catatonia or delirium, after 1–
  4); (2) pt substantially improved and shows no further improvement
  after another 2 or 3 Rxs; (3) no significant improvement after 6 consecutive bilateral Rxs; (4) unacceptable SEs (in practice, the most common SE leading to termination of treatments is postictal delirium that
  does not clear between Rxs); (5) a maximum of 20 Rxs during any
  given course of ECT (there is no *lifetime* maximum number of Rxs;
  some pts have done well with >1000 Rxs).

SIDE EFFECTS

Secondary to Stimulation per se: With stimulation there is a vagally
  mediated bradycardia, with, in some pts, an asystole lasting up to
  7 sec. In most pts, pretreatment with atropine (as above) moder-
  ates this to an acceptable degree; however, esp in pts on beta-
  blockers, prolonged asystole or bradycardia may occur.
Ictal: Significant tachycardia or hypertension may be treated with labetalol (Normodyne) 0.05–0.2 mg iv. Ventricular ectopy may also
  respond to labetalol; should it not, lidocaine 1–2 mg/kg iv may be
  given.
  Prolonged seizures (<120 sec) are *not* more effective and should be
  terminated with lorazepam (Ativan) 2 mg iv, followed, if necessary, by fosphenytoin (Cerebyx) in a dose of 15–20 mg phenytoin

equivalents/kg at a rate of 100–150 phenytoin equivalents/min, not to exceed 150 phenytoin equivalents/min.

Fractures are *very* rare, provided adequate muscle relaxation has been achieved. Compression fractures of the spine were most common in the past.

Postictal: Vomiting may occur immediately postictally; Rx with pro-chlorperazine (Compazine) 5 mg iv.

Postictal delirium is discussed above, under "Technique."

Agitation, which may be very severe, occurs in ~5%–10% of pts during the postictal delirium, and may be treated with lorazepam (Ativan) 2 mg iv or diazepam (Valium) 5–10 mg iv.

Headache is common, and responds to simple analgesics.

Myalgia, secondary to fasciculations with succinylcholine, is generally tolerable, with or without simple analgesics. When severe, fasciculations may be prevented by giving a curare preparation just before the succinylcholine.

Mania may be precipitated during the Rx of a depressive episode of bipolar disorder, and may be catastrophically severe. Thus, the first *hint* of mania is an indication to at least suspend further Rxs for the purpose of observation. Mania must be distinguished from the silly, noninfectious euphoric giddiness that occurs in some pts being treated for a depressive episode of major depression (particularly common in the elderly); mania is accompanied by pressure of speech and activity, increased energy, and decreased need for sleep, and these sx do not accompany the silly giddiness.

Epilepsy secondary to ECT, that is to say the appearance of recurrent unprovoked seizures in pts who never had seizures before ECT, is very rare. In all likelihood, such pts probably had a preexisting lesion (such as a mild degree of mesial temporal sclerosis, or a previously asymptomatic focal cortical dysplasia) that became active with ECT. Rx is with anticonvulsants, depending on the type of seizure.

Overall mortality with ECT is 0.01%, a figure that compares favorably with the risk of general anesthesia (0.04%). Most deaths are due to cardiovascular SEs, such as arrhythmias and hypertension.

Long-term memory loss, quite simply, has *never* been demonstrated as a SE of ECT; indeed, long-term studies, if anything, have shown an improvement in memory.

Postictal delirium, as noted above, is typical after ECT, and generally worsens in severity and duration with successive Rx. *During* the delirium, as with most deliria, there is both an anterograde and a partial retrograde amnesia. Pts are unable to fully recall events that occurred only minutes earlier and are also unable to recall events for a variable period of time before ECT. As the delirium clears, the retrograde amnesia "shrinks" and either disappears completely or becomes very short, encompassing perhaps events in the hospital before ECT was commenced. Concurrently, the anterograde deficit also gradually clears and eventually pts are able to recall, say, 3 words after 5 min; however, when pts look back, the period of time during which the delirium was present remains as a permanent "island" of amnesia, and years later, pts may not be able to fully recall the events that occurred during the delirium (e.g., actually having the Rx, receiving visitors during the course of Rx). Although in most pts the delirium fully clears within a few weeks after ECT is discontinued, in some pts a *subtle* degree of anterograde and partial retrograde amnesia may persist, long after the gross confusion has cleared, for up to 6 mo. Beyond 6 mo, however, there is *no* evidence of any further anterograde amnesia.

MANAGEMENT SUBSEQUENT TO ECT

With the exception of delirium, the neuroleptic malignant syndrome, and some cases of catatonia, all of the conditions treated by ECT are chronic, and as ECT is not a cure, ongoing Rx will be required to prevent a relapse.

Depression may be assumed to be Rx resistant to the medication used before ECT (provided that it was given an adequate trial in terms of dose and duration). If the depressive episode occurred as part of major depression, then treatment should proceed as in the algorithm presented in Figure 6.1-1. In pts with major depression that remains Rx resistant to medications, then maintenance ECT is appropriate, beginning at a frequency of 1 Rx/wk, and gradually reducing the frequency, if allowed by the clinical condition, over 1–3 mo to a frequency of 1/mo. If the depression was part of a bipolar disorder, proceed as outlined in 6.6. In pts with secondary depression, Rx must be individualized with reference to the underlying cause.

Mania, occurring as part of bipolar disorder or schizoaffective disorder, bipolar type, should be treated with 1 or a combination of mood stabilizers, as outlined in 6.6. In many cases, pts have not been compliant with 1 of these agents before the current mania, and thus, if there is evidence from hx that the pt had responded in the past, there is no reason to not simply start the same agent again.

Catatonia, if part of schizophrenia, should be treated with neuroleptics, as outlined in 4.1.

Schizophrenia should be treated with neuroleptics, as in 4.1 (importantly, there is no need to discontinue neuroleptics during a course of ECT).

Parkinson's disease should be treated with an optimum combination of antiparkinsonian medications. However, in most pts, it was precisely the failure of medications that led to ECT, and thus maintenance ECT is generally indicated, and should be titrated to the pt's symptomatology. Although some pts enjoy sustained remissions after a course of ECT, most require Rx q 2–3 wk. With such pts, one should also consider neurosurgical intervention (e.g., pallidotomy); however, it must be remembered that the risks of neurosurgery are greater than the risks of ECT.

Index

Abulia, in frontal lobe syndrome, 91
Acamprosate, in alcoholism, 98
Acquired immunodeficiency syndrome
    (AIDS), dementia in, 70
Adjustment disorders, 279–280
Adolescent rebelliousness, vs. conduct
    disorder, 44
Affect
  disturbances of, 19–20
  in frontal lobe syndrome, 91
Agitation, with electroconvulsive
    therapy, 319
Agnosia, 16
Agoraphobia, 173
Agraphia, 16
Akathisia, 268–270
  vs. caffeine-related disorders, 107
  neuroleptic-induced, 268–270, 274
  vs. restless legs syndrome, 234
Alcohol hallucinosis, 141–142
  vs. alcoholic paranoia, 140
Alcohol ingestion, violent behavior
    and, 288
Alcohol withdrawal syndrome, 99–101
  vs. generalized anxiety disorder, 181
  seizures in, 103
Alcoholic dementia, 78–79
  vs. inhalant-induced dementia, 80
Alcoholic paranoia, 139–141
Alcoholics Anonymous, 97
Alcohol-induced persisting amnestic
    disorder, 83–85
Alcoholism, 95–98
  vs. antisocial personality disorder,
    252

blackouts in, 98–99
vs. delusional disorder, 135
vs. major depression, 148
Wernicke's encephalopathy in,
    104
Alexia, 16
Alprazolam (Xanax), 295, 307
Alveolar hypoventilation syndrome,
    central, 232
Alzheimer's disease, 66–67
  vs. Pick's disease, 77
Amantadine (Symmetrel), 294, 302
Ambien (zolpidem), 296, 310
Amitriptyline (Elavil), 294
  in major depression, 150
  in opioid withdrawal, 116
Amnesia
  vs. delirium, 82
  dissociative, 82, 86, 197–198
  epileptic, 82
    vs. alcoholic blackouts, 99
  global, transient, 82, 85–86
    vs. alcoholic blackouts, 99
  with transient ischemic attack, 82
Amnestic disorders, 80–83
  vs. dementia, 62
Amoxapine (Asendin), 295
  in major depression, 151
Amphetamine-related disorders, 105–
    106
  vs. delusional disorder, 135
Anabolic steroid abuse, violent behav-
    ior and, 288
Anafranil (clomipramine). See Clomi-
    pramine

Anankastic personality disorder, 259–260

Anemia, iron deficiency pica and, 45

Anergia, 145

Aneurysm, of anterior communicating artery, 84

Anhedonia, 145

Animal phobia, 174–175

Anorexia nervosa, 217–219
  vs. body dysmorphic disorder, 195

Anosognosia, 16

Antabuse (disulfiram). See Disulfiram

Anterior communicating artery, aneurysm of, 84

Anticholinergics, 294, 301–302

Antidepressants, 294–295, 302–303
  drug interactions with, 304–305
  in generalized anxiety disorder, 181–182
  in major depression, 148–151
  in obsessive-compulsive disorder, 179
  in pain disorder, 192
  in panic disorder, 171–172
  serotonin syndrome and, 277

Antihistamines, 295, 308

Antisocial personality disorder, 251–252
  vs. narcissistic personality disorder, 257
  violent behavior and, 288

Anxiety attack, vs. panic attack, 171

Anxiety disorder(s), 170–184. See also specific disorders
  vs. caffeine-related disorders, 107
  generalized, 181–182
    vs. major depression, 147–148
    vs. posttraumatic stress disorder, 180
  secondary, 182–184

Anxiolytic-related disorders, 118–121

Aphasia, 16
  expressive, 31–32
  sensory, 32–33

Aphonia, conversion, 188

Apnea, sleep, 230–231

Apraxia, 16

Aprosodia, 16

Aricept (donepezil). See Donepezil

Artane (trihexyphenidyl), 294, 301–302

Arteriosclerotic parkinsonism, vs. Parkinson's disease, 73

Asendin (amoxapine). See Amoxapine

Astemizole, antidepressant drug interactions with, 305

Ataxia, conversion, 188

Athetosis, of tardive dyskinesia, 274

Ativan (lorazepam). See Lorazepam

Attention-deficit/hyperactivity disorder, 40–43
  vs. conduct disorder, 44

Auditory hallucinations, 22, 140
  in alcohol-induced psychotic disorder, 141

Autism (autistic disorder), 36–38
  etiology of, 37
  vs. reactive attachment disorder, 56
  vs. schizoid personality disorder, 249
  vs. schizotypal personality disorders, 250–251

Automatic obedience, 19

Avoidant personality disorder, 257–258
  vs. dependent personality disorder, 259
  vs. schizoid personality disorder, 249
  vs. social phobia, 176

Axonal injury, diffuse, in head trauma, 71–72

Basal ganglial lesions, vs. obsessive-compulsive disorder, 179

Behavior therapy
  in enuresis, 52–53
  in major depression, 148
  in separation anxiety disorder, 54

Benadryl (diphenhydramine), 295, 308
Benzodiazepines, 295, 304, 306
    antidepressant drug interactions
        with, 304
    in panic disorder, 172
    in violent behavior, 290
Benztropine (Cogentin), 294, 301–
        302
Bereavement, 281–282
Binswanger's disease, 69
    vs. Alzheimer's disease, 66
Bipolar disorder, 158–164
    vs. cyclothymia, 164
    vs. major depression, 147
    vs. postpartum psychosis, 137
    preventive treatment in, 164
    vs. schizoaffective disorder, 132
Bizarre affect, 20
Blackouts, 82, 98–99
Blindness, conversion, 188
Blood-injury phobia, 174–175
Body dysmorphic disorder, 194–195
    vs. hypochondriasis, 193
    vs. social phobia, 176
Borderline personality disorder, 253–
        255
    vs. cyclothymia, 165
    vs. histrionic personality disorder,
        256
    violent behavior and, 288
Bradykinesia, 262, 263
Brief psychotic disorder, 136–137
Briquet's syndrome, 185–187
Bulimia nervosa, 219–221
    vs. anorexia nervosa, 218–219
    vs. Kleine-Levin syndrome, 226
Bupropion (Wellbutrin), 295
    in attention-deficit/hyperactivity
        disorder, 42
    drug interactions with, 304–305
    in major depression, 151
Buspirone (BuSpar), 296, 309
    antidepressant drug interactions
        with, 305

Caffeine-related disorders, 106–107
Calculations
    in dementia, 62
    in diagnostic interview, 6
Cannabis-related disorders, 108–109
    vs. delusional disorder, 135
    vs. depersonalization disorder, 200
Carbamazepine (Tegretol), 293, 299
    in alcohol withdrawal syndrome,
        101
    in bipolar disorder, 162, 163
Cataplexy, 228, 229
    in narcolepsy, 227
Catapres (clonidine). See Clonidine
Catatonia, 86–89
    vs. dystonia, 267
    excited, 87
    vs. neuroleptic malignant syndrome,
        273
    vs. parkinsonism, 263
    vs. passive-aggressive personality
        disorder, 261
    stuporous, 86–87
    symptoms of, 18–19
Celexa (citalopram). See Citalopram
Central alveolar hypoventilation
        syndrome, 232
Chief complaint, 2–3
Chlordiazepoxide (Librium), 295,
        307
Chlorpromazine (Thorazine), 293
    in schizophrenia, 127
Chorea
    etiology of, 275, 276
    Huntington's, 75–76
    Sydenham's, vs. obsessive-compul-
        sive disorder, 178
    of tardive dyskinesia, 274
Cimetidine, antidepressant drug interac-
        tions with, 305
Circadian rhythm sleep disorder, 232–
        234
Circuit of Papez, focal lesions of, 84
Circumstantiality, 21

Cisapride, antidepressant drug interactions with, 305
Citalopram (Celexa), 294
  in major depression, 150
Clomipramine (Anafranil), 294
  in autism, 38
  in major depression, 151
Clonazepam (Klonopin), 295, 307
  in Tourette's disorder, 49
Clonidine (Catapres), 296, 309
  in Tourette's disorder, 49
  in opioid withdrawal, 116
Clozapine (Clozaril), 293
  in schizophrenia, 127, 129
Clumsiness, developmental, 30–31
Cocaine-related disorders, 105–106
  vs. delusional disorder, 135
Cogentin (benztropine), 294, 301–302
Cognitive akathisia, 268
Cognitive behavior therapy, in major depression, 148
Collateral information, 8–9
Color agnosia, 16
Compulsion, 22, 177
Compulsive personality disorder, 259–260
Conduct disorder, 43–44
Constipation, in encopresis, 49–51
Conversion disorder, 187–189
  vs. hypochondriasis, 193
  vs. pain disorder, 191
  vs. somatization disorder, 186
Coordination, developmental disorder of, 30–31
Cortical Lewy body disease, 74
  vs. Parkinson's disease, 73
Cranial nerves, assessment of, 14–15
Creutzfeldt-Jakob disease, 77–78
Criminality, vs. antisocial personality disorder, 252
Cross-dressing
  vs. gender identity disorder, 216
  vs. paraphilia, 214–215

Cyclothymia, 164–165
  vs. bipolar disorder, 161
  vs. borderline personality disorders, 254
Cylert (pemoline), 295, 306, 308

Deafness
  vs. autism, 38
  conversion, 188
Delirium, 57–61
  in alcohol withdrawal, 101–103
  vs. amnesia, 82
  vs. dementia, 62
  with electroconvulsive therapy, 317, 320
  etiology of, 57–60
  laboratory screen for, 60, 61
  vs. medical condition–related personality change, 90
  vs. schizophrenia, 125
  violent behavior and, 288
Delirium tremens, 101–103
Delusion(s), 23
  alcohol-induced psychotic disorder with, 139–141
  in diagnostic interview, 6, 10
  in Parkinson's disease, 72
  in schizophrenia, 122–123
Delusional disorder, 133–135
  vs. alcoholic paranoia, 140
  vs. paranoid personality disorder, 248
  vs. schizophrenia, 125
  subtypes of, 133–134
  violent behavior and, 289
Dementia, 61–65
  AIDS, 70
  alcoholic, 78–79
  vs. antisocial personality disorder, 252
  in Creutzfeldt-Jakob disease, 77–78
  vs. delusional disorder, 135
  etiology of, 62, 63–64
  head trauma and, 71–72

Dementia—*cont.*
  in Huntington's disease, 75–76
  inhalant-induced, 79
  vs. kleptomania, 244
  laboratory screen for, 65
  lacunar, 68–69
  vs. medical condition–related person-
    ality change, 90
  vs. mental retardation, 27
  multi-infarct, 67–68
  vs. paraphilia, 214
  in Parkinson's disease, 72, 73
  vs. Pick's disease, 77
  vs. postconcussion syndrome, 279
  vs. schizophrenia, 125
  violent behavior and, 288
Dementia pugilistica, vs. Parkinson's
    disease, 73
Depakote (divalproex). *See* Divalproex
Dependent personality disorder, 258–
    259
  vs. avoidant personality disorder,
    258
Depersonalization disorder, 200–201
Depression
  vs. anxiety disorder, 181
  vs. attention-deficit/hyperactivity dis-
    order, 41
  vs. bereavement, 181
  in bipolar disorder, 159, 163
  vs. cannabis-related disorders, 106
  vs. conduct disorder, 44
  vs. delusional disorder, 134
  vs. dementia, 64
  dementia syndrome of, 64
  vs. frontal lobe syndrome, 92
  vs. hallucinogen-related disorders,
    110
  in Huntington's disease, 76
  vs. hypochondriasis, 193
  major (unipolar), 145–154
    vs. agoraphobia, 173
    antidepressants for, 148–151
    vs. bipolar disorder, 160–161

  "normal," 147
  vs. obsessive-compulsive disorder,
    178
  vs. pain disorder, 191
  in Parkinson's disease, 74
  postpartum, 155–156
    vs. major depression, 147
  vs. posttraumatic stress disorder,
    180
  vs. schizoaffective disorder, 132
  secondary, 165–167
  vs. sexual desire disorder,
    hypoactive, 202
  vs. somatization disorder, 186–187
  suicidal behavior and, 283
Derealization, 200
Desipramine (Norpramin), 294
  in major depression, 150
Desmopressin acetate (DDAVP), in
    enuresis, 53
Desyrel (trazodone). *See* Trazodone
Developmental disorders
  of calculation, 29
  of coordination, 30–31
  of movement, 30–31
  of reading, 28–29
  of speech, 31–34
  of writing, 30
Dextroamphetamine (Dexedrine), 295,
    306, 308
  antidepressant drug interactions
    with, 305
  intoxication with, 105–106
Diagnostic interview, 1–10
  chief complaint in, 2–3
  collateral information and, 8–9
  conclusion of, 7–8
  difficult, 9–10
  directive portion of, 5–7
  nondirective portion of, 4–5
  rapport for, 2
  setting for, 1
  violent patient and, 9–10
Diazepam (Valium), 295, 307

Digoxin, antidepressant drug interactions with, 305
Diphenhydramine (Benadryl), 295, 308
Disfigurement
  vs. agoraphobia, 173
  vs. social phobia, 176
Disinhibition, in frontal lobe syndrome, 91
Dissociative amnesia, 82, 86, 197–198
Dissociative disorders, 197–201
Dissociative fugue, 198–199
Dissociative identity disorder, 199–200
Disulfiram (Antabuse), 296, 310
  in alcoholism, 97–98
Divalproex (Depakote), 293, 297–298
  in bipolar disorder, 161, 162
Donepezil (Aricept), 296, 309
  in Alzheimer's disease, 67
Dopaminergic agents, 294
Doxepin (Sinequan), 294
  in major depression, 151
Duty to warn, 291
Dysarticulation, 33–34
Dyscalculia, 29
Dysgraphia, 30
Dyskinesia, tardive, 274–276
  vs. Huntington's disease, 76
  in schizophrenia, 130
  vs. Tourette's disorder, 48
Dyslexia, developmental, 28–29
Dysmorphophobia (body dysmorphic disorder), 194–195
  vs. hypochondriasis, 193
  vs. social phobia, 176
Dyspareunia, 211–212
Dysthymia, 154–155
  vs. anxiety disorder, generalized, 181
  vs. avoidant personality disorder, 258
  vs. borderline personality disorders, 254
  vs. conduct disorder, 44
  vs. depression, major, 147

Dystonia, 265–267
  etiology of, 265, 266
  of tardive dyskinesia, 274

Eating disorders, 217–221
Echolalia, 19, 87
Echopraxia, 19, 87
Effexor (venlafaxine). See Venlafaxine
Ejaculation
  premature, 210
  retrograde, 209
Ekbom syndrome, 234–235
Elation, 20
Elavil (amitriptyline). See Amitriptyline
Eldepryl (selegiline). See Selegiline
Electroconvulsive therapy, 310–321
  contraindications to, 312–313
  course of, 318
  delirium after, 317
  evaluation for, 313
  follow-up for, 320–321
  indications for, 311
  maintenance, 320–321
  patient preparation for, 313–314
  side effects of, 318–320
  technique of, 315–317
Emotional incontinence, 20
Encephalitis lethargica, vs. obsessive-compulsive disorder, 179
Encopresis, 49–51
Enuresis, 51–53
Epilepsy, with electroconvulsive therapy, 319
Epileptic amnesia, 82
  vs. alcoholic blackouts, 99
Erectile dysfunction, 205–207
Erotomanic delusions, 23, 134
Eskalith (lithium). See Lithium
Euphoria, 20
Exhibitionism, 213
Explosive disorder, intermittent, 242–243
Expressive aphasia, 31–32

Factitious illness, 195–196
vs. conversion disorder, 189
vs. pain disorder, 191
vs. posttraumatic stress disorder, 180
vs. somatization disorder, 187
Female orgasmic disorder, 207–208
Female sexual arousal disorder, 204
Fentanyl-related disorders, 114–117
Fetal alcohol syndrome, 96
Fetishism, 213
Flattening, of affect, 19
Flight of ideas, 21
Flumazenil (Romazicon), 296, 310
in benzodiazepine-related respiratory depression, 120
Fluoxetine (Prozac), 294
in major depression, 150
Fluphenazine (Prolixin), 293
in schizophrenia, 127
Fluvoxamine (Luvox), 294
antidepressant drug interactions with, 304
in major depression, 150
Folie á deux, 138–139
Frontal lobe syndrome, 91–92
etiology of, 92
Frontotemporal dementia, vs. Pick's disease, 77
Frotteurism, 213
Fugue, dissociative, 198–199

Gait, assessment of, 15
Gambling, 245
Gender identity disorder, 215–216
Geschwind syndrome, 94
Gilles de la Tourette's syndrome, 47–49
Grandiose delusions, 23, 134
Gustatory hallucinations, 22

Hair pulling, 246–247
Haldol (haloperidol). See Haloperidol

Hallucinations, 22
alcohol-induced psychotic disorder with, 141
in diagnostic interview, 6, 10
gustatory, 22
hypnagogic, in narcolepsy, 227–228
in Parkinson's disease, 72
in schizophrenia, 122
Hallucinogen-related disorders, 109–111
vs. depersonalization disorder, 200
Haloperidol (Haldol), 293
in alcohol withdrawal syndrome, 102
in autism, 38
in delirium, 60
in Huntington's disease, 76
in Tourette's disorder, 49
in schizophrenia, 127
Haloperidol decanoate, in delusional disorder, 135
Head trauma
dementia and, 71–72
postconcussion syndrome with, 278–279
Hematoma, subdural
in head trauma, 71
vs. postconcussion syndrome, 279
Hemorrhage, subarachnoid, in head trauma, 71
Hepatocerebral degeneration, acquired, vs. Huntington's disease, 76
Heroin-related disorders, 114–117
Histrionic personality disorder, 255–256
vs. narcissistic personality disorder, 257
Homicidal ideation, in diagnostic interview, 5–6
Hoover's test, 188
Huntington's disease, 75–76, 275
Hydrocephalus
communicating, vs. postconcussion syndrome, 279
normal-pressure, vs. Alzheimer's disease, 67

Hydromorphone-related disorders, 114–117
Hydroxyzine (Vistaril), 295, 308
Hyperactivity, 17–18. *See also* Attention-deficit/hyperactivity disorder
Hypermetamorphosis, 93
Hyperorality, 93
Hyperphagia, vs. bulimia nervosa, 220
Hypersexuality, 93
Hypersomnia
  primary (idiopathic), 224–225
  vs. sleep apnea, 231
  recurrent, 225
Hyperthyroidism, vs. caffeine-related disorders, 107
Hypnagogic hallucinations, in narcolepsy, 227–228
Hypnic jerks, vs. nocturnal myoclonus, 235
Hypnotic-related disorders, 118–121
Hypochondriasis, 192–194
  vs. pain disorder, 191
  vs. somatization disorder, 186
Hypoglycemia
  vs. alcohol withdrawal syndrome, 100
  vs. depersonalization disorder, 201
Hypothyroidism
  antidepressant use and, 152
  vs. inhalant-induced dementia, 80
Hypoventilation syndrome, central alveolar, 232

Identity crisis, vs. borderline personality disorders, 254
Identity disorder
  dissociative, 199–200
  gender, 215–216
Imipramine (Tofranil), 294
  in enuresis, 53
  in major depression, 150
  in separation anxiety disorder, 54
Immobility, 19, 87

Inappropriate affect, 19
Incoherence, 21
Incubus, 236–237
Inderal (propranolol). *See* Propranolol
Inhalant-induced dementia, 79–80
Inhalant-related disorders, 111–112
Insight, assessment of, 14
Insomnia
  in depression, 145
  primary, 222–224
Interictal personality syndrome, 94
Intermittent explosive disorder, 242–243
  violent behavior and, 289
Intersex states, vs. gender identity disorder, 216
Interview. *See* Diagnostic interview
Iron deficiency anemia, pica and, 45
Irritability, 20

Jealous delusions, 23, 134, 139
Jet travel, circadian rhythm sleep disorder with, 232–234
Judgment, assessment of, 13–14

Kleine-Levin syndrome, 226
  vs. bulimia nervosa, 220–221
Kleptomania, 243–244
Klüver-Bucy syndrome, 92–93
Korsakoff's syndrome, 81, 83–85

Lability, of affect, 19
Lacunar dementia, 68–69
Language. *See* Speech
Late-luteal-phase disorder, 157–158
Leuprolide acetate (Lupron Depot), for paraphilia, 215
Levodopa-carbidopa, in Parkinson's disease, 73
Lewy body dementia, 74
  vs. Parkinson's disease, 73
Librium (chlordiazepoxide), 295, 296
Limbic encephalitis, paraneoplastic, 81

Lithium (Eskalith), 293, 298
  in autism, 38
  in bipolar disorder, 161–163
Looseness of associations, 21
  in schizophrenia, 123
Lorazepam (Ativan), 295, 307
  in alcohol withdrawal syndrome,
    100–101
Loxapine (Loxitane), 293
  in schizophrenia, 127
Ludiomil (maprotiline). *See* Maproti-
    line
Lupron Depot (leuprolide acetate), for
    paraphilia, 215
Luvox (fluvoxamine). *See* Fluvoxamine

Malingering, 195–196
  vs. conversion disorder, 189
  vs. pain disorder, 191
  vs. postconcussion syndrome, 279
  vs. posttraumatic stress disorder,
    180
  vs. somatization disorder, 187
Mania
  vs. antisocial personality disorder,
    252
  vs. attention-deficit/hyperactivity
    disorder, 41
  in bipolar disorder, 158–159, 160,
    161–163
  vs. conduct disorder, 44
  in cyclothymia, 164
  vs. delusional disorder, 135
  with electroconvulsive therapy, 319
  vs. frontal lobe syndrome, 92
  vs. hallucinogen-related disorders,
    110
  vs. intermittent explosive disorder,
    243
  vs. Kleine-Levin syndrome, 226
  vs. kleptomania, 244
  vs. pathologic gambling, 245
  vs. psychotic disorder, brief, 136
  vs. schizophrenia, 124

vs. schizophreniform disorder, 131
secondary, 168–169
violent behavior and, 287
Manic-depressive illness, 158–164. *See
    also* Bipolar disorder
Mannerisms, 18
  in schizophrenia, 123
Maprotiline (Ludiomil), 295
  in major depression, 151
Masochism, 213
Mathematics disorder, 29
Medroxyprogesterone acetate (Depo-
    Provera), for paraphilia, 215
Mellaril (thioridazine). *See* Thiorida-
    zine
Memory testing
  in amnestic disorders, 80
  in diagnostic interview, 6
Mental retardation, 25–27
  vs. attention-deficit/hyperactivity
    disorder, 41
  in autism, 36
  vs. conduct disorder, 44
  vs. dementia, 62, 64
  etiology of, 26, 27
  grades of, 25, 26
  vs. reactive attachment disorder, 56
  violent behavior and, 288
Mental status examination, 6–7
Meperidine-related disorders, 114–
    117
Mesoridazine (Serentil), 293
  in schizophrenia, 127
Methadone
  intoxication with, 114–117
  in opioid withdrawal, 116
Methamphetamine-related disorders,
    105–106
Methylphenidate (Ritalin), 295, 306,
    308
  antidepressant drug interactions
    with, 305
  in attention-deficit/hyperactivity
    disorder, 42

Mirtazapine (Remeron), 295
  drug interactions with, 304–305
  in major depression, 151
Mitral valve prolapse, panic disorder
      and, 171
Molindone (Moban), 293
  in schizophrenia, 127
Monoamine oxidase inhibitors
      (MAOI), 295
  antidepressant drug interactions
      with, 304
  in serotonin syndrome, 277, 278
Mood disorders, 20, 145–169. See
      also specific disorders
Mood stabilizers, 293, 297–299
Morphine-related disorders, 114–
      117
Motor akathisia, 268
Movement
  assessment of, 15
  developmental disorder of, 30–31
Multi-infarct dementia, 67–68
Multiple personality disorder, 199–
      200
Multiple system atrophy, vs. Parkin-
      son's disease, 73
Muteness, 19, 87
Mutism, selective (elective), 55
Myalgia, with electroconvulsive
      therapy, 319
Myoclonus
  nocturnal, 235–236
  vs. tremor, 272

Naloxone (Narcan), 296, 310
Naltrexone (ReVia), 296, 310
  in alcoholism, 98
  in autism, 38
Narcan (naloxone), 296, 310
Narcissistic personality disorder, 256–
      257
  vs. body dysmorphic disorder, 195
  vs. histrionic personality disorder,
      256

Narcolepsy, 227–229
  vs. primary hypersomnia, 225
  vs. sleep paralysis, 241
Nardil (phenelzine). *See* Phenelzine
Navane (thiothixene). *See* Thiothixene
Nefazodone (Serzone), 295
  drug interactions with, 304–305
  in major depression, 151
Negative symptoms, in schizophrenia,
      123
Negativism, 18, 87
Neologisms, 21
Neuroacanthocytosis, vs. Huntington's
      disease, 76
Neuroleptic(s), 200–201, 293–294
  akathisia with, 268–270, 274
    vs. restless legs syndrome, 234
  antidepressant drug interactions
      with, 304
  dystonia with, 265–267, 274
  parkinsonism with, 262–263
  in schizophrenia, 125–130
  tardive dyskinesia with, 274–276
  in violent behavior, 290
Neuroleptic malignant syndrome, 272–
      273
Nicotine-related disorders, 112–114
Night terrors, vs. nightmare disorder, 236
Nightmare disorder, 236–237
  vs. sleep terror disorder, 238
Nihilistic delusions, 23
No Suicide Contract, 286
Nocturnal myoclonus, 235–236
Normal-pressure hydrocephalus, vs.
      Alzheimer's disease, 67
Norpramin (desipramine). *See* Desipra-
      mine
Nortriptyline (Pamelor), 294
  in attention-deficit/hyperactivity
      disorder, 42
  in major depression, 150

Obedience, automatic, 19, 87
Obsession, 21, 177

INDEX

Obsessive-compulsive disorder, 177–179
  vs. obsessive-compulsive personality disorder, 260
Obsessive-compulsive personality disorder, 259–260
  vs. narcissistic personality disorder, 257
Oculogyric crisis, 267–268
Olanzapine (Zyprexa), 293
  in delusional disorder, 135
  in Huntington's disease, 76
  in schizophrenia, 127
Olfactory hallucinations, 22
Olivopontocerebellar degeneration, vs. inhalant-induced dementia, 80
Opioid withdrawal syndrome, 115, 116
Opioid-related disorders, 114–117
Orap (pimozide). See Pimozide
Orgasmic disorder
  female, 207–208
  male, 208–210
Orientation testing, in diagnostic interview, 7

Pain disorder, 189–192
  vs. conversion disorder, 189
  vs. hypochondriasis, 193
  vs. somatization disorder, 186
Pamelor (nortriptyline). See Nortriptyline
Panic disorder, 170–173
  with agoraphobia, 173
  vs. caffeine-related disorder, 107
  vs. cannabis-related disorder, 108
  vs. depersonalization disorder, 200
  vs. generalized anxiety disorder, 181
  nocturnal
    vs. nightmare disorder, 236
    vs. sleep terror disorder, 238
  vs. secondary anxiety disorder, 184
  vs. simple phobia, 174
Papez, circuit of, 84

Paralysis
  conversion, 188
  sleep, 240–241
    in narcolepsy, 227
Paraneoplastic limbic encephalitis, 81
Paranoia, alcoholic, 139–141
Paranoid personality disorder, 248–249
  vs. alcoholic paranoia, 140
  vs. delusional disorder, 135
  vs. passive-aggressive personality disorder, 261
  vs. schizophrenia, 125
  violent behavior and, 288
Paraphilias, 212–215
Parkinsonism, 262–264
  etiology of, 263, 264
Parkinson's disease, 72–74
  electroconvulsive therapy in, 321
Parnate (tranylcypromine). See Tranylcypromine
Paroxetine (Paxil), 294
  in major depression, 150
Passive-aggressive personality disorder, 260–261
Pavor nocturnus, 237–238
Paxil (paroxetine). See Paroxetine
Pedophilia, 213
Pemoline (Cylert), 295, 306, 308
Pentazocine-related disorders, 114–117
Periodic limb movement disorder of sleep, 235–236
Perphenazine (Trilafon), 293
  in schizophrenia, 127
Persecutory delusions, 23, 133, 139
Personality change
  vs. antisocial personality disorder, 252
  vs. kleptomania, 244
  medical condition–induced, 89–91
  vs. schizoid personality disorder, 249
  violent behavior and, 288

Personality disorder(s), 248–261
  antisocial, 251–252
  avoidant, 257–258
  borderline, 253–255
  dependent, 258–259
  histrionic, 255–256
  vs. medical condition–related personality change, 90
  narcissistic, 256–257
  obsessive-compulsive, 259–260
  paranoid, 248–249
  passive-aggressive, 260–261
  schizoid, 249–250
  schizotypal, 250–251
  suicidal behavior and, 284
Phencyclidine-related disorders, 117–118
  vs. hallucinogen-related disorders, 110
  violent behavior and, 288
Phenelzine (Nardil), 295
  in major depression, 151
Phenytoin, antidepressant drug interactions with, 305
Phobia
  vs. generalized anxiety disorder, 181
  social, 175–177
    vs. agoraphobia, 173
    vs. avoidant personality disorder, 258
    vs. simple phobia, 174
  specific (simple), 174–175
Phonologic disorder, 33–34
Physical examination, 8, 14
Pica, 45–46
Pick's disease, 76–77
Pickwickian syndrome, 232
Pimozide (Orap), 293
  in schizophrenia, 127
  in Tourette's disorder, 49
Postconcussion syndrome, 278–279
Postpartum blues, 156–157
Postpartum depression, 155–156
  vs. major depression, 147

Postpartum psychosis, 137–138
  vs. bipolar disorder, 161
  vs. brief psychotic disorder, 136
Posttraumatic stress disorder, 179–180
  vs. generalized anxiety disorder, 181
Posturing, 18, 87
Poverty, delusions of, 23
Poverty of speech, 21
Poverty of thought, 21
Premature ejaculation, 210
Premenstrual syndrome, 157–158
  vs. major depression, 147
Pressure of speech, 21
Prion diseases, 78
Progressive supranuclear palsy, vs. Parkinson's disease, 73
Prolixin (fluphenazine). See Fluphenazine
Propranolol (Inderal), 296, 308–309
  antidepressant drug interactions with, 305
Protriptyline (Vivactil), 294
  in major depression, 150
Proverbs testing
  in dementia, 61
  in diagnostic interview, 7
Prozac (fluoxetine). See Fluoxetine
Pseudodementia, 64
Pseudomemories, 23
Pseudoseizures, 188
Psychiatric evaluation
  affect disturbances in, 19–20
  catatonic symptoms in, 18–19
  delusions in, 23
  hallucinations in, 22
  hyperactivity in, 17–18
  interview for. See Diagnostic interview
  mannerisms in, 18
  mood disturbances in, 20
  psychomotor agitation in, 17
  psychomotor retardation in, 17
  report format for, 11–16
  speech disturbances in, 21

Psychiatric evaluation—*cont.*
  stereotypies in, 18
  thought disturbances in, 21
Psychic blindness, in Klüver-Bucy
    syndrome, 92
Psychomotor agitation, 17
Psychomotor retardation, 17
Psychosis
  postpartum, 137–138
    vs. bipolar disorder, 161
    vs. brief psychotic disorder, 136
  primary. *See* Schizoaffective disor-
      der; Schizophrenia
  secondary, 142–144
Psychotic disorder, brief, 136–137
Pyromania, 244–245

Quetiapine (Seroquel), 294
  in schizophrenia, 127

Reactive attachment disorder, 56
Reading disorder, 28–29
Receptive-expressive language disorder,
    mixed, 32–33
Referential delusions, 23
Reflexes, assessment of, 15–16
Remeron (mirtazapine). *See* Mirtaza-
    pine
REM-sleep behavior disorder, 240
Restless legs syndrome, 234–235
  vs. akathisia, 269
Restraints, in violent behavior, 291
Retardation, mental. *See* Mental
    retardation
Rett's syndrome (Rett's disorder), 38–
    40
ReVia (naltrexone). *See* Naltrexone
Rigidity, 19, 87, 262
Risperidone (Risperdal), 293
  in Huntington's disease, 76
  in schizophrenia, 127
Ritalin (methylphenidate). *See* Methyl-
    phenidate

Romazicon (flumazenil). *See* Fluma-
    zenil
Rum fits, 103
Rumination disorder, 46–47

Sadism, 213
Schizoaffective disorder, 131–133
  vs. bipolar disorder, 161
  vs. cyclothymia, 165
  vs. schizophrenia, 125
Schizoid personality disorder, 249–250
  vs. avoidant personality disorder,
      258
  vs. schizotypal personality disorders,
      250
  vs. social phobia, 176
Schizophrenia, 122–130
  vs. agoraphobia, 173
  vs. alcoholic paranoia, 140
  vs. anorexia nervosa, 218
  vs. autism, 38
  vs. borderline personality disorders,
      254
  vs. delusional disorder, 134
  etiology of, 124
  vs. gender identity disorder, 216
  vs. hallucinogen-related disorders,
      110
  vs. Klüver-Bucy syndrome, 93
  maintenance treatment in, 129
  vs. medical condition–related person-
      ality change, 90
  vs. mental retardation, 27
  neuroleptics for, 125–130. *See also*
      Neuroleptics
  vs. pain disorder, 191
  vs. paranoid personality disorder,
      248
  vs. paraphilia, 214
  vs. schizoaffective disorder, 132
  vs. schizoid personality disorder, 249
  vs. schizophreniform disorder, 130–
      131

vs. schizotypal personality disorders, 250
subtypes of, 123
suicidal behavior and, 283
tardive dyskinesia in, 130
treatment resistance in, 129
violent behavior and, 288
Schizophreniform disorder, 130–131
vs. brief psychotic disorder, 136
vs. schizophrenia, 124
Schizotypal personality disorder, 250–251
vs. schizoid personality disorder, 249
vs. social phobia, 176
Schneiderian First Rank symptoms, 24
Secondary psychosis, 142–144
Sedative-hypnotic withdrawal, vs. generalized anxiety disorder, 181
Sedative-related disorders, 118–121
Seizures
in alcohol withdrawal, 103
conversion, 188
vs. depersonalization disorder, 201
vs. hallucinogen-related disorders, 110
vs. intermittent explosive disorder, 243
nocturnal
vs. REM-sleep behavior disorder, 240
vs. sleep terror disorder, 238
vs. sleepwalking disorder, 239
vs. obsessive-compulsive disorder, 179
Selective (elective) mutism, 55
Selective serotonin receptor inhibitors, 294
antidepressant drug interactions with, 304
in serotonin syndrome, 277, 278
Selegiline (Eldepryl), 295

in Parkinson's disease, 73, 74
Senile dementia, of Lewy body type, 74
vs. Parkinson's disease, 73
Sensory aphasia, 32–33
Separation anxiety disorder, 53–55
Serentil (mesoridazine). See Mesoridazine
Seroquel (quetiapine). See Quetiapine
Serotonin syndrome, 276–278
etiology of, 277
Sertraline (Zoloft), 294
in major depression, 150
Serzone (nefazodone). See Nefazodone
Sexual aversion disorder, 203–204
Sexual disorders, 202–216
of aversion, 203–204
of dyspareunia, 211–212
of female arousal, 204
of female orgasm, 207–208
of hypoactive desire, 202–203
of male erection, 205–207
of male orgasm, 208–210
of paraphilias, 212–215
of premature ejaculation, 210
of vaginismus, 212
Shared psychotic disorder, 138–139
Sildenafil (Viagra), 207
Sin, delusions of, 23
Sinequan (doxepin). See Doxepin
Sleep apnea, 230–231
vs. primary hypersomnia, 225
Sleep disorders, 222–241. See also specific disorders
Sleep paralysis, 240–241
in narcolepsy, 227
Sleep starts, vs. nocturnal myoclonus, 235
Sleep terror disorder, 237–238
Sleep-drunkenness, vs. sleepwalking disorder, 239
Sleepwalking disorder, 238–239
vs. REM-sleep behavior disorder, 240

Smoking, cigarette, 112–114
Social phobia, 175–177
  vs. agoraphobia, 173
  vs. avoidant personality disorder, 258
  vs. simple phobia, 174
Somatic delusions, 23, 134
Somatization disorder, 185–187
  vs. conversion disorder, 189
  vs. hypochondriasis, 193
  vs. pain disorder, 191
Somnambulism, 238–239
  vs. REM-sleep behavior disorder, 240
Speaking, developmental disorder of, 31–32
Speech
  articulation disorder of, 33–34
  disturbances of, 21
  expressive disorder of, 31–32
  poverty of, 21
  receptive-expressive disorder of, 32–33
  stuttering disorder of, 35–36
Stauder's lethal catatonia, vs. neuroleptic malignant syndrome, 273
Stelazine (trifluoperazine). See Trifluoperazine
Stereotypies, 18
Steroid abuse, violent behavior and, 288
Stimulants, 295, 306, 308
  intoxication with, 105–106
    vs. cyclothymia, 165
    violent behavior and, 288
Strength, assessment of, 15
Stuttering, 35–36
Subarachnoid hemorrhage, in head trauma, 71
Subcortical arteriosclerotic encephalopathy, 69
  vs. Alzheimer's disease, 66
Subdural hematoma, in head trauma, 71

Suicidal behavior, 282–286
  risk factors for, 282–285
Suicidal ideation
  in alcoholism, 96
  in diagnostic interview, 5
Supranuclear palsy, progressive, vs. Parkinson's disease, 73
Sydenham's chorea, vs. obsessive-compulsive disorder, 178
Symmetrel (amantadine), 294, 302

Tactile agnosia, 16
Tactile hallucinations, 22
Tangentiality, 21
Tardive dyskinesia, 274–276
  vs. Huntington's disease, 76
  in schizophrenia, 130
  vs. Tourette's disorder, 48
Tegretol (carbamazepine). See Carbamazepine
Theft, vs. kleptomania, 244
Thiamine, in alcoholism, 97, 104
Thioridazine (Mellaril), 293
  in schizophrenia, 127
Thiothixene (Navane), 293
  in schizophrenia, 127
Thorazine (chlorpromazine). See Chlorpromazine
Thought
  disturbances of, 21
  poverty of, 21
Thought blocking, 21
Thyroid storm, vs. alcohol withdrawal syndrome, 100
Tics, in Tourette's disorder, 47–49
Tobacco use, 112–114
Tofranil (imipramine). See Imipramine
Tourette's disorder, 47–49
Transient global amnesia, 82, 85–86
  vs. alcoholic blackouts, 99
Transient ischemic attack, amnesia with, 82
Transsexualism, 215–216
Transvestic fetishism, 213

Tranylcypromine (Parnate), 295
  in major depression, 151
Trauma, postconcussion syndrome
  with, 278–279
Trazodone (Desyrel), 295
  drug interactions with, 304–305
  in major depression, 151
Tremor, 262, 270–272
  etiology of, 270, 271
Trichotillomania, 246–247
Trifluoperazine (Stelazine), 293
  in schizophrenia, 127
Trihexyphenidyl (Artane), 294, 301–
  302
Trilafon (perphenazine). See Perphenazine
Trimipramine, in major depression,
  150

Vaginismus, 212
Venlafaxine (Effexor), 295
  drug interactions with, 304–305
  in major depression, 151
Vertical gaze palsy, vs. oculogyric
  crisis, 268

Viagra (sildenafil), 207
Violent behavior, 286–291
Vistaril (hydroxyzine), 295, 308
Visual agnosia, 16
Visual hallucinations, 22
Vivactil (protriptyline). See Protripty-
  line
Voyeurism, 213

Warfarin, antidepressant drug interactions with, 305
Wellbutrin (bupropion). See Bupropion
Wernicke's encephalopathy, 83–85,
  104
Wilson's disease, vs. Huntington's
  disease, 76
Writing disorder, 30
  reading disorder and, 28

Xanax (alprazolam), 295, 307

Zoloft (sertraline). See Sertraline
Zolpidem (Ambien), 296, 310
Zyprexa (olanzapine). See Olanzapine

INDEX